Hormones in Normal and Abnormal Human Tissues

Hormones in Normal and Abnormal Human Tissues

Volume 3

Editors
K. Fotherby, S. B. Pal

Walter de Gruyter · Berlin · New York 1983

Editors
K. Fotherby, Ph. D., F.R.I.C.,
Department of Steroid Biochemistry
Royal Postgraduate Medical School
University of London
Ducane Road
London W 12 OHS, U. K.

S. B. Pal, D. Phil., Dr. rer. biol. hum., M. I. Biol.
Universität Ulm
Department für Innere Medizin
Steinhövelstrasse 9
D 7900 Ulm Donau
F. R. Germany

Library of Congress Cataloging in Publication Data

Hormones in normal and abnormal human tissues

Bibliography: v. 1, p.
Includes index.
1. Hormones. 2. Hormones, Ectopic.
I. Fotherby, K., 1927 – II. Pal, S. B., 1928 –
[DNLM: 1. Hormones. 2. Disease. WK 102 H8127]
QP571.H663 616.4 80-27070
ISBN 3-11-008616-6 (v. 3)

CIP-Kurztitelaufnahme der Deutschen Bibliothek

Hormones in normal and abnormal human tissues

ed. by K. Fotherby, S. B. Pal. – Berlin; New York: de Gruyter.
NE: Fotherby, Kenneth [Hrsg.]
Vol. 3 (1983).
ISBN 3-11-008616-6

 Printing: Gerike GmbH, Berlin. – Binding: Lüderitz & Bauer Buchgewerbe, Berlin. – Printed in Germany.

PREFACE

This volume is the last of the series of three providing literature reviews of hormones in human tissues. The range of topics covered in the series is extended by this part and includes articles especially devoted to ACTH and related peptides, erythropoietin, parathyroid hormones and renin. Volume 3 maintains the high standard of the two previous ones and we are grateful to the contributors to the series who have provided such excellent comprehensive reviews. As this is the last volume, the editors hope that endocrinologists, and research workers in general, will find the information presented in the series useful and time-saving.

K. Fotherby S. B. Pal

March 1983

CONTRIBUTORS

Numbers in parentheses indicate the page on which the authors' articles begin

W. Beischer, Universität Ulm, Department für Innere Medizin, 7900 Ulm (Donau), Federal Republic of Germany (1).

H. Dalheim, Department of Physiology, University of Munich, Pettenkoferstrasse 12, 8000 Munich 2, Federal Republic of Germany (251).

M. Finkelstein, Department of Endocrinology, Hebrew University-Hadassah Medical School, Jerusalem, Israel (45).

T. Fujita, Third Division, Department of Medicine, Kobe University School of Medicine, Kobe 650, Japan (169).

S. J. Gaskell, Tenovus Institute for Cancer Research, Welsh National School of Medicine, Heath, Cardiff CF4 4XX, U.K. (121).

P. C. Ghosh, Sheffield and Region Endocrine Investigation Centre, Jessop Hospital for Women, Sheffield S3 7RE, U.K. (157).

Y. Hirata, Third Division, Department of Medicine, Kobe University School of Medicine, Kobe 650, Japan (169).

M. B. Hodgins, Department of Dermatology, University of Glasgow, Scotland, U.K. (97).

I. C. M. Jacob, Department of Physiology, University of Munich, Pettenkoferstrasse 12, 8000 Munich 2, Federal Republic of Germany (251).

S. Matsukura, Third Division, Department of Medicine, Kobe University School of Medicine, Kobe 650, Japan (169).

H. W. Minne, Abteilung Innere Medizin VI, Endokrinologie, Universitätskliniken Heidelberg, Luisenstrasse 5, 6900 Heidelberg, Federal Republic of Germany (195).

M. A. S. Moore, Laboratories of Developmental Hematopoiesis, Sloan-Kettering Institute, 1250 First Avenue, New York 10021, U.S.A. (135).

L. M. Pelus, Laboratories of Developmental Hematopoiesis, Sloan-Kettering Institute, 1250 First Avenue, New York 10021, U.S.A. (135).

J. Pschorr, Department of Physiology, University of Munich, Pettenkoferstrasse 12, 8000 Munich 2, Federal Republic of Germany (251).

J. Rosenthal, Ulm University Medical Center, 7900 Ulm, Federal Republic of Germany (251).

G. W. Sang, Department of Pharmacology, Zhejiang Academy of Experimental Hygiene, Hangchow, China (215).

F. Sieber, Clayton Laboratories and Department of Medicine, The Johns Hopkins University School of Medicine, Baltimore, Maryland, U.S.A. (63).

J. L. Spivak, Clayton Laboratories and Department of Medicine, The Johns Hopkins University School of Medicine, Baltimore, Maryland, U.S.A. (63).

J. Weidenfeld, Laboratory of Experimental Endocrinology, Department of Neurology, Hadassah University Hospital, Jerusalem (45).

R. Ziegler, Abteilung Innere Medizin VI, Endokrinologie, Universitätskliniken Heidelberg, Luisenstrasse 5, 6900 Heidelberg, Federal Republic of Germany (195).

CONTENTS

PROINSULIN AND C-PEPTIDE IN HUMANS

W. Beischer
Universität Ulm, Department für Innere Medizin,
D-7900 Ulm (Donau), Federal Republic of Germany.

Introduction

A. Discovery of Proinsulin and C-Peptide

It was a question of great interest in the early 1960s whether the biosynthesis of the two chains of the insulin molecule occurs via a one-chain precursor or via combination of the separately synthesized A and B chains. Steiner et al. (1-4) proved the existence of proinsulin in studies on insulin biosynthesis with slices from beta-cell adenomas and with isolated pancreatic islets of the rat in vitro. In proinsulin the B chain of insulin is linked to the A chain by the "connecting peptide" consisting of 30 to 40 aminoacids. Proinsulin contributes less than 5% of the immunoreactive insulin extracted from islets, its conversion to insulin occurring within the islets. A large fragment of the "connecting peptide" appearing in addition to insulin on the conversion to proinsulin was called C-peptide (3, 5).

B. Chemistry of Proinsulin and C-Peptide

I a. Isolation of proinsulin

Since about 1950 it has been known that crystalline insulin preparations are heterogeneous on chromatography and electro-

Hormones in Normal and Abnormal Human Tissues, Vol. III

phoresis. Mirsky and Kawamura (6) confirmed the heterogeneity by gel electrophoresis. Proinsulin and proinsulin-like components (PLC) contribute to this heterogeneity of crystalline insulin (1, 2). Thus, crystalline insulin is the most important source for the isolation of proinsulin. The technique for the isolation of proinsulin from crystalline insulin started with a gel filtration step followed by ion exchange chromatography (7-12). The authors reported that for different species, between 1.4% and 3% of crystalline insulin appeared in the position of proinsulin on gel filtration. The yield of a fairly pure human proinsulin was less than 0.005% of the crystalline human insulin, lower than in animal species.

I b. Isolation of C-peptide

C-peptide does not appear as an impurity of crystalline insulin since it is not precipitated on salting out insulin with sodium chloride (15%). A crude C-peptide is obtained by precipitation with acids and organic solvents from an acid-ethanol extract of the pancreas. Further purification is effected by gel filtration, ion exchange chromatography and preparative electrophoresis. Details of two different isolation methods have been described (13, 14, 15) as well as later modifications (10, 12, 16). Yields for the C-peptides from different species varied between 24 mg/kg pancreas for bovine C-peptide (15) and 0.9 mg/kg pancreas for human C-peptide (14). While Steiner et al. (15) reported on equimolar contents of insulin and C-peptide in bovine pancreas (17), Markussen et al. (14) found only 11% of the amount of C-peptide expected on the basis of equimolarity with insulin in human pancreas. The authors discuss higher losses by purification due to difficulties in identification and by post-mortem autolysis. C-peptide fragments in purified extracts of human pancreas (12, 17, 18) are not artifacts and also appear as secretion products (19).

II a. Primary structure of proinsulin

The primary structures of proinsulin and C-peptide were determined by the classical techniques of enzymatic hydrolysis. The sequence analysis of the isolated fragments was carried out by stepwise Edman degradation and dansylation from the NH_2-terminal end and by treatment with carboxypeptidases from the COOH-terminus. A semi-micro adaptation of the Edman degradation procedure allowing the total sequence analysis of the intact C-peptide has been described (20).

The primary structure of proinsulin was only determined in the case of the porcine (8) and the bovine products (21). In 1971 Steiner et al. (15) showed the identity of a peptide isolated from bovine pancreas in equimolar amounts with insulin with the C-peptide portion of proinsulin from crystalline insulin. In bovine and porcine proinsulin two Arg residues link the B chain of insulin and a Lys and an Arg residue the A chain to the C-peptide. The structure of proinsulin from other species was inferred from the known structures of insulin and C-peptide and by analogy to that of beef and pig. Only in man (10) and rat (11, 22) were the comparison of the sequences of insulin and C-peptide with an amino acid analysis of proinsulin performed, suggesting that in these species also Arg-Arg and Lys-Arg dipeptides link insulin and C-peptide.

II b. Primary structure of C-peptide

The primary structures are known for eleven mammalian (man, 10, 18; monkey, 20; pig, 8, 23; beef, 4, 21, 24; sheep, 20; horse, 25; dog, 20; rat, 22, 25; guinea pig, 26, 27; chinchilla, 28 and rabbit, 16) and one avian (duck, 29) C-peptide.

The number of amino acids in C-peptides from different species varies between 23 and 31. The peptides of different species show much greater amino acid variations than the corresponding insulins. However, all C-peptides start with an acidic amino acid (Glu, Asp) followed by an aliphatic amino acid in position 2 (Ala, Val, Leu) and by glutamic acid in position 3 and end with glutamin. Leu in position 21 is the third amino acid common to all C-peptides whose structure has so far been elucidated. All known C-peptides are acidic compounds.

III. Conformation of proinsulin and C-peptide

Because of difficulties in crystallizing proinsulin it was not possible until recently to get precise information on its three dimensional structure by X-ray studies (30). The conformation of free insulin and of the insulin moiety in proinsulin are very similar, if not identical (31).

There is no general agreement about the conformation of C-peptide. Most likely the C-peptide molecule shows a random coil structure at its NH_2-end, a β-turn in the middle causing a refolding along its own axis and some ordered structure at the COOH-end (32).

IV. Intermediates between proinsulin and insulin

Several substances with a structure between proinsulin and insulin were isolated from crystalline bovine (7, 21, 33) and porcine insulin (23, 34) and from islet tissue of the anglerfish (35). The existence of intermediates of the conversion of proinsulin to insulin was shown in a variety of biosynthetic studies (5, 36-41). It appears likely that at least some of the isolated substances are identical with some of the biosynthetic intermediates.

The mechanism of the conversion of proinsulin to insulin *in vivo* is not fully understood; available facts and hypotheses have been summarized (42, 43) and some further details are given below (pp. 9-10).

The possible existence of C-peptide fragments *in vivo* has already been mentioned above.

V. Biochemical relevance of proinsulin and C-peptide

The important question arises as to the role of proinsulin and of its C-peptide moiety in the biosynthesis of insulin. The essential feature for the correct conformation of the disulfide bridges between the B and A chains of insulin is a covalent linkage between the chains. This is obvious from the poor reduction-reoxidation yields following any interruption between the insulin chains (23, 33, 44). The correct formation of the disulfide bridges in vitro does not at all depend on the nature of the link between B and A chain as shown by studies with chemically synthesized "miniproinsulins" (45-49). It was recently shown that Insulin-like Growth Factor I (IGF I, corresponding to NSILA I) is a structural analogue to proinsulin (50). However, the connecting peptide part of the molecule consists of only 12 amino acids not related to C-peptide.

Precursors were also discovered for other hormones showing a single chain peptide structure (51). Progress in molecular biology helped to explain this observation and led to a more general interpretation of the prehormone concept. According to this concept, hormones, like other secretory products (52, 53), start with a presequence of amino acids (preproinsulin, 54) which initiates the binding of the ribosomes translating the mRNA endoplasmic reticulum. The distance between mRNA and cisternal space of the endoplasmic reticulum might very well necessitate a minimum length of 65 to 70 amino acids and thus a prohormone in case of hormones with a shorter sequence (42, 55, 56). More information concerning insulin biosynthesis and its regulation is expected from recent progress in gene research and technology (56-61).

C. Radioimmunoassay of Proinsulin and C-Peptide

I. Techniques available

Shortly after the discovery of proinsulin, its presence in human serum or plasma was shown by determining the distribution of immunoreactive insulin (IRI) in the individual fractions after gel filtration (62, 63). Until recently no better technique was available to measure proinsulin.

Melani, Rubenstein, Oyer and Steiner (64) were the first to describe a radioimmunoassay for human C-peptide applying an antiserum against natural human C-peptide raised in guinea pigs. The assay had to be improved further for direct determination of immunomeasurable C-peptide (IMCP) (synonymous: immunoreactive C-peptide (IRCP) or C-peptide immunoreactivity (CPR)) in serum or plasma (65). The antibodies of other radioimmunoassays for IMCP in man, including our own, were raised against synthetic preparations of human connecting peptide or C-peptide in rabbits (66), goats (67) and guinea pigs (68). Further radioimmunoassays were developed in Japan, one of which gained widespread distribution as a commercially available kit (Daiichi Radioisotope Laboratories, Tokyo).

Due to difficulties in raising antisera against C-peptide, Heding and coworkers set up a radioimmunoassay with antiserum raised against a crude preparation of human proinsulin (17, 69). However, the authors measured C-peptide specifically by separating proinsulin and C-peptide as the first step of their assay. In a batch technique insulin and proinsulin are immobilized by Sepharose bound antibodies against insulin; C-peptide is determined in the supernatant (69).

In the Sepharose-insulin antibody-proinsulin complex, the proinsulin preserves its ability to bind antibodies against its C-peptide moiety. This is the basis of Heding's (70) technique to determine proinsulin. This elegant method provides optimal sensitivity and precision and is more economical than previous methods (for a similar technique cf. 71). Of the foregoing techniques, one method for measuring proinsulin after destruction of insulin by a specific protease, must be mentioned because it gained some practical relevance besides the gel filtration technique (72).

II. Problems encountered

Table 1 illustrates the great variation of the IMCP concentrations in fasting subjects of normal weight. While the IMCP concentrations are rather homogeneously distributed over the range between 0.29 and 1.17 nmolar, IMI only varies between 0.048 and 0.07 nmolar, apart from our own concentration which was determined using a double antibody kit (Insik-1, CEA-IRE-Sorin).

Table 1. Fasting concentrations of immunomeasurable C-peptide (IMCP) and insulin (IMI). (from 147. Concentrations are shown in the different scales being used (nmolar corresponds to pmol/ml). The underlined data were taken from each reference. To calculate alternative concentrations a molecular weight of 3025 was taken for C-peptide and 5808 for insulin and 1 ng insulin was taken as equivalent to 25 μU).

IMCP n molar ng/ml	IMI n molar ng/ml μU/ml	IMCP/IMI	n	Reference
0,43 ± 0,10 ? 1,30 ± 0,30 ?	(0,05) (0,29) (7,20)	(8,6)	9	65
0,29 ± 0,07 SEM 0,88 ± 0,21 SEM	(0,06) (0,36) (9,00)	(4,8)	20	66
0,37 ± 0,071 SD 1,12 ± 0,21 SD	0,048 ± 0,33 SD 0,28 ± 0,19 SD 7,00 ± 4,80 SD	7,7	14	146
1,17 ± 0,35 SD 3,54 ± 1,05 SD	0,06 ± 0,04 SD 0,36 ± 0,21 SD 9,00 ± 5,30 SD	19,5	6	133
0,60 ± 0,13 SD 1,80 ± 0,40 SD	0,111 ± 0,034 SD 0,64 ± 0,20 SD 16,1 ± 5,00 SD	5,4	25	75
0,81 ± 0,32 SD 2,45 ± 0,96 SD	0,07 ± 0,04 SD 0,39 ± 0,24 SD 9,70 ± 6,00 SD	11,6	19	203
0,79 ± 0,28 SD 2,40 ± 0,85 SD	– – –	4,3	130	165

As stated by Yalow and Berson (73): "The validity of the assay depends on the identical immunoreactivity of standard and unknown in their ability to compete against binding of the labelled hormone...". This assumption is not fulfilled for the radioimmunoassay of C-peptide as shown by a lack in total identity of dilution curves for the standard and the unknown material (66, 69, 74-76). As a consequence the results for IMCP in serum are influenced by the individual antiserum (76-79) and also by the individual tracer and even the tracer fraction applied (78, 79).

Three factors may contribute to the non-identical immunoreactivity of the standard and the unknown. Firstly, synthetic human C-peptides used most commonly as standard preparations may be slightly chemically different from the natural product.

Secondly, cross-reactivity with proinsulin is to be expected with any antiserum suitable for measuring C-peptide. Here it is important to differentiate between free and antibody bound proinsulin in serum, both of which will interfere with the C-peptide determination. Heding and her coworkers have produced fascinating data on the relevance of free proinsulin under physiological and pathological conditions (80). These results should be kept in mind when evaluating IMCP concentrations.

Human proinsulin bound to antibodies against insulin may very seriously influence the IMCP concentrations in serum of insulin treated diabetics (65, 81, 82). According to our own experience (78) and that of others (83, 84) the pretreatment of these sera with polyethyleneglycol (PEG) was very effective in precipitating the bound proinsulin enabling the C-peptide to be estimated in the supernatant. It is to be recommended that all sera of insulin treated diabetics be pretreated with polyethylene-glycol, as according to our own experience, proinsulin will interfere in almost 50% of these patients.

Thirdly, C-peptide fragments were isolated especially from human pancreas (see above) and Kuzuya and coworkers (76) presented convincing evidence for C-peptide fragments in serum.

Whether such C-peptide fragments in serum arise as an artefact on storage or whether they are secreted and correspond to the fragments isolated from pancreas remains to be established.

The aim of accurately estimating C-peptide concentrations in human body fluids by radioimmunoassay is unattainable in case C-peptide and C-peptide fragments appear together. Similar considerations apply to the radioimmunological determination of other peptide hormones.

D. Proinsulin and C-Peptide in Islet Tissue

I. In healthy and diabetic subjects

Paul Langerhans discovered the pancreatic islets in 1869 and twenty years later Minkowsky and von Mering observed the occurrence of diabetes after pancreatectomy in dogs (85). Initially, the islets of Langerhans were assumed to produce a secretion important for carbohydrate metabolism (86). Zülzer (87) showed in 1908 that the injection of pancreatic extracts clearly improved the diabetic state in a dog. However, the era of insulin availability did not begin before 1921, when Banting and Best again extracted the blood glucose lowering "insulin" or "isletin", as it was first called, from the pancreas (88).

The observation that a correlation existed between the histologically verified β-cell granulation and extractable insulin of the pancreas (89-92) was the first step towards a subcellular localization of insulin production. Due to the discovery of proinsulin and great progress in molecular biology our knowledge about the subcellular course of insulin biosynthesis greatly improved (42, 43, 51-53, 55, 56, 93, 94) and can be summarized as follows. The process starts in the cytoplasm with the translation of mRNA. This mRNA does not code for the proinsulin itself but for pre-proinsulin, a precursor of the prohormone. The pre-peptide most likely mediates the interaction of the large ribosomal subunit with the membrane of the rough endoplasmic reticulum. This biosynthetic mechanism very likely applies for all secretory peptide products of any cell. The pre-peptide is rapidly cleaved off the secretory product before completion of the polypeptide chain. Proinsulin is transferred to the Golgi apparatus of the β-cell within microvesicles. About 30 minutes elapse between the beginning of protein synthesis and the appearance of proinsulin in the Golgi region. From the Golgi apparatus immature secretion granules are formed which maturate on their way to the plasma membrane of the cell surface. The conversion of proinsulin into insulin and C-peptide is initiated in the Golgi apparatus or in newly formed secretion granules and continues during the process of maturation of the granules. The half time for the conversion of proinsulin to insulin in the β-cells is about one hour.

The enzymatic conversion of proinsulin to insulin and C-peptide has not been clarified in detail. Appropriate mixtures of pancreatic trypsin and carboxypeptidase B can quantitatively convert proinsulin to intermediate forms and finally to insulin in vitro. This combination of enzymes might also exist in vivo with the trypsin-like activity being bound to the granule membrane (38, 51, 95). On the other hand, a soluble enzyme not identical with trypsin (96), cathepsin B (97) and chymotrypsin (19, 23) were also suggested to effect or take part in the conversion of proinsulin to insulin. The action of chymotrypsin might create C-peptide fragments as they were isolated from pancreatic extracts.

Much information on the morphology, physiology and biochemistry of the release of insulin, C-peptide and proinsulin from the β-cells has accumulated during the past years. Several symposia, reviews and monographs have dealt with the subject (98-103).

The finding of Steiner (2) that proinsulin or a proinsulin-like component (PLC) contributes less than 5% of the immunomeasurable insulin in pancreatic islets of the rat was confirmed for PLC in the pancreas of other species including the human pancreas (17, 104-106). The percentage of PLC was also confirmed for the pancreas of diabetic humans containing measurable amounts of IRI (107). The presence of C-peptide in the pancreas and its generally equimolar relation to pancreatic insulin has already been discussed in relation to the isolation of C-peptide from pancreatic glands (p. 2). C-peptide was also determined as C-peptide immunoreactivity (CPR) in crude extracts of human pancreas (107, 108). Tasaka and coworkers (107) reported between 8.76 to 25.65 μg CPR/g wet weight in non-diabetic and 0 to 14.84 μg CPR/g wet weight in diabetic pancreas. These results reach the order of magnitude reported by Steiner et al. (15) for the yield of purified C-peptide from bovine pancreas (p. 2). The molar CPR/IRI ratios in the pancreatic extracts were found to be less than one (107, 108). Factors like a smaller yield of C-peptide on extraction as compared to insulin (107, 109), a different cross-reactivity of proinsulin with CPR and IRI and the occurrence of C-peptide fragments must be considered to explain the variation from the postulated equimolarity.

Grube (110) has successfully applied our antiserum against synthetic human C-peptide (67) for staining normal human β-cells with different immunocytochemical techniques (110, 111).

II. In patients with insulinomas

Of special interest in abnormal human tissues are the morphological and biochemical findings in insulinomas. This subject was extensively studied and reviewed by Creutzfeldt and coworkers (112, 113) who reported on 40 human insulinomas.
A variable number of tumour cells contained abnormal or no β-granules. Four ultrastructural types of tumour cells could be differentiated on the grounds of varying granulation. In general the IRI concentration in the tumour was lower and the percentage of PLC higher than in islet tissue of normal pancreas from the same patient and from patients without insulinoma.
With the insulinomas, the tumours with β-cell granules contained the most IRI and the smallest PLC percentage whilst virtually

agranular tumours contained the least IRI and the highest PLC percentage, the tumours with more or less atypical β-granules being in between. They concluded that a defective storage capacity for insulin seems to be the major functional abnormality of insulinoma cells. This conclusion was further substantiated by the results of <u>in vitro</u> studies on the rate of proinsulin and insulin turnover in human insulinomas carried out by the same authors (114, 115). These experiments demonstrated that insulinoma tissue as compared to normal islet tissue showed a much faster release of newly synthesized proinsulin, a clearly higher ratio of IRI release to IRI content and a much higher proportion of IRI in the cytoplasm compared to other subcellular fractions.

Creutzfeldt et al. (113) stressed the concomitant occurrence of gastrinomas and insulinomas in the same patient and of insulin containing cells in gastrinomas and suggested that cells with atypical granules occurring in insulinomas, gastrinomas, Verner-Morrison tumours and glucagonomas corresponded to, or were derived from, a stem cell which was the primitive precursor of the gastrointestinal endocrine system.

Ohneda, Sakai and Goto (108) confirmed a higher content of CPR in insulinomas with typical β-granules compared to tumours with atypical β-granules and usually observed a rather heterogeneous pattern of CPR on gel filtration including immunoreactive substances smaller than C-peptide.

The simultaneous occurrence of several intestinal hormones in the same islet tumour was proved by immunohistology and by radioimmunoassay of tumour extracts (e.g. 116-120). In general, the clinical symptoms depend on the hormone which is predominantly elevated in plasma. Fujiya et al. (120) described a patient with an insulinoma-gastrinoma,somatostatinoma-pancreatic polypeptidoma. In the resected surrounding pancreas of this patient the authors found islet proliferation and budding islets from the ductal epithelium. Insulin, glucagon and somatostatin producing cells were demonstrated in the acinar ductal epithelium by immunohistology. These results again point to the existence of a pluripotent stem cell from which all tumour cells originate.

The islet cells were grouped into hypothetical cell systems concerning their origin. Some types of islet cells at least are typical APUD (amine precursor uptake and decarboxylation) cells according to the definition of Pearse and thus derive either from ectoderm or from neuroectoderm (121, 122). The term apudoma has been widely applied for tumours arising from apud cells (123). The APUD cell concept is in total disagreement with the hypothesis by which all peptide hormones are regarded as derivatives of the primitive foregut entoderm (124, 125). A more functional paraneuron concept was proposed by Fujita and includes also the pancreatic β-cell (126, 127).

E. Metabolism of Proinsulin and C-Peptide

It is generally agreed that the half-disappearance time in plasma is longer and the metabolic clearance rate (MCR) lower for proinsulin and C-peptide than for insulin, although there is much variation in the results. Studies in man were reviewed by Faber, Kehlet, Madsbad and Binder (128).

The most important organ for the metabolism of insulin is the liver (129). Porcine and bovine proinsulin and C-peptide showed an almost negligible clearance in perfusion experiments of rat liver (130, 131). In vivo studies in pigs showed an extraction of endogenous C-peptide by the liver about 50% lower than that of insulin (132). Simultaneous determinations of insulin, proinsulin and C-peptide in the peripheral and portal circulation in man confirmed the smaller extraction of proinsulin and C-peptide in the liver (133, 134).

The kidney is known to play an important role in the metabolism of low molecular weight proteins. The contribution of the renal extraction to the MCR was 33% for insulin, 55% for proinsulin and 68% for C-peptide. These results were obtained in rats in vivo with peptides of bovine origin (135). An inverse correlation between renal clearance and molecular size of β-cell peptides was observed on perfusion of rat kidneys (136). Both experimental studies concluded that peritubular extraction contributed to renal clearance of C-peptide, insulin and proinsulin.

F. Proinsulin and C-Peptide in the Circulation of Healthy Subjects

Steiner (2) reported small quantities of proinsulin in medium in which rat islets had been incubated. Further _in vitro_ studies confirmed this finding, excluded the possibility of an artefact and characterized proinsulin secretion (137-140).

Rubenstein, Cho and Steiner (68) and Roth, Gorden and Pastan (62) were the first to demonstrate the presence of proinsulin in the circulation of man. The extensive literature concerning this subject has been reviewed recently (72, 141).

There is general agreement that the proinsulin portion in the fasting state is negligible with IMCP but not with IMI. The concentrations in 46 nondiabetics in the fasting state (142) were IRI: 0.054 ± 0.027 pmol/ml (8.8 ± 4.3 µU/ml), C-peptide: 0.39 ± 0.12 pmol/ml and proinsulin: 0.014 ± 0.009 pmol/ml. After β-cell stimulation in healthy subjects the proinsulin portion is not negligible for either IMI or IMCP. Proinsulin comprises more than 50% of IRI and more than 25% of C-peptide three hours after an oral glucose load (80). Further studies are needed to fully elucidate the contribution of proinsulin to IMI and IMCP.

An equimolar release of insulin and C-peptide by isolated islets of the rat has been reported (5, 143) and is the basis of the interpretation of clinical and experimental C-peptide determinations. It has been contended recently (144, 145). The simultaneous secretion of insulin and C-peptide from the pancreas was confirmed but much higher concentrations of immunoreactive insulin than C-peptide were found in pancreatic venous blood of the dog as well as in the perfusate of the isolated rat pancreas. A different sensitivity and specificity of the respective antisera was discussed but the authors concluded that C-peptide was secreted in much smaller amounts than insulin. It is important to define clearly the equimolarity of insulin and C-peptide secretion of the β-cells in future experiments. Indirect evidence for an equimolar secretion of insulin and C-peptide was found by comparing immunomeasurable insulin (IMI) and C-peptide (IMCP) in the pancreatico-duodenal vein in the pig (17) and in the portal vein in man (75, 133, 134).

In case of an equimolar secretion of insulin and C-peptide by the β-cells, C-peptide should be a suitable second indicator to monitor β-cell secretion. In insulin treated diabetics it should offer an unique chance to follow-up the residual β-cell secretion capacity.

Under all conditions of β-cell stimulation, a correlation between the course of IMCP and IMI in the circulation was observed (65, 66, 133, 146, 147). However, not only the basal concentration but also its increase were greater for IMCP than for IMI, this being particularly noticeable with long acting stimulators such as glibenclamide-glucose (75). Today there is general agreement that C-peptide or IMCP is a more reliable indicator of the secretion of the β-cells than insulin (75, 133, 146).

Renal or liver disease influences the reliability of both indicators of β-cell secretion. According to the metabolic role of both organs, C-peptide (IMCP) and proinsulin are mainly raised in renal failure while hepatic damage causes hyperinsulinism. However, our own results in patients before and after mesocaval shunt surgery suggest that hypersecretion of the β-cells also occurs in liver diseases (78).

G. Proinsulin and C-Peptide in the Circulation of Diabetics

I. Occurrence of proinsulin in diabetes

The idea that the occurrence of more biologically less active proinsulin instead of insulin might explain the diabetic condition in general, did not prove true. In diabetics not treated with insulin and showing raised basal and stimulated IMI concentrations, the absolute proinsulin concentrations were shown to be raised with a normal proinsulin/IMI ratio (70, 148-154). On the contrary, in diabetics not treated with insulin and showing subnormal basal and stimulated IMI concentrations, increased proinsulin/IMI and proinsulin/IMCP ratios were observed (70, 155, 156). Heding (70) found an increase in the proinsulin/IMI ratio only after β-cell stimulation. All authors speculate that the exhausted β-cell on permanent stimulation releases more proinsulin.

However, a hypersecretion of proinsulin or related intermediates with proinsulin/IMI ratios up to 92% was not associated with diabetes in 18 patients from 4 generations of an American family (157, 158).

In insulin treated diabetics human proinsulin may be the major portion of IMCP (65, 82, 159) and may be detected in serum even in cases of undetectable C-peptide (142, 160). It is an open issue as to how much a preferential release of proinsulin by the β-cell (78,82) and a more passive accumulation of the prohormone bound to antibodies against insulin (81) contribute to the high proinsulin levels. The preferential release of proinsulin could be favoured by the stress exerted on the exhausted β-cell, as discussed above, and/or by the appearance of antibodies to insulin in the circulation (69, 82, 161-163).

Thus, to our actual knowledge, a relationship does exist between diabetes and the occurrence of proinsulin. This relationship suggests that raised proinsulin portions are more likely a consequence,than a cause of diabetes.

II. Occurrence of C-peptide and IMCP

The occurrence of C-peptide even in totally duodeno-pancreatectomized patients (78, 164-166) is most likely due to the necessity and difficulty in choosing a suitable zero serum for the radioimmunoassay. For practical purposes the maximum IMCP in pancreatectomized patients (0.3 ng/ml, corresponding to 0.099 nmol/ml in our assay) must be taken as the limit of detection.

Eleven children between 1.5 and 14.5 years of age presenting with blood glucose concentrations between 223 and 1167 mg/dl and ketonuria showed undetectable IMCP only in two cases and IMCP concentrations above the fasting level of healthy volunteers in two other cases. These findings are in agreement with those of others (167). Measurable, but subnormal IMCP fasting concentrations, were found in ten of 25 patients between 7 and 21 years of age diabetic for a period of 19 to 178 months (75). The risk of undetectable IMCP concentrations increased with the duration of the disease. It is now generally accepted that the great majority of insulin dependent, ketosis prone diabetics show detectable IMCP concentrations at diagnosis and shortly after, and that IMCP decreases with the duration of diabetes and occurs more frequently when manifested at a later age (163, 164, 168-171).

The decrease of β-cell function with time was confirmed in follow-up studies which suggested that two types of diabetes could be differentiated, one with slow and one with rapid loss of residual beta-cell function (167, 172, 173).

Most diabetics not dependent on insulin, although some of them are treated with it, and not at risk of severe ketosis, show a normal or raised fasting IMCP level (75, 146, 159, 165). C-peptide is a valuable indicator of β-cell function not only in diabetics but also in their newborn children (174, 175).

After an acute onset, the juvenile type diabetes often enters a remission phase or "honeymoon period" (176). Determinations of IMCP proved that the remission phase is due to recovery of residual β-cell function (177). However, this recovery is by no means total. While fasting IMCP concentrations are normal or even raised during the remission phase, the stimulation capacity of the β-cells is reduced and altered (75, 178, 179). The β-cell secretion responded best to an arginine infusion (0.5 g/kg over 30 min), showed some response to an oral glucose load (1.75 g/kg) and responded very weakly or not at all to an i.v. glucose load (0.33 g/kg) even if repeated after 60 min (178, 179). These observations are of pathophysiological interest and might be of therapeutic relevance.

III. Clinical relevance of C-peptide in diabetes

1. Residual β-cell secretion and diabetes therapy. Glucose together with the sulfonylurea glibenclamide exerts a powerful and long acting stimulation of the β-cell secretion *in vitro* (180) and *in vivo* (181). A standardized intravenous glibenclamide-glucose load was suggested as a prediction test to decide between insulin and sulfonylurea therapy (182, 183). The prediction at this time was based on the evaluation of blood glucose (BG) during the test. By determining IMCP the relationship between the residual β-cell secretion and the therapeutic need was examined. Our first results showed a lack of stimulation capacity in 20 insulin dependent patients and a preserved stimulation capacity in 20 patients successfully treated with sulfonylureas (184, 185). By discrimination analysis we examined which of 14 parameters relating to BG, IMCP and IMI correlated best with the therapeutic need of 122 patients treated with insulin and 116 treated orally (186). All parameters relating to IMCP were important, the maximal absolute rise of IMCP during the first 40 min of the test (total duration 180 min) being the most relevant parameter. The therapeutic decision thus depends essentially on the "Sekretionsstarre" (187) or the "insulinogenic reserve" (188).

The most relevant BG parameter was the fasting BG. Taking $\Delta_{max}IMCP_{0-40min}$ and the fasting BG together, about 90% of the patients were correctly treated with insulin and sulfonylurea. Therapy also influenced residual β-cell secretion. In adult type diabetics, some recovery of β-cell secretion was observed after changing from sulfonylurea to insulin (189-191). In juvenile type diabetics strict metabolic control seems to be an important prerequisite for a preserved β-cell secretion later (192-194).

2. Residual β-cell secretion and diabetes control. In 28 insulin requiring diabetics aged 14 to 74 years, blood glucose, urine glucose and acetonuria as well as the blood glucose concentrations and the mean blood glucose (MBG) of a continuously registered 24-hour BG profile were measured as well as the mean IMCP from 23 determinations during the 24-hour profile as an index of residual β-cell function (185). The individual mean IMCP concentrations correlated inversely with the MBG. The 14 patients with the higher mean IMCP concentration showed better control according to clinical criteria and a lower mean level of BG during the 24-hour profile compared to the 14 patients with lower mean IMCP concentrations. Patients with higher mean IMCP concentrations required less insulin daily, six were adequately treated with only one injection daily while the other 22 had two injections.

Many authors have concluded that diabetes control and stability are positively correlated to the extent of residual β-cell secretion (e.g. 164, 168, 195). Even if there is doubt as to whether the chosen criteria for diabetes control and stability were fulfilled by all the reports, there is overwhelming evidence for the positive influence of residual β-cell secretion and only very few papers did not record it (170, 196, 197). Several of the studies also found a lesser requirement of insulin in cases with more IMCP. Our own data suggest that the treatment with a single daily insulin injection can only be successful in patients with a preserved residual β-cell secretion.

3. Residual β-cell secretion and retinopathy. From the abovementioned 238 patients tested with glibenclamide-glucose i.v. 110 were selected on the basis of an examination with the fundus camera within one month of the test, a normal serum creatinine level and a history of diabetes after the age of 30 (198).

Table 2 shows the clinical data of the selected patients. The study confirmed the well-known strong dependency of a retinopathy on the duration of diabetes. As IMCP parameters, e.g.

Table 2. Summary of clinical data from 110 diabetic patients

		range	median
diabetes duration (years):		0-35	9
age at onset (years):		30-77	50
body weight (% of normal):		63-185	102
retinopathy	with	n = 44	
	without	n = 66	
therapy	diet only	n = 2	
	diet + sulfonylurea	n = 70	
	diet + insulin	n = 38	
sex	female	n = 58	
	male	n = 52	

the integrated stimulation area during glibenclamide-glucose test, depended on the duration of diabetes this might indirectly suggest a dependency of retinopathy on IMCP. A further indirect hint for such a dependency is the relationship between diabetes control and IMCP on the one hand (see above), and diabetes control and retinopathy (199) on the other. Direct evidence for a relationship between retinopathy and IMCP was also found. Only twelve of 56 patients with a duration of diabetes less than 10 years showed a retinopathy while this occurred in 32 of 54 patients with a diabetes duration of 10 years and more. No correlation between IMCP parameters and retinopathy was found for the patients with less than 10 years duration of diabetes. However, the higher frequency of retinopathy with less IMCP for the patients with more than 10 years duration of diabetes was statistically significant (chi square test, $p<0.01$) if the residual β-cell secretion was expressed by the maximal absolute increase of IMCP during the first 40 minutes of the glibenclamide-glucose test (Table 3). From Table 3 it can also be seen that ΔIMCP/40min had no influence on the severity of the retinopathy, graded as +, up to five microaneurysms; ++, minimal changes, soft and hard exudates, bleeding; +++, proliferations. The only report of a relationship between retinopathy and residual β-cell secretion examined 64 patients with long-term juvenile diabetes (170) and showed a higher prevalence of severe retinopathy in IMCP non-secretors than in secretors.

It is of interest that the rapid stimulation capacity of residual β-cell secretion as expressed by the $\Delta IMCP_{0-40\ min}$ value is the most relevant parameter for the therapeutic need as well as for the prevention of retinopathy.

Table 3. Distribution of 54 diabetics with ≥ 10 years duration of the disease according to retinopathy and stimulation increment of immunomeasurable C-peptide (IMCP) at 40 min. following glibenclamide-glucose i.v.

		ΔIMCP/40 min.(ng/ml)		
		≤1,0	>1,0	total
retinopathy	ø – +++	31	23	54
	ø	8	14	22
	+ – +++	23	9	32
	+	10	4	14
	++	12	5	17
	+++	1	ø	1

H. C-Peptide and Proinsulin in Other Body Fluids

The significance of measuring C-peptide in urine was described by Rubenstein (200) who also described the presence of proinsulin in urine (63) and gave some technical details on its determination (201). However, the measurement of insulin as well as proinsulin in urine has gained almost no practical relevance. Urine contains greater amounts of C-peptide than of insulin. Reliable methods to determine C-peptide in diluted urine samples were described by several authors (202-204). In our experience, measurements of C-peptide in urine are less precise than in serum.

Kuzuya et al. (205) found 81 $\pm$ 36 μg CPR in urine per day in normal subjects. However, the results varied depending on the authors, as in the case of serum or plasma (cf. Table 1). CPR in urine and serum correlated well apart from uremia (203) and rare unexplained exceptions (206). There is general agreement that CPR determinations in urine are suitable to document β-cell secretion capacity in diabetes and for reasons of practicability especially in diabetic children (e.g. 203-205, 207-209).

The occurrence of CPR was also reported in cerebrospinal fluid, ascites and pleural effusions (144, 202). Our studies showed IMCP to occur in human pancreatic juice obtained by direct endoscopic cannulation of the Papilla of Vater in eight patients without known pancreatic disease (210). Material cross-reacting with antisera against insulin, glucagon, gastrin, pancreatic polypeptide and somatostatin was also found in pancreatic juice in concentrations corresponding to plasma levels. The physiologic relevance of pancreatic hormones in pancreatic juice has not been elucidated. Both insulin and C-peptide appear in amniotic fluid (211) and are of prognostic value in fetal macrosomia.

I. C-Peptide and Proinsulin in the Differential Diagnosis of Hypoglycemia

Several reports in literature confirm the diagnostic role of C-peptide in factitious hypoglycemia by revealing the discrepancy between BG, β-cell secretion as expressed by IMCP and the serum IMI concentration (213-218).

We observed a very interesting case of factitious hypoglycemia (212). A 35 year old nurse and nun presented with characteristic symptoms of fasting hypoglycemia. IMI was extremely high in the patient's serum, in the presence of antibodies to insulin, while IMCP was in the normal range. It was furthermore suspicious of a factitious hypoglycemia by exogenous insulin injection that BG fell, IMI rose and IMCP remained constant on injection of 1 g tolbutamide i.v. The final proof of insulin self-injection was the demonstration that proinsulin in the patient's serum did not cross-react with our antiserum against human C-peptide and therefore was not of human origin. The patient confessed when confronted with this fact.

According to our experience the only use of C-peptide in the diagnosis of insulinoma is to exclude a factitious hypoglycemia, except for the more hypothetical case of an insulinoma in an insulin-treated diabetic patient.

The frequently described and recommended elegant insulin suppression test (219-224) can be falsely negative (220, 223, 224) and therefore cannot replace the much more time-consuming fasting test, extended to 72 hours if necessary. In the whole literature, to our knowledge, there is only a single case report of a negative 72 hours fasting test in an insulinoma patient (225).

The occurrence of raised absolute and relative (to IMI and IMCP) proinsulin concentrations in insulinoma patients is well known (for a review see 226). However, according to the literature and our own unpublished experience, proinsulin and its percentage of IMI and IMCP may also be normal in surgically proven insulinomas. It is most interesting in this respect that Heding, applying her new and very sensitive technique to measure proinsulin (70), reported raised proinsulin concentrations in 31 insulinoma cases compared to 47 healthy controls (80). This means that raised proinsulin levels might well be pathognomonic in patients with insulinomas.

J. Biological Activity of Proinsulin and C-Peptide

I. Proinsulin

The results of a large number of studies have been reviewed (72, 227, 228) and can be summarized as follows: Only insulin-like effects of proinsulin have been reported and in general the multiple insulin-like effects were less potent than those of insulin. However, differences in biological potency of insulin and proinsulin showed great variations depending on the effects examined. As to its hypoglycaemic effect _in vivo_, proinsulin also differs qualitatively from insulin, showing a retarded and prolonged effect. The majority of results are against a peripheral transformation of proinsulin to insulin.

The possibility of a biological role for proinsulin in the regulation of metabolism was stressed by Steiner (51); the problem is still an open issue. The observation of a relatively pronounced effect of proinsulin on the DNA synthesis of fibroblasts (229) and the similarities of proinsulin and IGF I (50) point to preferential anabolic growth-related effects of the prohormone. This interesting subject deserves further scientific investigation.

II. C-peptide

No effect of C-peptide and no influence on the effects of insulin and proinsulin were observed on examining CO_2 and lipid production from glucose and lipolysis in fat tissue (reviewed by 70, 228).

Several authors observed an inhibition of β-cell secretion by C-peptide in vitro in rats (230-233). However, the results differ as to the relative potency of rat C-peptides I and II and of human C-peptide and in respect to the effective concentrations. Further studies must confirm the interesting phenomenon and examine its physiologic relevance.

Most recent findings suggest that C-peptide might be a candidate for the suspected negative feedback between the endocrine pancreas and the release of gastric inhibitory polypeptide (GIP). Further studies are required to confirm the physiologic relevance of this regulating mechanism (234).

References

1. Steiner, D.F., Oyer, P.E.: The biosynthesis of insulin and a probable precursor of insulin by a human islet cell adenoma. Proc. natn. Acad. Sci. 57, 473-480 (1967).
2. Steiner, D.F.: Evidence for a precursor in the biosynthesis of insulin. Trans. N.Y. Acad. Sci. 30, 60-68 (1967).
3. Steiner, D.F., Cunningham, D., Spigelman, L., Aten, B.: Insulin biosynthesis: Evidence for a precursor. Science 157, 697-700 (1967).
4. Steiner, D.F., Clark, J.L., Nolan, C., Rubenstein, A.H., Margoliash, E., Aten, B., Oyer, P.E.: Proinsulin and the biosynthesis of insulin. Recent Prog. Horm. Res. 25, 182-207 (1969).
5. Clark, J.L., Steiner, D.F.: Insulin biosynthesis in the rat: Demonstration of two proinsulins. Proc. natn. Acad. Sci. U.S.A. 62, 278-285 (1969).
6. Mirsky, I.A., Kawamura, K.: Heterogeneity of crystalline insulin. Endocrinology 78, 1115-1119 (1966).
7. Steiner, D.F., Hallund, O., Rubenstein, A.H., Cho, S., Bayliss, C.: Isolation and properties of proinsulin, intermediate forms, and other minor components from crystalline insulin. Diabetes 17, 725-736 (1968).
8. Chance, R.E., Ellis, R.M., Bromer, W.W.: Porcine proinsulin: Characterization and amino acid sequence. Science 161, 165-167 (1968).
9. Schmidt, D.D., Arens, A.: Proinsulin vom Rind. Isolierung, Eigenschaften und seine Aktivierung durch Trypsin. Hoppe-Seyler's Z. physiol. Chem. 349, 1157-1168 (1968).

10. Oyer, P.E., Cho, S., Peterson, J.D., Steiner, D.F.: Studies on human proinsulin. Isolation and amino acid sequence of the human pancreatic C-peptide. J. biol. Chem. 246, 1375-1386 (1971).

11. Sundby, F., Markussen, J.: Rat proinsulins and C-peptides. Europ. J. Biochem. 25, 147-152 (1972).

12. Kuzuya, H., Chance, R.E., Steiner, D.F., Rubenstein, A.H.: On the preparation and characterization of standard materials for a natural human proinsulin and C-peptide. Diabetes 27 (Suppl. 1), 161-169 (1978).

13. Sundby, F., Markussen, J.: Preparative method for the isolation of C-peptides from ox and porc pancreas. Horm. Metab. Res. 2, 17-20 (1970).

14. Markussen, J., Sundby, F., Smyth, D.G., Ko, A.: Preparation of human C-peptide. Horm. Metab. Res. 3, 229-232 (1971).

15. Steiner, D.F., Cho, S., Oyer, P.E., Terris, S., Peterson, J.D., Rubenstein, A.H.: Isolation and characterization of proinsulin C-peptide from bovine pancreas. J. biol. Chem. 246, 1365-1374 (1971).

16. Chance, R.E., Hoffmann, J.A., Johnson, M.G., Wolfe, T.M., Blix, P.M., Rubenstein, A.H.: Studies on rabbit C-peptide. In: "Proinsulin, Insulin, C-Peptide", Eds. Baba, S., Kaneko, T., Yanaihara, N., Excerpta Medica ICS No. 468, Amsterdam, pp. 99-106 (1979).

17. Heding, L.G., Larsen, U.D., Markussen, J., Jørgensen, K.H., Hallund, O.: Radioimmunoassays for human, porc and ox C-peptides and related substances. Horm. Metab. Res. Suppl. Ser. No.5, 40-44 (1974).

18. Ko, A.S., Smyth, D.G., Markussen, J., Sundby, F.: The amino acid sequence of human proinsulin. Europ. J. Biochem. 20, 190-199 (1971).

19. Tager, H.S., Emdin, S.O., Clark, J.L., Steiner, D.F.: Studies on the conversion of proinsulin to insulin. II. Evidence for a chymotrypsin-like cleavage on the connecting peptide region of insulin precursors in the rat. J. biol. Chem. 248, 3476-3482 (1973).

20. Peterson, J.D., Nehrlich, S., Oyer, P.E., Steiner, D.F.: Determination of the amino acid sequence of monkey, sheep, and dog proinsulin C-peptides by a semi-micro Edman degradation procedure. J. biol. Chem. 247, 4866-4871 (1972).

21. Nolan, Ch., Margoliash, E., Peterson, J.D., Steiner, D.F.: The structure of bovine proinsulin. J. biol. Chem. 246, 2780-2795 (1971).

22. Markussen, J., Sundby, F.: Rat-proinsulin C-peptides. Europ. J. Biochem. 25, 153-162 (1972).

23. Chance, R.E.: Chemical, physical, biological and immunological studies on porcine proinsulin and related polypeptides. In: Proceedings 7th IDF Congress, Eds. Rodriguez, R.R., Vallance-Owen, J., Excerpta Medica ICS No.231, Amsterdam, pp. 292-305 (1970).

24. Salokangas, A., Smyth, D.G., Markussen, J., Sundby, F.: Bovine proinsulin: Amino acid sequence of the C-peptide isolated from pancreas. Europ. J. Biochem. 20, 183-189 (1971).

25. Tager, H.S., Steiner, D.F.: Primary structure of the proinsulin connecting peptides of the rat and the horse. J. biol. Chem. 247, 7936-7940 (1972).

26. Smyth, D.G., Markussen, J., Sundby, F.: The amino acid sequence of guinea pig C-peptide. Nature 248, 151-152 (1974).

27. Massey, D.E., Smyth, D.G.: Guinea pig proinsulin. Primary structure of the C-peptide isolated from pancreas. J. biol. Chem. 250, 6288-6290 (1975).

28. Snell, C.R., Smyth, D.G.: Proinsulin: A proposed three-dimensional structure. J. biol. Chem. 250, 6291-6295 (1975).

29. Markussen, J., Sundby, F.: Isolation and amino-acid sequence of the C-peptide of duck proinsulin. Europ. J. Biochem. 34, 401-408 (1973).

30. Low, B.W., Fullerton, W.N., Rosen, L.S.: Insulin/proinsulin a new crystalline complex. Nature 248, 339-340 (1974).

31. Frank, B.H., Pekar, A.H., Veros, A.J.: Insulin and proinsulin conformation in solution. Diabetes 21 (Suppl. 2) 486-491 (1972).

32. Vogt, H.P., Wollmer, A., Naithani, V.K., Zahn, H.: The conformational potential of porcine proinsulin C-peptide. Hoppe-Seyler's Z. physiol. Chem. 357, 107-116 (1976).

33. Markussen, J., Heding, L.G.: Separation of the double-chain bovine intermediates of the proinsulin-insulin conversion. I. Chemical, immunological, circular dichroism, and biological characterization. Int. J. Pept. Protein Res. 8, 597-606 (1976).

34. Chance, R.E.: Amino acid sequence of proinsulins and intermediates. Diabetes 21, (Suppl. 2) 461-467 (1972).

35. Yamaji, K., Tada, K., Trakatellis, A.C.: On the biosynthesis of insulin in anglerfish islets. J. biol. Chem. 247, 4080-4088 (1972).

36. Sorenson, R.L., Steffes, M.W., Lindall, A.W.: Subcellular localization of proinsulin to insulin conversion in isolated rat islets. Endocrinology 86, 88-96 (1970).

37. Clark, W.R., Rutter, W.J.: Synthesis and accumulation of insulin in the fetal rat pancreas. Develop Biol. 29, 468-481 (1972).

38. Kemmler, W., Steiner, D.F., Borg, J.: Studies on the conversion of proinsulin to insulin. III. Studies in vitro with crude secretion granule fraction isolated from rat islets of Langerhans. J. biol. Chem. 248, 4544-4551 (1973).

39. Tung, A.K., Yip, C.C.: Biosynthesis of insulin in bovine fetal pancreatic slices: The incorporation of tritiated leucine into a single-chain proinsulin, a double-chain intermediate, and insulin in subcellular fractions. Proc. natn. Acad. Sci. U.S.A. 63, 442-449 (1969).

40. Grant, P.T., Reid, K.B.: Biosynthesis of an insulin precursor by cod islet tissue and the occurrence of intermediates in the conversion to insulin. Biochem. J. 109, 32P (1968).

41. Noe, B.D., Baste, C.A., Bauer, G.E.: Studies on proinsulin and proglucagon biosynthesis and conversion at the subcellular level. II. Distribution of radioactive peptide hormones and hormone precursors in subcellular fractions after pulse-chase incubation of islet tissue. J. Cell Biol. 74, 589-604 (1977).

42. Steiner, D.F., Kemmler, W., Clark, J.L., Oyer, P.E., Rubenstein, A.H.: The biosynthesis of insulin. In: "Handbook of Physiology", Section 7, Vol. I, Eds. Steiner, D.F., Freinkel, N., American Physiological Society, Washington D.C., pp. 175-198 (1972).

43. Steiner, D.F., Kemmler, W., Tager, H.S., Rubenstein, A.H.: Molecular events taking place during intracellular transport of exportable proteins. The conversion of peptide hormone precursors. Adv. Cytopharmacol. 2, 195-205 (1974).

44. Geiger, R., Wissmann, H., Weidenmüller, H.L., Schröder, H.G.: Rekombination der A- und B- Ketten von Schweine-Insulin in Anwesenheit von synthetischem C-Peptid des Schweine-Proinsulins. Z. Naturforsch. (B) 24, 1489-1490 (1969).

45. Brandenburg, D., Wollmer, A.: The effect of a non-peptide interchain crosslink on the reoxidation of reduced insulin. Hoppe-Seyler's Z. physiol. Chem. 354, 613-627 (1973).

46. Robinson, S.M.L., Beetz, I., Loge, O., Lindsay, D.G.: Spaltung und Rückbildung der Disulfidbrücken an intramolekular vernetzten Insulinen. Tetrehedron Letters 12, 985-988 (1973).

47. Geiger, R., Obermeier, R.: Insulin synthesis from natural chains by means of reversible bridging compounds. Biochem. biophys. Res. Commun. 55, 60-66 (1973).

48. Busse, W.D., Carpenter, F.H.: Carbonylbis (L-methionine p-nitrophenyl ester). A new reagent for the reversible intramolecular cross-linking of insulin. J. Amer. chem. Soc. 96, 5947-5948 (1974).

49. Markussen, J.: Proteolytic degradation of proinsulin and of intermediate forms: Application to synthesis and biosynthesis of insulin. In: "Proinsulin, Insulin, and C-Peptide", Eds. Baba, S., Kaneko, T., Yanaihara, N., Excerpta Medica ICS No. 468, Amsterdam, pp. 50-61 (1979).

50. Rinderknecht, E., Humbel, R.E.: The amino acid sequence of human insulin-like growth factor I and its structural homology with proinsulin. J. biol. Chem. 253, 2769-2776 (1978).

51. Steiner, D.F.: Peptide hormone precursors: Biosynthesis, processing, and significance. In: "Peptide Hormones", Ed. Parsons, J.A., Macmillan Press, London, pp. 49-64 (1976).

52. Blobel, G., Dobberstein, B.: Transfer of proteins across membranes. I. Presence of proteolytically processed and unprocessed nascent immunoglobulin light chains on membrane-bound ribosomes of murine myeloma. J. Cell Biol. 67, 835-851 (1975).

53. Blobel, G., Dobberstein, B.: Transfer of proteins across membranes. II. Recognition of functional rough microsomes from heterologous components. J. Cell Biol. 67, 852-862 (1975).

54. Chan, S.J., Keim, P., Steiner, D.F.: Cell-free synthesis of rat pre-proinsulins: Characterization and partial amino acid sequence determination. Proc. natn. Acad. Sci. U.S.A. 73, 1964-1968 (1976).

55. Patzelt, C., Chan, S.J., Duguid, J., Hortin, G., Keim, P., Henrikson, R.L., Steiner, D.F.: Biosynthesis of polypeptide hormones in intact and cell free systems. In: "Regulatory Proteolytic Enzymes and their Inhibitors", Vol. 47, Symposium A6, Ed. Schambye, P., Pergamon Press, Oxford, pp. 69-78 (1978).

56. Steiner, D.F., Duguid, J.R., Patzelt, C., Chan, S.J., Quinn, P., Labrecque, A., Hastings, R.: New aspects of insulin biosynthesis.In: "Proinsulin, Insulin, C-Peptide", Eds. Baba, S., Kaneko, T., Yanaihara, N., Excerpta Medica ICS No. 468, Amsterdam, pp. 9-19 (1979).

57. Permutt, M.A., Biesbroeck, J., Chyn, R., Boine, I., Szczesna, E., Mc Williams, D.: Isolation of biologically active messenger RNA: Preparation from fish pancreatic islets by oligo (2'-deoxythymidylic acid) affinity chromatography. In: "Polypeptide Hormones: Molecular and Cellular Aspects", Ciba Foundation Symposium 41, Elsevier/Excerpta Medica, Amsterdam, pp. 97-116 (1976).

58. Ullrich, A., Shine, J., Chirgwin, J., Pictet, R., Tischer, E., Rutter, W.J., Goodman, H.M.: Rat insulin genes: Construction of plasmids containing the coding sequence. Science 196, 1313-1319 (1977).

59. Duguid, F.R., Steiner, D.F.: Identification of the major polyadenylated transcription products and the genes active in the synthesis in a rat insulinoma. Proc. natn. Acad. Sci. U.S.A. 75, 3249-3253 (1978).

60. Okamoto, H., Nose, K., Itoh, N., Sei, T., Yamamoto, H.: Translational control of proinsulin in pancreatic islets. In: "Proinsulin, Insulin, C-Peptide", Eds. Baba, S., Kaneko, T., Yanaihara, N., Excerpta Medica ICS No. 468, Amsterdam, pp. 27-35 (1979).

61. Ullrich, A., Shine, J., Seeburg, P.H., Tischer, E., Pictet, R.L., Cordell, B., Bell, G.I., Chirgwin, J.M., Rutter, W.J., Goodman, H.M.: The structure and expression of the insulin gene. In: "Proinsulin, Insulin, C-Peptide", Eds. Baba, S., Kaneko, T., Yanaihara, N., Excerpta Medica ICS No. 468, Amsterdam, pp. 20-26 (1979).

62. Roth, J., Gorden, P., Pastan, I.: "Big insulin": A new component of plasma insulin detected by immunoassay. Proc. natn. Acad. Sci. U.S.A. 61, 138-145 (1968).

63. Rubenstein, A.H., Cho, S., Steiner, D.F.: Evidence for proinsulin in human urine and serum. Lancet 1, 1353-1355 (1968).

64. Melani, F., Rubenstein, A.H., Oyer, P.E., Steiner, D.F.: Identification of proinsulin and C-peptide in human serum by a specific immunoassay. Proc. natn. Acad. Sci. U.S.A. 67, 148-155 (1970).

65. Block, M.B., Mako, M.E., Steiner, D.F., Rubenstein, A.H.: Circulating C-peptide immunoreactivity, studies in normals and in diabetic patients. Diabetes 21, 1013-1026 (1972).

66. Kaneko, T., Oka, H., Munemura, M., Oda, T., Yamashita, K., Suzuki, S., Yanaihara, N., Hashimoto, T., Yanaihara, C.: Radioimmunoassay of human proinsulin C-peptide using synthetic human connecting peptide. Endocrinol.jap. 21, 141-145 (1974).

67. Beischer, W., Keller, L., Maas, M., Schiefer, E., Pfeiffer, E.F.: Human C-peptide. Part I: radioimmunoassay. Klin. Wschr. 54, 709-715 (1976).

68. Faber, O.K., Markussen, J., Naithani, V.K., Binder, C.: Production of antisera to synthetic benzyloxycarbonyl-C-peptide of human proinsulin. Hoppe-Seyler's Z. physiol. Chem. 357, 751-757 (1976).

69. Heding, L.G.: Radioimmunological determination of human C-peptide in serum. Diabetologia 11, 541-548 (1975).

70. Heding, L.G.: Specific and direct radioimmunoassay for human proinsulin in serum. Diabetologia 13, 467-474 (1977).

71. Rainbow, S.J., Woodhead, J.S., Yue, D.K., Luzio, S.D., Hales, C.N.: Measurement of human proinsulin by an indirect two-site immunoradiometric assay. Diabetologia 14, 264 (1978).

72. Kitabchi, A.E.: Proinsulin and C-peptide. Metabolism 26, 547-587 (1977).

73. Berson, S.A., Yalow, R.S.: Measurement of hormones. 2. Radioimmunoassay. In: "Methods in Investigative and Diagnostic Endocrinology", vol. 2A, part I, Eds. Berson, S.A., Yalow, R.S., North Holland Publishing Comp., Amsterdam, p. 85 (1973).

74. Yanaihara, N., Hashimoto, T., Yanaihara, C., Sakagami, M., Steiner, D.F., Rubenstein, A.H.: Synthesis of human connecting peptide derivatives and their immunological properties. Biochem. biophys. Res. Commun. 59, 1124-1130 (1974).

75. Beischer, W., Heinze, E., Keller, L., Raptis, S., Kerner, W., Pfeiffer, E.F.: Human C-peptide, Part II. Clinical studies. Klin. Wschr. 54, 717-725 (1976).

76. Kuzuya, H., Blix, P.M., Horwitz, D.L., Rubenstein, A.H., Steiner, D.F., Faber, O.K., Binder, C.: Heterogeneity of circulating human C-peptide. Diabetes 27,(Suppl. 1)184-191 (1978).

77. Faber, O.K., Binder, C., Markussen, J., Heding, L.G., Naithani, V.K., Kuzuya, H., Blix, P., Horwitz, D.L., Rubenstein, A.H.: Characterization of seven C-peptide antisera. Diabetes 27, (Suppl. 1) 170-177 (1978).

78. Beischer, W.: Proinsulin und C-Peptid. Habilitationsschrift, Ulm (1980).

79. Beischer, W., Hartweg, D., Maas, M., Keller, L., Pfeiffer, E.F.: The radioimmunoassay of peptide hormones, in special of C-peptide: A critical evaluation. Hoppe-Seyler's Z. physiol. Chem. (submitted for publication).

80. Heding, L.G., Faber, O., Kasperska-Czyzykowa, T., Sestoft, T., Turner, R.: Radioimmunoassay of proinsulin and hyperproinsulin states. In: "Proinsulin, Insulin, C-Peptide", Eds. Baba, S., Kaneko, T., Yanaihara, N., Excerpta Medica ICS No. 468, Amsterdam, pp. 255-261 (1979).

81. Fink, G., Cresto, J.C., Gutman, R.A., Lavine, R.L., Rubenstein, A.H., Recant, L.: Plasma proinsulin-like material in insulin treated diabetics. Horm. Metab. Res. 6, 439-443 (1974).

82. Beischer, W., Keller, L., Heinze, E., Kerner, W., Jonatha, E.M., Pfeiffer, E.F.: The relevance of extremely high serum C-peptide concentrations in three cases of juvenile diabetes mellitus. In: "C-Peptide", Eds. Beyer, J., Krause, U., Naegele, W., Schnetztor Verlag, Konstanz, pp. 169-183 (1977).

83. Kuzuya, H., Blix, P.M., Horwitz, D.L., Steiner, D.F., Rubenstein, A.H.: Determination of free and total insulin and C-peptide in insulin-treated diabetics. Diabetes 26, 22-29 (1977).

84. Oyama, H., Horino, M., Nakashima, Y., Tenku, A., Matsumura, S.: Free C-peptide immunoreactivity in insulin treated patients. Endocrinol. jap. 24, 223-237 (1977).

85. Mering, J., von Minkowsky, O.: Diabetes mellitus nach Pankreasexstirpation. Naunyn-Schmiedebergs Arch. exp. Path. Pharmak. 26, 371 (1889/90).

86. Languesse, E.L.: Sur la formation des îlots de Langerhans dans le pancréas. C. r. Séanc. Soc. Biol. 45, 819 (1893).

87. Zülzer, G., Dohrn, M., Marxner, H.: Neuere Untersuchungen über den experimentellen Diabetes. Dtsch. Med. Wschr. 34, 1380 (1908).

88. Banting, F.G., Best, C.H., Macleod, J.J.R.: Pancreatic extracts in the treatment of diabetes mellitus. Canad. med. Ass. J. 12, 141-146 (1922).

89. Hartroft, W.S.: The islets of Langerhans in man visualized by phase contrast microscopy. Proc. Am. Diabetes Assoc. 10, 46-61 (1950).

90. Wrenshall, G.A., Bogoch, A., Ritchie, R.C.: Extractable insulin of pancreas. Diabetes 1, 87-107 (1952).

91. Bell, E.T.: The incidence and significance of degranulation of the beta-cells in the islets of Langerhans. Diabetes 2, 125-129 (1953).

92. Hartroft, W.S., Wrenshall, G.A.: Correlation of beta-cell granulation with extractable insulin of the pancreas. Studies in adult human diabetics and nondiabetics. Diabetes 4, 1-7 (1955).

93. Howell, S.L., Kostianovsky, M., Lacy, P.E.: Beta-cell formation in isolated islets of Langerhans. A study by electron microscopic radioautography. J. Cell Biol. 42, 695-705 (1969).

94. Orci, L., Lambert, A.E., Kanazawa, Y., Amherdt, M., Rouiller, C., Renold, A.: Morphological and biochemical studies of B-cell of fetal rat endocrine pancreas in organ culture. Evidence for (pro)insulin biosynthesis. J. Cell Biol. 50, 565-582 (1971).

95. Sun, A.M., Lin, B.J., Haist, R.E.: Studies on the conversion of proinsulin to insulin in isolated islets of Langerhans in the rat. Can. J. Physiol. Pharmacol. 51, 175-182 (1973).

96. Yip, C.C.: A bovine pancreatic enzyme catalyzing the conversion of proinsulin to insulin. Proc. natn. Acad. Sci. U.S.A. 68, 1312-1315 (1971).

97. Puri, R.B., Anjaneyulu, K., Kidwai, J.R., Mohan Rao, V.K.: In vitro conversion of proinsulin to insulin by cathepsin B and role of C-peptide. Acta Diab. Lat. 15, 243-250 (1978).

98. Schatz, H.: Insulin. Biosynthese und Sekretion. Thieme Verlag, Stuttgart (1976).

99. Ostlund, R.E.: Contractile proteins and pancreatic beta-cell secretion. Diabetes 26, 245-252 (1977).

100. Brown, J.C., Otte, S.C.: Gastrointestinal hormones and the control of insulin secretion. Diabetes 27, 782-787 (1978)

101. Zawalich, W.S.: Intermediary metabolism and insulin secretion from rat islets of Langerhans. Diabetes 28, 252-260 (1979).

102. Maier, V.: Die isolierte Langerhanssche Insel. Biosynthese und Sekretion von Insulin in vitro. Thieme Verlag, Stuttgart, (1980), p. 169.

103. Malaisse, W.J., Tjäldal, I.B.: Biochemistry and Biophysics of the Pancreatic B-Cell. Horm. Metab. Res. Suppl. Series No. 10, Thieme Verlag, Stuttgart (1980).

104. Rastogi, G.K., Letarte, J., Fraser, T.R.: Proinsulin content of pancreas in human fetuses of healthy mothers. Lancet I, 7-9 (1970).

105. Lockwood, D.H., Misbin, R.I.: Proinsulin content of adult and fetal pancreatic tissue extracted after rapid freezing in situ. Horm. Metab. Res. 4, 232-234 (1972).

106. Hayashi, M., Floyd, J.C., Pek, S., Fajans, S.S.: Insulin, proinsulin, glucagon and gastrin in pancreatic tumours and in plasma of patients with organic hyperinsulinism. J. clin. Endocrinol. Metab. 44, 681-694 (1977).

107. Tasaka, Y., Takei, M., Iwatani, M., Odagiri, R., Hirata, Y.: Content of C-peptide, insulin and proinsulin-like components in diabetic human pancreas and their relation to the stability of blood sugar levels. In: "Proinsulin, Insulin, C-Peptide", Eds. Baba, S., Kaneko, T., Yanaihara, N., Excerpta Medica ICS No. 468, Amsterdam, pp. 239-245 (1979).

108. Ohneda, A., Sakai, T., Goto, Y.: C-peptide in patients with insulinoma. In: "Proinsulin, Insulin, C-Peptide", Eds. Baba, S., Kaneko, T., Yanaihara, N., Excerpta Medica ICS No. 468, Amsterdam, pp. 380-385 (1979).

109. Oyama, H., Tenku, A., Katika, K., Matsumura, S., Nishida, S., Horino, M.: Recovery of human C-peptide by acid-ethanol extraction. Endocrinol. jap. 25, 493-498 (1978).

110. Grube, D.: Immunoreactivites of Gastrin (G-) cells. II. Histochemistry 66, 149-167 (1980).

111. Grube, D., Weber, E.: Immunoreactivity of Gastrin (G-) cells. I. Histochemistry 65, 223-237 (1980).

112. Creutzfeldt, W., Arnold, R., Creutzfeldt, C., Deuticke, U., Frerichs, H., Track, N.S.: Biochemical and morphological investigations of 30 human insulinomas. Diabetologia 9, 217-231(1973).

113. Creutzfeldt, W., Creutzfeldt, C., Frerichs, H., Track, N.S., Arnold, R.: Histochemistry, ultrastructure and hormone content of human insulinomas. Horm. Metab. Res. Suppl. Series No. 6, 7-18 (1976).

114. Creutzfeldt, C., Track, N.S., Creutzfeldt, W.: In vitro studies of the rate of proinsulin and insulin turnover in seven human insulinomas. Europ. J. clin. Invest. 3, 371-384 (1973).

115. Track, N.S., Creutzfeldt, C., Creutzfeldt, W.: Human insulinoma tissue: in vitro studies of proinsulin/insulin biosynthesis and release. Horm. Metab. Res. Suppl. Series No. 6, 19-25 (1976).

116. Murray-Lyon, I.M., Eddleston, A.L., Williams, T.: Treatment of multiple hormone producing malignant islet-cell tumour with streptozotocin. Lancet 2, 895-898 (1968).

117. Larsson, L.I., Grimelius, L., Hakanson, R., Rehfeld, J.F., Stadil, F., Holst, J., Angerwall, L., Sundler, F.: Mixed endocrine pancreatic tumors producing several peptide hormones. Am. J. Path. 79, 271-284 (1975).

118. Arnold, R., Creutzfeldt, C., Creutzfeldt, W.: Multiple hormone production of endocrine tumours of the gastro-intestinal tract. In: "Endocrinology", Vol. 2, Ed. James, V.H.T., Excerpta Medica, Amsterdam, pp. 448-452 (1977).

119. Abe, K., Yamaguchi, K., Adachi, I., Yanaihara, N.: Multiple hormone production in islet-cell tumors. In: "Proinsulin, Insulin, C-Peptide", Eds. Baba, S., Kaneko, T., Yanaihara, N., Excerpta Medica ICS No. 468, Amsterdam, pp. 473-479 (1979).

120. Fujiya, H., Toyota, T., Umezu, M., Goto, Y., Yanaihara, N.: Immunohistological study of endocrine pancreatic tumors. In: "Proinsulin, Insulin, C-Peptide", Eds. Baba, S., Kaneko, T., Yanaihara, N., Excerpta Medica ICS No. 468, Amsterdam, pp. 386-393 (1979).

121. Pearse, A.G.E.: The cytochemistry and ultrastructure of polypeptide hormone-producing cells of the APUD series and the embryologic, physiologic and pathologic implications of the concept. J. Histochem. Cytochem. 5, 303-313 (1969).

122. Pearse, A.G.E.: Evolutionary and developmental relationships among the cells producing peptide hormones. In: "Peptide Hormones", Ed. Parsons, J.A., Macmillan Press, London and Basingstoke, pp. 32-46 (1976).

123. Welbourn, R.B.: Current status of the Apudomas. Ann. Surg. 185, 1-12 (1977).

124. Adelson, J.W.: Enterosecretory proteins. Nature 229, 321-325 (1971).

125. Weinstein, B.: A generalized homology correlation for various hormones and proteins. Experimentia 28, 1517-1522 (1972).

126. Fujita, T.: The gastro-enteric endocrine cell and its paraneuric nature. In: "Chromaffin, Enterochromaffin and Related Substances", Eds. Coupland, R.E., Fujita, T., Elsevier, Amsterdam, pp. 191-208 (1976).

127. Fujita, T., Kobayashi, S., Serizawa, Y.: The insulin producing B-cell as a paraneuron. In: "Proinsulin, Insulin, C-Peptide", Eds. Baba, S., Kaneko, T., Yanaihara, N., Excerpta Medica ICS No. 468, Amsterdam, pp. 327-334 (1979).

128. Faber, O.K., Kehlet, H., Madsbad, S., Binder, C.: Kinetics of human C-peptide in man. Diabetes 27,(Suppl. 1) 207-208 (1978).

129. Field, J.B.: Insulin extraction by the liver. In: "Handbook of Physiology", Section 7, Vol. 1, Eds. Steiner, D.F., Freinkel, N., American Physiological Society, Washington D.C., pp. 505-513 (1972).

130. Stoll, R.W., Touber, J.L., Menahan, L.A., Williams, R.H.: Clearance of porcine insulin, proinsulin, and connecting peptide by the isolated rat liver. Proc. Soc. exp. Biol Med. 133, 894-896 (1970).

131. Rubenstein, A.H., Pottenger, L.A., Mako, M., Getz, G.S., Steiner, D.F.: The metabolism of proinsulin and insulin by the liver. J. clin. Invest. 51, 912-921 (1972).

132. Kühl, C., Faber, O.K., Hornnes, P., Jensen, S.L.: C-peptide metabolism and the liver. Diabetes 27, (Suppl. 1) 197-200 (1978).

133. Horwitz, D.L., Starr, J.I., Mako, M.E., Blackard, W.G., Rubenstein, A.H.: Proinsulin, insulin and C-peptide concentrations in human portal and peripheral blood. J. clin. Invest. 55, 1278-1283 (1975).

134. Rövenstrunck, U., Beischer, W., Loeprecht, H., Raptis, S., Pfeiffer, E.F.: Hepatic clearance of insulin and C-peptide. In: "C-Peptide", Eds. Beyer, J., Krause, U., Naegele, W., Schnetztor Verlag, Konstanz, pp. 41-49 (1977).

135. Katz, A.J., Rubenstein, A.H.: Metabolism of proinsulin, insulin and C-peptide in the rat. J. clin. Invest. 52, 1113-1121 (1973).

136. Rabkin, R., Ross, B.D., Mako, M.E., Rubenstein, A.H.: The handling of insulin, proinsulin and C-peptide by the isolated rat kidney. Diabetes 27, (Suppl. 1) 192-196 (1978).

137. Burr, I.M., Stauffacher, W., Balant, L., Renold, A.E., Grodsky, G.: Dynamic aspects of proinsulin release from perifused rat pancreas. Lancet 2, 882-883 (1969).

138. Lazarus, N.R., Tanese, T., Gutman, R., Recant, L.: Synthesis and release of proinsulin and insulin by human insulinoma tissue. J. clin. Endocrinol. Metab. 30, 273-281 (1970).

139. Sando, H., Grodsky, G.M.: Dynamic synthesis and release of insulin and proinsulin from perfused islets. Diabetes 22, 354-360 (1973).

140. Track, N.S., Frerichs, H., Creutzfeldt, W.: Release of newly synthesized proinsulin and insulin from granulated and degranulated isolated rat pancreatic islets. The effect of high glucose concentrations. Horm. Metab. Res. Suppl. Series No. 5, 97-103 (1974).

141. Rubenstein, A.H., Steiner, D.F., Horwitz, D.L., Mako, M.E., Block, M.B., Starr, J.I., Kuzuya, H., Melani, F.: Clinical significance of circulating proinsulin and C-peptide. Recent Prog. Horm. Res. 33, 435-475 (1976).

142. Heding, L.G.: Insulin, C-peptide and proinsulin in non-diabetic and insulin treated diabetics. Characterization of the proinsulin in insulin treated diabetics. Diabetes 27, (Suppl. 1) 178-183 (1978).

143. Rubenstein, A.H., Clark, J.L., Melani, F., Steiner, D.F.: Secretion of proinsulin by pancreatic β-cells and its circulation in blood. Nature 224, 697-699 (1969).

144. Kaneko, T.: Clinical and experimental studies on C-peptide. In: Proceedings IXth IDF Congress, Ed. Bajaj, J.S., Excerpta Medica ICS No. 413, Amsterdam, pp. 142-148 (1977).

145. Kaneko, T., Kaneto, A., Yanaihara, N., Yasuda, H., Suzuki, S., Oka, H., Oda, T.: Insulin and C-peptide in animals. In: "Proinsulin, Insulin, C-Peptide", Eds. Baba, S., Kaneko, T., Yanaihara, N., Excerpta Medica ICS No. 468, Amsterdam, pp. 138-147 (1979).

146. Heding, L.G., Rasmussen, S.M.: Human C-peptide in normal and diabetic subjects. Diabetologia 11, 201-206 (1975).

147. Beischer, W.: Normales Verhalten von Insulin, Proinsulin und C-Peptid im Blut. In: "Die Bedeutung der C-Peptidbestimmung für die Diagnostik", Eds. Grüneklee, D., Herzog, W., Schnetztor Verlag, Konstanz, pp. 22-48 (1979).

148. Gorden, P., Roth, J.: Circulating insulins. "Big" and "little". Arch. intern. Med. 123, 237-247 (1969).

149. Gorden, P., Roth, J.: Plasma insulin: Fluctuations in the "big" insulin component in man after glucose and other stimuli. J. clin. Invest. 48, 2225-2234 (1969).

150. Melani, F., Rubenstein, A.H., Steiner, D.F.: Human serum proinsulin. J. clin. Invest. 49, 497-507 (1970).

151. Rosenbloom, A.L., Starr, J.I., Juhn, D., Rubenstein, A.H.: Serum proinsulin in children and adolescents with chemical diabetes. Diabetes 24, 753-757 (1975).

152. Phelps, R.L., Bergenstal, R., Freinkel, N., Rubenstein, A.H., Metzger, B.E., Mako, M.: Carbohydrate metabolism in pregnancy: XIII. Relationships between plasma insulin and proinsulin during late pregnancy in normal and diabetic subjects. J. clin. Invest. 42, 1085-1091 (1975).

153. Burghen, G.A., Etteldorf, J.N., Trouy, R.L., Kitabchi, A.E.: Insulin and proinsulin in normal and chemical diabetic children. J. Pediat. 89, 48-53 (1976).

154. Kühl, C.: Serum proinsulin in normal and gestational diabetic pregnancy. Diabetologia 12, 295-300 (1976).

155. Gorden, P., Hendricks, C.M., Roth, J.: Circulating proinsulin-like component in man: increased proportion in hypoinsulinemic states. Diabetologia 10, 469-474 (1974).

156. Mako, M.E., Starr, J.I., Rubenstein, A.H.: Circulating proinsulin in patients with maturity onset diabetes. Am. J. Med. 63, 865-869 (1977).

157. Gabbay, K.H., De Luca, K., Fischer, J.N., Mako, M.E., Rubenstein, A.H.: Familial hyperproinsulinaemia. An autosomal defect. New Engl. J. Med. 294, 911-915 (1976).

158. Gabbay, K.H., Bergenstal, R.M., Wolff, J., Mako, M.E., Rubenstein, A.H.: Familial hyperproinsulinemia: Partial characterization of circulating proinsulin-like material. Proc. natn. Acad. Sci. U.S.A. 76, 2281-2285 (1979).

159. Block, M.B., Mako, M.E., Steiner, D.F., Rubenstein, A.H.: Diabetic ketoacidosis: Evidence for C-peptide and proinsulin secretion following recovery. J. clin. Endocrinol. Metab. 35, 402-406 (1972).

160. Heding, L.G., Ludvigsson, J.: Human proinsulin in insulin-treated juvenile diabetics. Acta paediat. (Uppsala)(Suppl.) 270, 48-52 (1977).

161. Logothetopoulos, J., Bell, E.G.: Histological and autoradiographic studies of the islets of mice injected with insulin antibody. Diabetes 15, 205-211 (1966).

162. Grodsky, G.M., Feldman, R., Toreson, W.E., Lee, J.C.: Diabetes mellitus in rabbits immunized with insulin. Diabetes 15, 579-585 (1966).

163. Ludvigsson, J., Heding, L.G.: C-peptide in children with juvenile diabetes. Diabetologia 12, 627-630 (1976).

164. Hendriksen, C., Faber, O.K., Drejer, J., Binder, C.: Prevalence of residual beta-cell function in insulin treated diabetics evaluated by the plasma C-peptide response to intravenous glucagon. Diabetologia 13, 280-288 (1977).

165. Krause, U., Cordes, U., Beyer, J.: C-Peptid. Sekretion und Stoffwechsel bei unterschiedlichen Funktionszuständen und Störungen der B-Zellen der Langerhansschen Inseln. Dtsch. med. Wschr. 102, 785-790 (1977).

166. Nelson, R.L., Baldus, W.P., Rubenstein, A.H., Go, V.L., Service, F.J.: Pancreatic alpha-cell function in diabetic hemochromatosis. J. clin. Endocrinol. Metab. 49, 412-426 (1979).

167. Ludvigsson, J., Heding, L.G.: Beta-cell function in children with diabetes. Diabetes 27, (Suppl. 1) 230-234 (1978).

168. Grawjer, L.A., Pildes, R.S., Horwitz, D.L., Rubenstein, A.H.: Control of juvenile diabetes mellitus and its relationship to endogenous insulin secretion as measured by C-peptide. Pediatrics 90, 42-49 (1977).

169. Faber, O.K., Binder, C.: β-Cell function and blood glucose control in insulin dependent diabetics within the first month of insulin treatment. Diabetologia 13, 263-268 (1977).

170. Eff, Ch., Faber, O.K., Deckert, T.: Persistent insulin secretion, assessed by plasma C-peptide in long-term juvenile diabetics with low insulin requirement. Diabetologia 15, 169-172 (1978).

171. Madsbad, S., Faber, O.K., Binder, C., Nair, Mc P., Christiansen, C., Transbøl, L.: Prevalence of residual beta-cell function in insulin-dependent diabetics in relation to age at onset and duration of diabetes. Diabetes 27, (Suppl. 1) 262-264 (1978).

172. Faber, O.K., Binder, C.: Plasma C-peptide during the first year of insulin-dependent diabetes mellitus. In: Proceedings IXth IDF Congress, Ed. Bajaj, J.S., Excerpta Medica ICS No. 413, Amsterdam, pp. 149-154 (1977).

173. Binder, C., Faber, O.K.: Residual beta-cell function and its metabolic consequences. Diabetes 27, (Suppl. 1) 226-229 (1978).

174. Block, M.B., Pildes, R.S., Mossabhoy, N.A., Steiner, D.F., Rubenstein, A.H.: C-peptide immunoreactivity (CPR): A new method for studying infants of insulin-treated diabetic mothers. Pediatrics 53, 923-928 (1974).

175. Sosenko, I.R., Kitzmiller, J.L., Loo, S.W., Blix, P.M., Rubenstein, A.H., Gabbay, K.H.: The infant of the diabetic mother. Correlation of increased cord C-peptide levels with macrosomia and hypoglycemia. New Engl. J. Med. 301, 859-862 (1979).

176. Pirart, J., Lavaux, J.P.: Remission in diabetes. In: "Handbuch des Diabetes Mellitus", Ed. Pfeiffer, E.F., J. Lehmann, München, vol. 2, pp. 443-502 (1971).

177. Block, M.B., Rosenfield, R.L., Mako, M.E., Steiner, D.F., Rubenstein, A.H.: Sequential changes in beta-cell function in insulin treated diabetic patients assessed by C-peptide immunoreactivity. New Engl. J. Med. 288, 1144-1148 (1973).

178. Heinze, E., Beischer, W., Keller, L., Winkler, G., Teller, W.M., Pfeiffer, E.F.: C-peptide during the remission phase of juvenile diabetes. Diabetes 27, 670-676 (1978).

179. Vetter, K., Heinze, E., Beischer, W., Teller, W.: Studies on the C-peptide secretion during the remission in diabetic children. Acta Paediat. Belg. 33, 67 (1980).

180. Fussgänger, R.D., Goberna, R., Hinz, M., Jaros, P., Karsten, C., Pfeiffer, E.F., Raptis, S.: Comparative studies on the dynamics of insulin secretion following HB 419 and tolbutamide on the perfused isolated rat pancreas and the perifused isolated pieces and islets of rat pancreas. Horm. Metab. Res. Suppl. Series No. 1, 34-40 (1969).

181. Raptis, S., Rau, R.M., Schröder, K.E., Faulhaber, J.D., Pfeiffer, E.F.: Comparative study of insulin secretion following repeated administration of glucose, tolbutamide and glibenclamide (HB 419) in diabetic and non-diabetic human subjects. Horm. Metab. Res. Suppl. Series No.1, 65-72 (1969).

182. Pfeiffer, E.F., Raptis, S.: Controlled extension of oral antidiabetic therapy on former insulin dependent diabetics by means of the combined i.v. glibenclamide-glucose-response-test. Diabetologia 8, 41-47 (1972).

183. Pfeiffer, E.F., Raptis, S., Schröder, K.E.: Einmalige intravenöse Glibenclamid-Glukose-Belastung als Vorhersagetest. Dtsch. med. Wschr. 99, 1281-1294 (1974).

184. Beischer, W., Raptis, S., Keller, L., Maas, M., Beischer,B., Feilen, K., Pfeiffer, E.F.: Humanes C-Peptid. Teil III: Sekretionsdynamik der Beta-Zellen erwachsener Diabetiker nach Glibenclamid-Glukose i.v. Klin. Wschr. 56, 111-120 (1978).

185. Beischer, W., Kerner, W., Raptis, S., Keller, L., Beischer, B., Pfeiffer, E.F.: Insulin therapy in relation to circulating C-peptide levels. Diabetes 27, (Suppl. 1) 235-240 (1978).

186. Dittus, E., Beischer, W., Keller, L., Maas, M.: The therapeutic relevance of the fast beta-cell stimulation capacity. Diabetologia 19, 270 (1980).

187. Pfeiffer, E.F., Pfeiffer, M., Ditschuneit, H., Chang-Su Ahn: Über die Bestimmung von Insulin im Blute am epididymalen Fettanhang der Ratte mit Hilfe markierter Glukose. II. Experimentelle und klinische Erfahrungen. Klin. Wschr. 37, 1239-1245 (1959).

188. Seltzer, H.S., Smith, S.W.: Plasma insulin activity after glucose. Diabetes 8, 417 (1959).

189. Beischer, W., Keller, L., Heinze, E., Raptis, S., Tamás, Gy., Thum, Ch., Pfeiffer, E.F.: Nachweis von körpereigener Insulinreserven beim insulinbehandelten Diabetiker mittels C-Peptid-Bestimmung. Therapiewoche 26, 1936-1947 (1976).

190. Turner, R.C., Holman, R.R.: Beta-cell function during insulin or chlorpropamide treatment of maturity onset diabetes mellitus. Diabetes 27, (Suppl. 1) 241-246 (1978).

191. Regal, H., Ogris, E., Lageder, H., Sochor, H., Irsigler, K.: β-Cell function: Can it be improved by strict diet or insulin therapy ? Giorn. It. Chim. Cl. 4, (Suppl. 1) 113-126 (1979).

192. Ludvigsson, J., Heding, L.G., Larsson, Y., Leander, E.: C-peptide in juvenile diabetics beyond the postinitial remission period. Acta paediat. (Uppsala) 66, 177-184 (1977).

193. Ludvigsson, J., Hägglöf, B., Holmgren, G.: Early remission in juvenile diabetes in relation to symptoms and treatment at onset. In: Proceedings Xth IDF Congress, Eds. Waldhäusl, W., Alberti, K.G.M.M., Excerpta Medica ICS No. 481, Amsterdam, p. 145 (1979).

194. Mirouze, J., Selan, J.L., Pham, T.C., Mendoza, E., Orsetti, A.: Sustained insulin-induced remissions of juvenile diabetes by means of an external artificial pancreas. Diabetologia 14, 223-227 (1978).

195. Gonen, B., Rubenstein, A.H., Horwitz, D.L., Blix, P.M.: Clinical significance of C-peptide. In: "Proinsulin, Insulin, C-Peptide", Eds. Baba, S., Kaneko, T., Yanaihara,N., Excerpta Medica ICS No. 468, Amsterdam, pp. 246-253 (1979).

196. Ikeda, Y., Ando, N., Minami, N., Ide, Y.: B-cell function of insulin-dependent young onset diabetics assessed by C-peptide immunoreactivity. Diabetologia 11, 351-352 (1975).

197. Bruni, B., Gamba, S., Barbero, P.L., Regis, G., Turco, G.L.: Residual β-cell function in long-term insulin-dependent diabetics. Giorn. It. Chim. Cl. 4, (Suppl. 1) 157-162 (1979).

198. Beischer, W., Pfeiffer, M., Beischer, B., Dittus, E.: Retinopathy and residual beta-cell function. In: Proceedings Xth IDF Congress, Eds. Waldhäusl, W., Alberti, K.G.M.M., Excerpta Medica ICS No. 481, Amsterdam, p. 18 (1979).

199. Tchobroutsky, G.: Relation of diabetic control to development of microvascular complications. Diabetologia 15, 143-152 (1978).

200. Rubenstein, A.H.: The significance of immunoassayable insulin in urine. JAMA 209, 254-256 (1969).

201. Rubenstein, A.H., Mako, M.E., Welbourne, R.B. Melani, F., Steiner, D.F.: Measurement of proinsulin, C-peptide and insulin in serum and urine. In: "Laboratory Diagnosis of Endocrine Diseases", Eds. Sunderman, F.W., Sunderman, F.W. jr., W.H. Green, St. Louis, pp. 354-366 (1970).

202. Kaneko, T., Munemura, M., Oka, H., Oda, T., Suzuki, S., Yasuda, H., Yanaihara, N., Nakagawa, S., Makabe, K.: Demonstration of C-peptide immunoreactivity in various body fluids and clinical evaluation of the determination of urinary C-peptide immunoreactivity. Endocr. jap. 22, 1144-1148 (1975).

203. Kuzuya, T., Matsuda, A., Saito, T., Yoshida, S.: Human C-peptide immunoreactivity in blood and urine - Evaluation of a radioimmunoassay method and its clinical applications. Diabetologia 12, 511-518 (1976).

204. Horwitz, D.L., Rubenstein, A.H., Katz, A.I.: Quantitation of human pancreatic beta-cell function by immunoassay of C-peptide in urine. Diabetes 26, 30-35 (1977).

205. Kuzuya, T., Matsuda, A., Sakamoto, Y., Tanabshi, S., Kajinuma, H.: C-peptide immunoreactivity (CPR) in urine. Diabetes 27, (Suppl. 1) 210-215 (1978).

206. Horwitz, D.L.: Insulin secretory responses to various food components: a factor in dietary management of diabetes. In: Proceedings Xth IDF Congress, Eds. Waldhäusl, W., Alberti, K.G.M.M., Excerpta Medica ICS No. 481, Amsterdam, p. 96 (1979).

207. Grüneklee, D., Hedtmann, A.: Immunoassay of C-peptide in urine of patients with idiopathic diabetes and after pancreatectomy.In: "C-Peptide", Eds. Beyer, J., Krause, U., Naegele, W., Schnetztor Verlag, Konstanz, pp. 161-166 (1977).

208. Kuzuya, T., Matsuda, A., Sakamoto, Y.: Further studies on urine C-peptide immunoreactivity in diabetic patients. In: "Proinsulin, Insulin, C-Peptide", Eds. Baba, S., Kaneko, T., Yanaihara, N., Excerpta Medica ICS No. 468, Amsterdam, pp. 174-182 (1979).

209. Hürter, P., Zick, R., Mitzkat, H.J.: Die Bedeutung der C-Peptid Bestimmung im 24-Std.-Urin für die Behandlung diabetischer Kinder und Jugendlicher. In: "Die Bedeutung der C-Peptidbestimmung für die Diagnostik", Eds. Grüneklee, D., Herzog, W., Schnetztor Verlag, Konstanz, pp. 117-125 (1979).

210. Bieger, W.P., Fölsch, U., Malfertheiner, P., Henrichs, I., Etzrodt, H., Pfeiffer, E.F.: Concentrations of pancreatic hormones in human pancreatic juice. J. clin. Endocrinol. Metab. (in press).

211. Andreani, D., Falluca, F., Russo, A., Maldonato, A., Caccano, C., Lamalfa, G., Gado, de E., Pachi, A.: Insuline, peptide C et glucagon dans le liquide amniotique des femmes enceintes normales et diabétiques. Journée Annu. Diabétol. Hôtel-Dieu, Publ. Flammarion, Paris, pp. 93-101 (1979).

212. Beischer, W., Keller, L., Schürmeyer, E., Raptis, S., Thum, Ch., Pfeiffer, E.F.: Insulin, Proinsulin und C-Peptid im Serum bei Hypoglycaemia factitia. Verh. dtsch. Ges. inn. Med. vol. 81, J.F. Bergmann, München, pp. 1493-1495 (1975).

213. Couropmitree, C., Freinkel, N., Nagel, T.C., Horwitz, D.L., Metzger, B., Rubenstein, A.H., Hahnel, R.: Plasma C-peptide and diagnosis of factitious hypoglycemia. Study of an insulin-dependent diabetic patient with "spontaneous" hypoglycemia. Ann. intern. Med. 82, 201-204 (1975).

214. Service, F.J., Rubenstein, A.H., Horwitz, D.L.: C-peptide analysis in diagnosis of factitial hypoglycemia in an insulin-dependent diabetic. Mayo Clinic Proc. 50, 697-701 (1975).

215. Scarlett, J.A., Mako, M.E., Rubenstein, A.H., Blix, P.M., Goldman, J., Horwitz, D.L., Tager, H., Jaspan, J.B., Stjernholm, M.R., Olefsky, J.M.: Factitious hypoglycemia, diagnosis by measurement of serum C-peptide immunoreactivity and insulin-binding antibodies. New Engl. J. Med. 297, 1029-1032 (1977).

216. Safrit, H.F., Young, C.W.: Factitious hypoglycemia. New Engl. J. Med. 298, 515 (1978).

217. Kurtz, A.B., Harrington, M.G., Matthews, J.A., Nabarro, J.D.: Factitious hypoglycemia and antibody mediated resistance to beef insulin. Diabetologia 16, 65-67 (1979).

218. Stellon, A., Townell, N.L.: C-peptide assay for factitious hyperinsulinism. Lancet II, 148-149 (1979).

219. Horwitz, D.L., Rubenstein, A.H.: Insulin suppression. Lancet II, 1021 (1974).

220. Service, F.J., Horwitz, D.L., Rubenstein, A.H., Kuzuya, H., Mako, M.E., Reynolds, C., Molnar, G.D.: C-peptide suppression test for insulinoma. J. Lab. clin. Med. 90, 180-186 (1977).

221. Senator, G.B., Rainbow, S.J., Greenwood, R.H., Mahler, R.F., Woodhead, J.S., Hales, C.N.: Plasma C-peptide measurement in the diagnosis of pancreatic insulinoma with special reference to insulin induced hypoglycaemia. In: "C-Peptide", Eds. Beyer, J., Krause, U., Naegele, W., Schnetztor Verlag, Konstanz, pp. 185-196 (1977).

222. Cordes, U., Krause, U., Beyer, J.: C-peptide determination in insulinoma diagnostics. In: "C-Peptide", Eds. Beyer, J., Krause, U., Naegele, W., Schnetztor Verlag, Konstanz, pp. 197-208 (1977).

223. Turner, R.C., Heding, L.G.: Plasma proinsulin, C-peptide and insulin in diagnostic suppression tests for insulinomas. Diabetologia 13, 571-577 (1977).

224. Beischer, W., Kerner, W., Raptis, S., Herfarth, C., Pfeiffer, E.F.: Automie der Hormonsekretion beim Insulom. Verh. dtsch. Ges. inn. Med. vol. 83, J.F. Bergmann, München, pp. 1410-1413 (1977).

225. Rayfield, E.J., Pulini, M., Golub, A., Rubenstein, A.H., Horwitz, D.L.: Nonautonomous function of a pancreatic insulinoma. J. clin. Endocrinol. Metab. 43, 1307-1311 (1976).

226. Rubenstein, A.H., Mako, M.E., Starr, J.I., Juhn, D.J., Horwitz, D.L.: Circulating proinsulin in patients with islet cell tumors. In: Proceedings VIIIth IDF Congress, Eds. Malaisse, W.I., Pirart, I., Vallance-Owen, J., Excerpta Medica ICS No. 312, Amsterdam, pp. 736-752 (1974).

227. Rubenstein, A.H., Melani, F., Steiner, D.F.: Circulating proinsulin: Immunology, measurement, and biological activity. In: "Handbook of Physiology" Section 7, Vol. 1, Eds. Steiner, D.F., Freinkel, N., American Physiological Society, Washington D.C., pp. 515-528 (1972).

228. Kitabchi, A.E., Duckworth, W.C., Stentz, F.B., Yu, S.: Properties of proinsulin and related polypeptides. Crc. Crit. Rev. Biochem. 1, 59-94 (1972).

229. Nissley, S.P., Rechler, M.M., Moses, A.C., Short, P.A., Podskalny, J.M.: Proinsulin binds to a growth peptide receptor and stimulates DNA synthesis in chick embryo fibroblasts. Endocrinology 101, 708-716 (1977).

230. Toyota, T., Abe, K., Kudo, M., Kimura, K., Goto, Y.: Inhibitory effects of synthetic rat C-peptide I on insulin secretion in the isolated perfused rat pancreas. Tohoku J. Exp. Med. 117, 79-83 (1975).

231. Yasuda, H., Suzuki, S., Yamashita, K., Kaneko, T., Oka, H., Oda, T., Yanaihara, N.: Inhibition of insulin release by synthetic rat C-peptide II in isolated rat islets. Endocrinol. jap. 23, 271-273 (1976).

232. Wojcikowsky, Cz., Fussgänger, R.D., Pfeiffer, E.F.: Inhibition of insulin and glucagon secretion of the isolated perfused rat pancreas by synthetic human and rat C-peptide. In: "C-Peptide", Eds. Beyer, J., Krause, U., Naegele, W., Schnetztor Verlag, Konstanz, pp. 75-88 (1977).

233. Klier, M.: Die Wirkung von C-peptid auf die Insulinsekretion und Biosynthese isolierter Langerhansscher Inseln der Ratte. Dissertation, Ulm (1978).

234. Dryburgh, J.R., Hampton, S.M., Marks, V.: Endocrine pancreatic control of the release of gastric inhibitory polypeptide. A possible physiological role for C-peptide. Diabetologia 19, 397-401 (1980).

PERCEPTIONS ON THE ETIOLOGY OF THE POLYCYSTIC OVARY SYNDROME

M. Finkelstein and J. Weidenfeld*
Department of Endocrinology, Hebrew University-Hadassah Medical School, Jerusalem, Israel

Introduction

At the meeting of the Central Association of the Obstetricians and Gynecologists, November 1 to 3, 1934, New Orleans, La. Drs. Irving F. Stein and Michael L. Leventhal read a paper, which was subsequently published in The American Journal of Obstetrics and Gynecology under the title "Amenorrhea Associated with Bilateral Polycystic Ovaries" (1). The authors noted that "cyst formation in the follicular apparatus of the ovary is very common and is regarded to some extent as a physiologic process. When these structures are visible to the naked eye, they are regarded as cysts, when not, they are called follicles. When this process becomes excessive, persistent or progressive, the ovary becomes enlarged, tense, tender and painful, and produces what has been termed "cystic degeneration of the ovary", and is usually bilateral. The exact cause of this formation is still in doubt. Formerly, it was regarded as the result of inflammatory change due to either local infection or that from some distant focus. More recent observations and experiments point to an endocrine causal relationship of the polycystic changes in the ovaries. "... In some patients, there was observed a distinct tendency toward masculinizing changes. Atypical rhomboid hairy escutcheon, hair on the face, arms and legs, and coarse skin was noted. No voice changes have been observed by us.

---

* Present address: Laboratory of Experimental Endocrinology, Dept.of Neurology, Hadassah University Hospital, Jerusalem

Hormones in Normal and Abnormal Human Tissues, Vol. III

The external genitals in most patients were normal, but in some, the labia minora and clitoris were markedly hypertrophied. Libido is apparently not affected by the changes noted in the ovaries".

This classic description of the condition prompted many physicians and scientists to refer to it as the Stein Leventhal syndrome, and this term was in general use until the early 1960's, when the descriptive part of Drs. Stein and Leventhal title pertaining to polycystic ovaries replaced the reference to the author's names.

Although little has since been added to the original description of the polycystic ovary syndrome (POS), it has been noted by many authors that some of the characteristics of the syndrome are shared by other irregularities originating either in the ovary or in the adrenal cortex, or even in other unidentified sources (2-6). Moreover, even in fully verified cases of POS it was not always possible to correlate the histologic appearance of the ovary with the clinical symptoms of the patient. Thus in some cases the thecal growth may be minimal with no luteinization and a corpus luteum or luteinized follicle cyst may be present (7).

Since many of the somatic and the functional changes seen in this syndrome pertain to irregularities in the action of sex hormones, it was quite natural that a search for the defect concentrated around the secretion and metabolism of the sex hormones and their trophic hormones. The high hopes, which were attached to these investigations, faded when a vast amount of data on the concentration of urinary and blood gonadotropins (8-10), androgens (3, 8) and estrogens (6, 8, 11) showed that not a single one of these hormones was specifically present in concentrations different from the normal or from other forms of "idiopathic" hirsutism and amenorrhea (12). Similarly, *in vivo* stimulation or inhibition of the secretion of sex hormones or their precursors by the adrenal or the ovarian glands provided no clues, which might link the various symptoms of the syndrome with a specific defect either in the steroid hormone producing glands or in their peripheral metabolism (6, 8, 10, 11-15).

The following inadequacies residing in the hypothalamo-pituitary system, the adrenal cortex or the ovary, have been observed or suspected by various authors to be operative in the development of the conditions ascribed to the syndrome.

Hypothalamus-Pituitary

According to Berger (6) elevated radioimmunoassayable LH levels in an anovulatory patient, comparable with those found during a LH peak or during the climacteric in association with normal radioimmunoassayable FSH values, are diagnostic of the characteristic form of POS. However, spontaneous ovulation or a rise in circulating LH stimulating the ovulatory events may blur the picture. Moreover, in approximately 10% of POS patients, basal levels and the pulsative pattern of LH release are similar to those of normal menstruating women (3). The primary involvement of the pituitary in the etiology of POS was suspected on the basis of an increased pituitary sensitivity to LHRH, which manifests itself by an elevated LH secretion along with a diminished secretion of FSH (3, 6, 10, 16-18). However, this dual pituitary response is probably due not to an intrinsic deficiency of the gland in POS, but is rather caused by the chronically elevated estrogen levels (see below), which at one and the same time augment the pituitary sensitivity to LHRH with respect to LH secretion and inhibit the FSH secretion (19). Such a course of events would eliminate the hypothalamic-pituitary system as an etiologic factor in POS. On the other hand, a premature discharge of LH following LHRH-stimulation has been considered to be the primary defect in some POS patients (20).

Ovary

The characteristic feature of ovarian function in POS is the hyper-production of androgen (21-23) and a low production of estrogen (21, 24, 25). Paradoxically, this ovarian deficiency is accompanied by increased levels of circulating estrogen, mainly estrone (26). The high ovarian androgen production, with concomitant low estrogen synthesis could at first sight, be easily explained by a glandular deficiency in the aromatase system, which slows down the transformation of androstenedione to estrone. This defect is, however, questionable in view of the results of Erickson et al (27), which showed that stimulation with FSH of granulosa cells from ovaries of POS patients resulted in a pronounced increase in estrogen production. This confirms the results of earlier in vivo studies, in which excretion of urinary estrogens increased markedly after treatment of POS patient with FSH (28-30), and suggests that FSH stimulates the aromatase enzyme complex contained in the ovary. On the other hand, the aromatase complex present in peripheral tissues seems to be independent of FSH stimulation, and thus the extragonadal production of estrogen arising from ovarian androstenedione or testosterone, not only is not synchronized with the secretion of the hypothalamo-pituitary hormones, but in fact interferes with their cyclic production (10, 26).

Although the sites of extragonadal production of estrogens have not been fully explored, much attention has been lately given to the aromatization of steroid precursors by the hypothalamus as well as by other brain areas (31, 32). It is possible that in POS an increased availability of androgenic precursors accelerates the aromatization in these tissues and that the resulting local increment of estrogens influences the regulation of ovarian steroid biosynthesis by the hypothalamo-pituitary unit (33). This remains to be proven, however. All of the above evidence clearly shows that factors within the ovaries must be responsible for the physiopathology of POS; it does not, however, answer the question of whether they are intrinsic to the ovaries, or whether they are secondary to aberrations in other sites.

Adrenal Cortex

The fact that most of the steroid hormones or metabolites, which were frequently found to be increased in POS patients normally originate from both the ovary and the adrenal cortex, gave rise to the supposition of adrenal involvement in POS (8, 12, 14).

In order to identify the origin of the implicated steroids, "specific" stimulators or inhibitors of either the gonadal or the adrenal cortex secretion were administered to POS patients and to normal menstruating volunteers. In spite of many promising reports based on ACTH stimulation or corticosteroid inhibition (3, 6, 8, 34), the bulk of evidence was against an adrenal involvement in POS (3, 6, 8). Conflicting results, which were obtained by estimating steroid concentrations in adrenal vein blood (35-37) and which, in many cases, showed an elevation of dehydroepiandrosterone, but not of testosterone, androstenedione and dihydrotestosterone, suggested involvement of the adrenal cortex secondary to an ovarian disturbance. However, the frequent amelioration of POS symptoms, by ovarian wedge resection, especially relating to the regulation of the menstrual cycle and to ovulation, seems irreconcilable with the concept of adrenal involvement. Thus the balance of the opposing views leaned to ovarian dysfunction until Cox and Shearman (38) discovered that an unusual adrenal steroid metabolite, thought to be pathognomonic to a certain form of congenital adrenal hyperplasia (defective C-21 hydroxylation, 39-43) is excreted in the urine of an overwhelming majority of POS patients. This steroid was identified as pregnanetriolone (39), a metabolite of 21-deoxycortisol (44). The unexpected direct evidence of a metabolic deviation pertaining to steroid biosynthesis in the adrenal cortex in an otherwise ovarian disease prompted Shearman and Cox to name the condition "The Enigmatic Polycystic Ovary" (8).

In the following we shall try to correlate the data and theories relating to POS in an attempt to solve the enigma.

Ovarian and Adrenal Steroid Biosynthesis

The physiologic precursor of steroid hormones is cholesterol. Both in the ovary (Fig. 1) and the adrenal cortex (Fig. 2) cholesterol is enzymatically cleaved to pregnenolone by a mitochondrial cytochrome P_{450} dependent enzyme system. However, the ovarian reaction is initiated by FSH and subsequently regulated by LH, whereas the adrenal reaction is under the control of ACTH (45-46). So far it has not been established whether the ovarian and adrenal enzyme complexes cleaving the cholesterol side-chain are identical or different. The conversion of pregnenolone to progesterone, of pregnenolone to 17-hydroxypregnenolone and of progesterone to 17-hydroxyprogesterone, are common to both glands and are apparently independent of tropic hormone stimulation. On the contrary, the aromatization step (reaction "f" in Fig. 1), which converts either androstenedione or testosterone

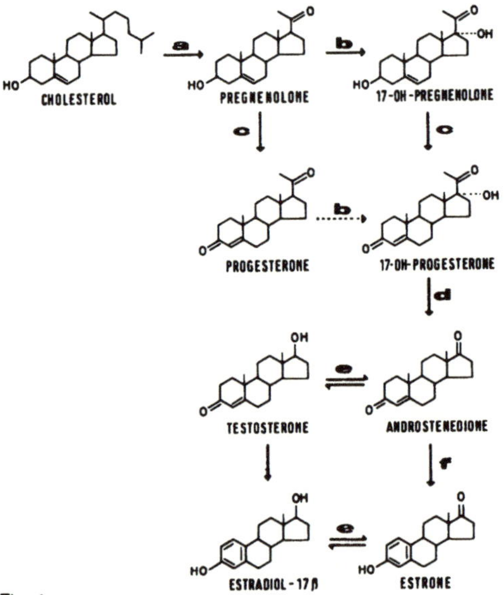

Fig. 1
MAJOR PATHWAY OF HUMAN OVARIAN STEROID BIOSYNTHESIS

a - Side-chain cleavage; b - 17-hydroxylase;
c - 3β-ol-dehydrogenase, $\Delta^{5,4}$ isomerase; d - 17,20-lyase
e - 17β-ol-oxidoreductase; f - aromatization

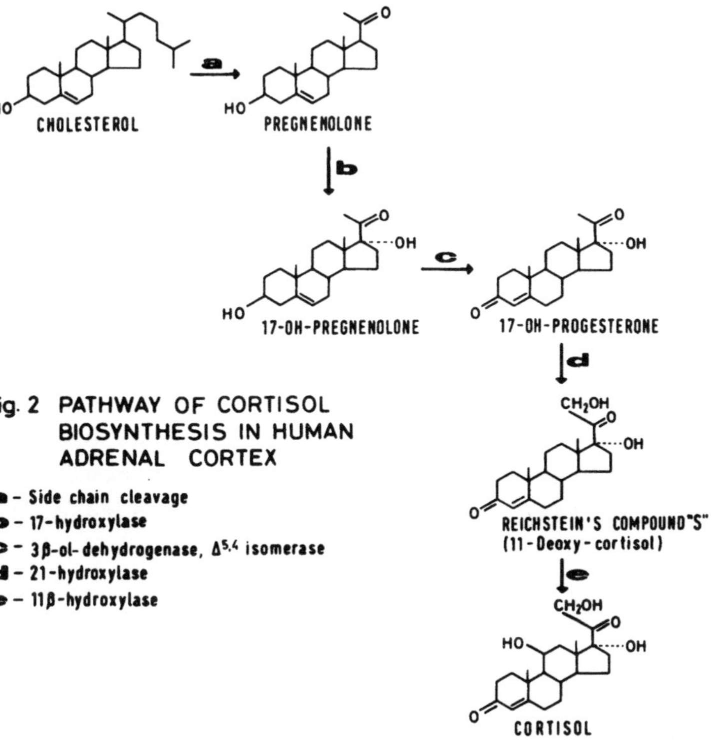

Fig. 2 PATHWAY OF CORTISOL BIOSYNTHESIS IN HUMAN ADRENAL CORTEX

a - Side chain cleavage
b - 17-hydroxylase
c - 3β-ol-dehydrogenase, $\Delta^{5,4}$ isomerase
d - 21-hydroxylase
e - 11β-hydroxylase

to estrogens, is in man normally specific to the gonads and FSH dependent (47). Similarly, the C-21 and the C-11β hydroxylases are specific to the adrenal cortex, but only the 11β-hydroxylation has been shown to be ACTH dependent (48, 49). This specificity and dependency is the quid pro quo (albeit not perfectly understood) for the dual relationship between the tropic hormones and their respective target glands; the products of the tropic hormone dependent reactions are the most efficient natural inhibitors (<u>via</u> the hypothalamus-pituitary) of their own production, thus giving rise to the feed-back system between the tropic and target glands. Figures 1 and 2 illustrate schematically the pathways of the ovarian and adrenal steroid biosynthesis.

Ovarian aberration of steroid production in POS

Any one of the pathways is susceptible to pre- or post-natal influences, which may change the course of events in the biosynthesis of either the ovarian or adrenalcortical hormones, or both of these, resulting in physiologic and somatic abnormalities specific to hypo or hyper states, depending on the aberration.

Prenatal defects, which are believed to have a genetic basis and which affect the steroidogenetic enzymes of the adrenal cortex lead to a series of conditions,which have been classified as congenital adrenal hyperplasia (CAH) (50-52). In the most common form of CAH, in which the C-21 hydroxylation of 17-hydroxyprogesterone is deficient, the production of cortisol is impaired and 21-deoxycortisol is formed instead. Its urinary metabolite has been isolated and identified as pregnanetriolone (3α,17α,20α-trihydroxy-5β-pregnan-11-one, 43). Because of the oxygen function at C-11 this compound was believed to derive exclusively from the adrenal cortex. This supposition was strengthened by the observation that, while the urinary excretion of pregnanetriolone can be inhibited by the administration of cortisol or its analogues to CAH patients (43), estrogens have no effect (unpublished results).

Soon after the identification of pregnanetriolone in urine of POS patients (38), the presence of the steroid was independently recognized (43). It has subsequently been observed in all POS patients investigated (over 100 cases, 53, 54 and unpublished results). Stimulation with ACTH increased, and treatment with cortisol derivatives decreased excretion of the compound (53-55). Paradoxically, several POS patients responded with uterine bleeding after three days treatment ACTH (54). It is noteworthy that patients, who responded favourably to wedge resection by restoration of regular menstrual cycles, ovulation or pregnancy, ceased to excrete detectable amounts of pregnanetriolone (8, 53, 56). This alleviation usually lasted as long as relief from the clinical conditions continued and, in the majority of patients, return of the characteristic symptoms of the syndrome was heralded by a renewed excretion of pregnanetriolone (43). A partial unriddling of the source of pregnanetriolone (adrenal vs. ovarian) was achieved after bilaterally ovariectomy of a POS patient who ceased to excrete pregnanetriolone even after ACTH stimulation (55). This result was highly suggestive of an ovarian involvement in the abnormal 11β-hydroxylation. It could, however, be interpreted to suggest a secondary involvement, by which an unknown ovarian product changes adrenal biosynthesis, so that 17-hydroxyprogesterone would be abnormally hydroxylated at position C-11 (Fig. 3, reaction "a"). The final and decisive proof of an ovarian enzymic aberration in POS was demonstrated when it was shown that homogenates and mitochondria of polycystic ovaries contained an 11β-hydroxylase specific to 21-deoxysteroids; this enzyme is absent from normal ovaries (57, 58).

Considering that normally the ovary contains neither a C-21 steroid hydroxylase nor an 11β-C-21 steroid hydroxylase, the presence in POS of an ovarian 11β-hydroxylase with affinity for 17-hydroxypregnenolone or 17-hydroxyprogesterone but not for 11-deoxycortisol, implicated two types of 11β-C-21 steroid hydroxylase: one, aberrant with affinity for 20-methylsteroids (such as 17-hydroxypregnenolone or 17-hydroxyprogesterone) and functioning in CAH and POS (Fig. 3, reaction "a") and the other normal, with affinity for 21-hydroxysteroids (like 11-deoxycortisol) (Fig. 2, reaction "e") and residing exclusively in the adrenal cortex. Rare exceptions have been described where malignant tumors of the gonads contained 11β-C-21 steroid hydroxylase (59).

Possible factors (genetic or congenital) causative to the etiology of POS

The finding of the aberrant 11β-hydroxylase supplements a previous observation that the ovarian stroma of POS patients encloses mesothelium-like cells, which normally have not been distinguished in the ovaries (55, 57, 58, 60). Although we have not proven that the abnormal 11β-21-deoxysteroid hydroxylase is

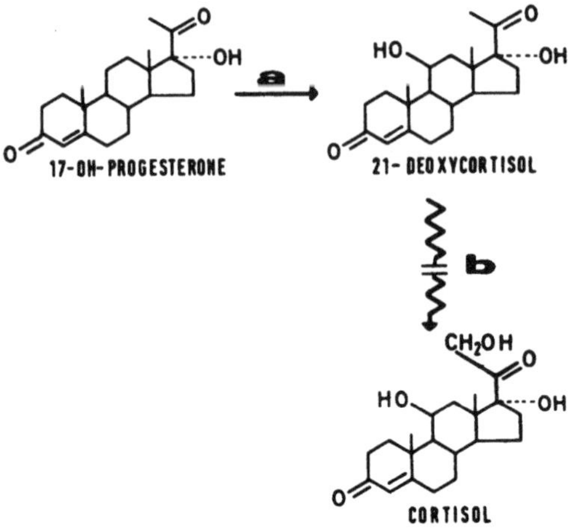

Fig. 3 AN ABERRANT 11β-HYDROXYLASE FUNCTIONING IN CONGENITAL ADRENAL HYPERPLASIA AND IN POLYCYSTIC OVARY SYNDROME

a - Aberrant 11β-hydroxylase
b - 21-hydroxylase

located in the mesothelium-like cells, it seems a possibility. If this were so, the common defect in CAH and in POS relating to the secretion of 21-deoxycortisol could derive from imperfections in the pre-natal development of either the adrenal cortex or the ovary, which could influence the maturation of either gland. In principle, the defect could be either inherited or acquired, but, whereas there is a good evidence that CAH conforms to Mendelian laws, whereby the trait is transmitted from heterozygous parents (51, 61, 62), there is no solid proof for inheritance in POS. The lack of evidence in POS may be, in part, due to the fact that the condition is recognizable only in the females, so that the Mendelian pattern is not noticed.

However, there is a further probability that the multitude of symptoms encompassed in the "polycystic ovary syndrome" evolves from a diversified etiology, so that certain POS patients are genetically affected, whereas in others, the disposition is due to incidental errors in differentiation of the gonads and the adrenal cortex. The latter possibility deserves a special consideration. Normally, the adrenal cortex and the follicular cells are derived from the common primordial embryonic tissue, the mesodermal coelomic epithelium. The primordial adrenal cortical cells proliferate from this embryonic tissue in the 6th week of gestation. The primordial follicular cells penetrate during the 7th week of gestation and produce the so-called sex cords, the cells of which differentiate into follicular elements. It may be presumed that, in contrast to the normal sequence of events, development of the ovaries in certain cases of POS is disturbed by a misplaced penetration of the primordial coelomic epithelial cells. This displacement could result from either a migration early in the 6th week of gestation of the undifferentiated cells from the prospective adrenocortical site into the gonadal ridge, or from the persistence of the primitive coelomic cells in the future germinal epithelium, which later migrate with the "cords" into the ovary. In either case, the "inadequate" cells do not mature, perhaps because of the alien environment and thus retain their primitive characteristics, one being the 11β-C-21 deoxysteroid hydroxylase, otherwise highly specific to the most common type of CAH. Hence, due to imperfection in enzyme-substrate specificity, the normal pathway of ovarian steroid biosynthesis is changed and ovarian disorders ensue.

Originally, we postulated that the 21-hydroxylation defect in CAH results from a decreased activity of an adrenal 21-hydroxylase, but several subsequent findings mitigated against this. Instead, we proposed that in most cases of the above form of CAH, the defect arises from an aberrant 11β-hydroxylase specific for 21-deoxysteroids, by action of which 11β-hydroxylated 21-deoxy compounds are formed, which are poor substrates for 21-hydroxylase (63).

As we have discussed earlier, a genetic basis for the occurrence of POS has been frequently considered in the past.

If the presence of the aberrant 11β-steroid hydroxylase is applied to such consideration, certain alternative assumptions must be made.

1. The steroidogenic enzymes of the ovary are coded for independently of the enzymes of the adrenal cortex, so that enzymes exhibiting the same functions may be not fully identical.
2. In CAH the aberrant adrenal enzyme may derive from a mutation in structural gene, thereby modifying the substrate affinity of the enzyme.
3. In POS the probability of a mutation of a structural gene giving rise to an aberrant ovarian 11β-hydroxylase is low, because normally ovary does not contain any 11β-C-21 steroid hydroxylase.
4. The structural gene for the irregular C-11β hydroxylase is intrinsic to the ovary, but is expressed only in POS patients. Modification in a regulator gene, whereby a repressor is not generated, increases the production of the aberrant enzyme.

From the above considerations it follows that POS must be a congenital ailment and that a genetic etiology remains a probability.

With regard to the abnormal production of C-21-deoxycortisol, there is no evidence to link it with the various symptoms characteristic of POS. It is quite possible that the compound is void of any physiological activity and that it is produced in parallel with some other, hormonally active 11β-hydroxysteroids. It is equally possible that 21-deoxycortisol produced by the ovaries competes with cortisol for the hypothalamic-pituitary receptors and thus leaves some of the ACTH secretion unopposed. This unbalanced secretion of ACTH may account for the irregularities in adrenal steroid secretion so often observed in POS.

Whether this approach will bring us closer to solving the enigma of POS, or whether it merely introduces a new factor, "the hidden meaning of which is to be discovered or guessed"

(Webster New International Dictionary 1934, cited by Shearman and Cox) (8), remains to be determined by further investigations.

Acknowledgements

This investigation was generously supported by the Steiner Family Endowment Fund, Vancouver, B.C., and the Max London Foundation, Johnstown, Pa.

References

1. Stein, I.F., Leventhal, M.L.: Amenorrhea associated with bilateral polycystic ovaries. Am. J. Obstet. Gynec. 29, 181-191 (1935).
2. Aiman, J., Nalick, R.H., Jacobs, A., Porter, J.C., Edman, C.D., Vellios, F., MacDonald, P.C.: The origin of androgen and estrogen in a virilized postmenopausal woman with bilateral benign cystic teratomas. Obstet. and Gynec. 49, 695-704 (1977).
3. Yen, S.S.C.: The polycystic ovary syndrome. Clin. Endocr. 12, 177-207 (1980).
4. Sizonenko, P.C., Schindler, A.M., Kohlberg, I.J., Paunier,L.: Gonadotrophins, testosterone and oestrogen levels in relation to ovarian morphology in 11β-hydroxylase deficiency. Acta Endocrinol. 71, 539-550 (1972).
5. Lavric, M.V.: Galactorrhea and amenorrhea with polycystic ovaries. Am. J. Obstet. Gynec. 104, 814-817 (1969).
6. Berger, M.J.: Conceptual Advances in the Polycystic Ovary Syndrome. In: "Progress in Gynecology", Eds. Taymor, M.L., Green, T.H., Grune and Stratton, New York, Vol. VI, pp.237-246 (1975).
7. Leventhal, M.L., Scommegna, A.: Multiglandular effect of the Stein-Leventhal syndrome. Am. J. Obstet. Gynec. 87, 445-454 (1963).
8. Shearman, R.P., Cox, R.I.: The enigmatic polycystic ovary. Obstet. gynec. Surv. 21, 1-33 (1966).
9. Jeffcoate, T.N.A.: The androgenic ovary with special reference to Stein-Leventhal syndrome. Am. J. Obstet. Gynec. 88, 143-156 (1964).

10. Rebar, R.W., Judd, H.L., Yen, S.S.C., Rakoff, J., Van Den Berg, G., Naftolin, F.: Characterization of the inappropriate gonadotropin separation in polycystic ovary syndrome. J. clin. Invest. 57, 1320-1329 (1976).

11. Ichii, S., Forchielli, E., Perloff, W.H., Dorfman, R.L.: Determination of plasma estrone and estradiol. Anal. Biochem. 5, 422-425 (1963).

12. Mahesh, V.S., Greenblatt, R.B.: Steroid secretion in the normal and polycystic ovary. Recent Progr. Horm. Res. 20, 341-394 (1964).

13. Givens, J.R., Andersen, R.N., Wiser, W.L., Fish, S.A.: Dynamics of suppression and recovery of plasma FSH, LH, androstenedione and testosterone in polycystic ovarian disease using an oral contraceptive. J. clin. Endocrinol. Metab. 38, 727-735 (1974).

14. Abraham, G.E., Chakmakjian, Z.H., Buster, J.E., Marshall, J.R.: Ovarian and adrenal contributions to peripheral androgens in hirsute women. Obstet. and Gynec. 46, 169-173 (1975).

15. Goldzieher, J.W.: Perspectives in Polycystic Ovarian Diseases.In: "Endocrine Causes of Menstrual Disorders", Ed. Givens, J.R., New-York Medical Publishers, Inc., New-York, pp. 307-332 (1978).

16. Berger, M.J., Taymor, M.L., Patton, W.C.: Gonadotropin levels and secretory pattern in patients with typical and atypical polycystic ovarian disease. Fertil.and Steril. 26, 619-626 (1975).

17. Duignan, N.M., Shaw, R.W., Rudd, B.T., Holder, G., Williams, J.W., Butt, W.R., Logan-Edwards, R., London, D.R.: Sex hormones levels and gonadotropin release in the polycystic ovary sndrome. Clin. Endocr. 4, 287-295 (1975).

18. Shaw, R.W., Duignan, N.M., Butt, W.R., Logan-Edwards, R., London, D.R.: Modification by sex steroids of LHRH response in the polycystic ovary syndrome. Clin. Endocr. 5, 495-502 (1976).

19. Yen, S.S.C., Lasley, B.L., Wang, C.F., Leblanc, H., Siler, T.M.: The operating characteristics of the hypothalamic-pituitary system during the menstrual cycle and observations of biological action of somatostatin. Recent Progr. Horm. Res. 31, 321-363 (1975).

20. Kendeel, F.R., Butt, W.R., London, D.R., Lynch, S.S., Logan-Edwards, R., Rudd, B.T.: Oestrogen amplification of LH-RH response in the polycystic ovary syndrome. Clin. Endocr. 9, 429-441 (1978).

21. Horton, R., Neisler, J.: Plasma androgens in patients with polycystic ovary syndrome. J. clin. Endocrinol. Metab. 28, 479-484 (1968).

22. Bardin, C.W., Hembree, W.C., Lipsett, M.B.: Suppression of testosterone and androstenedione production rates with dexamethasone in women with idiopathic hirsutism and polycystic ovaries. J. clin. Endocrinol. Metab. 28, 1300-1306 (1969).

23. Abraham, G.E., Buster, J.E.: Peripheral and ovarian steroids in ovarian hyperthecosis. Obstet. and Gynec. 47, 583-585 (1976).

24. Axelrod, L.R., Goldzieher, J.W.: Enzymatic inadequacies in human polycystic ovaries. Archs Biochem. Biophys. 95, 547-548 (1961).

25. Spaeth, D.G., Osawa, T.: Estrogen biosynthesis. III. Stereospecificity of aromatization by normal and diseased human ovaries. J. clin. Endocrinol. Metab. 38, 783-786 (1974).

26. Siiteri, P.C., MacDonald, P.C.: Role of Extraglandular Estrogen in Human Endocrinology. In: "Handbook of Physiology: Endocrinology", Eds. Greep, R.O., Astwood, E., American Physiological Society, Washington, D.C., Vol. II, pp. 615-629 (1973).

27. Erickson, G.P., Hsueh, A.J.W., Quigley, M.E., Rebar, R.W., Yen, S.S.C.: Functional studies of aromatase activity in human granulosa cells from normal and polycystic ovaries. J. clin. Endocrinol. Metab. 49, 514-519 (1979).

28. Gemzell, C.A., Diczfalusy, E., Tillinger, E.G.: Human pituitary follicle-stimulating hormone. I. Clinical effect of a partially purified preparation. Ciba Found. Coll. Endocr. 13, 191-209 (1950).

29. Crooke, A.C., Butt, W.R., Palmer, R., Morris, R., Logan-Edwards, R., Taylor, C.W., Short, R.V.: Effect of human pituitary-follicle-stimulating hormone and chorionic gonadotrophin in Stein-Leventhal syndrome. Brit. med. J. 1, 1119-1123 (1963).

30. Shearman, R.P., Cox, R.I.: Clinical and chemical correlations in the Stein-Leventhal syndrome. Amer. J. Obstet. Gynec. 92, 747-754 (1965).

31. Naftolin, F., Ryan, K.J., Petro, Z.: Aromatization of androstenedione by the anterior hypothalamus of adult male and female rats. Endocrinology 90, 295-298 (1972).

32. Selmonoff, M.K., Brodkin, L.D., Weiner, R.I., Siiteri, P.K.: Aromatization and 5α-reduction of androgens in discrete hypothalamic and limbic regions of the male and female rat. Endocrinology 101, 841-848 (1977).

33. McEwen, B.S., Davis, P.G., Parsons, B., Pfaff, D.W.: The brain as a target for steroid hormone action. Ann. Rev. Neurosci. 2, 65-112 (1979).

34. Lachelin, G.C.L., Barnett, N., Hopper, B.R., Brink, G., Yen, S.S.C.: Adrenal function in normal women and women with polycystic ovary syndrome. J. clin. Endocrinol. Metab. 49, 892-898 (1979).

35. Kirschner, M.A., Jacobs, J.B.: Combined ovarian and adrenal vein catherization to determine the site of androgen overproduction in hirsute women. J. clin. Endocrinol. Metab. 33, 199-209 (1971).

36. Stahl, N.L., Teeslink, C.R., Greenblatt, R.B.: Ovarian, adrenal and peripheral testosterone levels in the polycystic ovary syndrome. Am. J. Obstet. Gynec. 117, 194-200 (1973).

37. Kirschner, M.A., Zucker, I.R., Jespersen, D.: Idiopathic hirsutism - an ovarian abnormality. New Engl. J. Med. 294, 637-640 (1976).

38. Cox, R.I., Shearman, R.P.: Abnormal excretion of pregnanetriolone and Δ^5-pregnenetriol in the Stein-Leventhal syndrome. J. clin. Endocrinol. Metab. 21, 586-590 (1961).

39. Finkelstein, M., von Euw, J., Reichstein, T.: Isolierung von 3α,17,20α-trioxy-pregnanon (11) aus pathologischen menschlichen Harn. Helv. chim. Acta 36, 1266-1277 (1953).

40. Finkelstein, M., Goldberg, S.: A test for qualitative and quantitative estimation of pregnane-3α,17,20α-triol-11-one in urine and its significance in adrenal disturbances. J. clin. Endocrinol. Metab. 17, 1062-1070 (1957).

41. Cox, R.I., Finkelstein, M.: Pregnane-3α,17,20α-triol and pregnane-3α,17,20α-triol-11-one excretion by patients with adrenocortical dysfunction. J. clin. Invest. 36, 1726-1735 (1957).

42. Fukushima, D.K., Gallagher, T.F.: Steroid isolation studies in congenital adrenal hyperplasia. J. biol. Chem. 229, 85-92 (1957).

43. Finkelstein, M.: Pregnanetriolone, an Abnormal Urinary Steroid. In: "Methods in Hormone Research", (2nd ed.), Ed. Dorfman, R.I., Academic Press, New-York, Vol. I., pp. 451-487 (1968).

44. Fukushima, D.K., Bradlow, H.L., Hellman, L., Gallagher, T.F.: Further studies of 21-deoxyhydrocortisone-4-C^{14} in man. J. clin. Endocrinol. Metab. 19, 393-402 (1959).

45. Richards, J.A.: Hormonal control of ovarian follicular development: A 1978 perspective. Recent Progr. Horm. Res. 35, 343-373 (1979).

46. Hechter, O., Zaffaroni, A., Jacobsen, R.P., Levy, H., Jeanloz, R.W., Schenker, W., Pincus, C.: The nature and the biogenesis of the adrenal secretory product. Recent Progr. Horm. Res. 6, 215-246 (1951).

47. Dorrington, J.H., Armstrong, D.T.: Effects of FSH on gonadal functions. Recent Progr. Horm. Res. 35, 301-342 (1979).

48. Ganguly, A., Meikle, A.W., Tyler, F.H., West, C.D.: Assessment of 11β-hydroxylase activity with plasma corticosterone, deoxycorticosterone, cortisol and deoxycortisol: role of ACTH and angiotensin. J. clin. Endocrinol. Metab. 44, 560-568 (1977).

49. Milner, A.J., Viller, D.B.: Steroidogenetic and morphologic effects of ACTH on human fetal adrenal cells grown in tissue culture. Endocrinology 87, 596-601 (1970).

50. Wolf, S.: Female pseudohermaphroditism with adrenocortical failure in identical twins. Arch. Dis. Childh. 29, 132-135 (1954).

51. Childs, B., Grumbach, M.M., Van Wick, J.J.: Virilizing adrenal hyperplasia, a genetic and hormonal study. J. clin. Invest. 35, 213-222 (1956).

52. Schneeberg, N., Steinberg, A., Malan, M.M., Chernoff, B., Yap, C.L.: Congenital virilizing hyperplasia in identical twins. J. clin. Endocrinol. Metab. 19, 203-212 (1959).

53. Finkelstein, M., Shoenberg, J., Maschler, I., Halperin, G.: An attempt to unify concepts of C-21 steroids producing pathways in certain adrenal and ovarian disorders. In: "Research on Steroids", Eds. Cassano, C., Finkelstein, M., Klopper, A., Conti, C., North-Holland, Amsterdam, Vol.III, pp. 223-248 (1968).

54. Finkelstein, M.: The sclerocystic ovary and steroid synthesis. In: Proceedings IV International Congress of Endocrinology, Washington, 1972, Eds. Scow, R.O., Ebling, F., Henderson, I.W., Excerpta Medica International Congress Series No. 273, Endocrinology, Amsterdam, pp. 845-850 (1973).

55. Finkelstein, M.: Mechanism of involution of congenital adrenal hyperplasia and polycystic ovary syndrome. In: "First Postgraduate Course on Mechanism of Hormone Action", Ed. De Salcedo, I., Livraria Gruz, Porto, pp. 188-204 (1972).

56. Travaglini, F., Faglia, G.: Pregnanetriolone excretion in Stein-Leventhal syndrome. Acta Endocrinol. 68, 826-832 (1971).

57. Maschler, I., Salzberger, M., Finkelstein, M.: 11β-Hydroxylase with affinity to C-21-deoxysteroids from ovaries of patients with polycystic ovary syndrome. J. clin. Endocrinol. Metab. 41, 999-1002 (1973).

58. Maschler, I., Salzberger, M., Finkelstein, M.: Ovarian enzymatic divergence in patients with polycystic ovary syndrome excreting urinary pregnanetriolone. Acta Endocrinol. 82, 366-379 (1976).

59. Engel, F.L., McPherson, H.T., Fetter, S.F., Baggett, B., Engel, L.L., Carter, P., Fielding, L.L., Savard, K., Dorfman, R.I.: Clinical morphological and biochemical studies on a malignant testicular tumor. J. clin. Endocrinol. Metab. 24, 528-542 (1964).

60. Nebel, L., Safriel, O.J., Salzberger, M., Finkelstein, M.: Coelomic mesothelium-like cells in the ovarian stroma of patients with the polycystic ovary syndrome (Stein-Leventhal syndrome). Amer. J. Obstet. Gynec. 11, 755-772 (1971).

61. Grumbach, M.M., Barr, M.L.: Cytologic tests of chromosomal sex in relation to sexual anomalies in man. Recent Progr. Horm. Res. 14, 255-334 (1958).

62. Prader, A., Anders, G.J., Habick, H.: Zur Genetic der Congenitalen Adrenogenitalen Syndrome. Helv. paediat. Acta 17, 271-284 (1962).

63. Finkelstein, M., Shaefer, J.M.: Inborn errors of steroid biosynthesis. Physiol. Rev. 59, 353-406 (1979).

ERYTHROPOIETIN

J. L. Spivak and F. Sieber
Clayton Laboratories and Department of Medicine, The Johns Hopkins University School of Medicine, Baltimore, Maryland, U.S.A.

Red blood cell production is a complex process which is regulated by erythropoietin, a hormone produced in the kidney (1) and to a lesser extent in the liver (2). Many aspects of the physiology of erythropoietin remain unknown, but progress in this area has accelerated recently owing to the purification of the hormone (3) and the development of sensitive techniques for studying its mechanism of action (4, 5, 6). In this paper, we review the physiology of erythropoietin based on data derived from both clinical and laboratory investigations with emphasis on the information gained from the application of new technology.

Erythropoietin is a sialoglycoprotein with a molecular weight under denaturing conditions of approximately 33,000 (7). It is heat stable and retains its biologic activity after exposure to 4M guanidine (8), 8M urea, 0.1M mercaptoethanol and acidic (pH 3.5) or alkaline (pH 10.0) conditions (9). Iodination results in a loss of biologic activity (3); desialation does not impair biologic activity but enhances clearance of the hormone from the plasma (10).

The cells within the kidney responsible for the production of erythropoietin have not been identified. Production of the hormone is governed by the balance between tissue oxygen demands and tissue oxygen supply. Tissue hypoxia stimulates erythropoietin production; a surfeit of oxygen suppresses it. The oxygen sensor is thought to be located within the kidney but neither its anatomic location nor the mechanism by which tissue oxygenation is coupled with erythropoietin synthesis and secretion has been established.

Hormones in Normal and Abnormal Human Tissues, Vol. III

In man, the plasma erythropoietin concentration increases within 12 hours after exposure to an hypoxic environment, reaching peak levels by 24 hours (11, 12). Thereafter, in spite of continued exposure and before a compensatory erythropoiesis occurs, the concentration of erythropoietin in the plasma falls to levels undetectable by bioassay (12). The physiologic significance of the initial burst of erythropoietin synthesis is unclear but it can be inhibited by blunting the respiratory alkalosis associated with acute hypoxia (13). It is tempting to speculate that the decline in hormone production with continued hypoxia represents a resetting of the threshold of the renal oxygen sensor. Alternatively, circulatory and respiratory adaptation might improve tissue oxygenation sufficiently to reduce the stimulus for erythropoietin production.

Erythropoietin production is influenced by other factors in addition to tissue oxygenation. These include hypercarbia (14), endotoxin (15) and protein deprivation (16) which depress production of the hormone, and androgens (17), thyroid hormone (18), prostaglandins (19) and cyclic nucleotides (20) which enhance it. Estrogens (21) and prolactin (22) have been reported to influence erythropoietin production but these reports require confirmation. The inhibitory effect of endotoxin and protein deprivation on erythropoietin production could explain in part the anemias associated with inflammation, infection and malignancy. The ability of androgens to stimulate erythropoietin production and cause erythrocytosis is well recognized (23). It remains to be established if the effects of prostaglandins or cyclic nucleotides observed experimentally are of physiologic significance.

Whether erythropoietin is synthesized in an active form (24) or is activated in plasma after secretion from the kidney (25, 26) is a matter of controversy. Attempts to isolate erythropoietin from the kidney have met with limited success (27, 28). If there is renal storage of the hormone, it is not large, since inhibitors of RNA and protein synthesis inhibit secretion of erythropoietin by the kidney in response to an hypoxic stimulus (29).

Studies of the effect of total or partial hepatectomy in anephric animals suggest that the hormone is also produced to a small extent in the liver (2, 30). Extrarenal erythropoietin is immunologically similar to renal erythropoietin (31), and is probably responsible for the basal level of erythropoiesis observed in anephric patients (32, 33). Extrarenal erythropoietin production, like renal erythropoietin production, is subject to modulation by androgens (34) but is insensitive or unresponsive to alterations in tissue oxygenation (35) and is of an insufficient magnitude to maintain an adequate level of erythropoiesis by itself.

Extrarenal erythropoietin production is most likely a legacy of ontogeny, with the switch to renal production of the hormone occurring in the neonatal period (36). In the fetus, erythropoiesis is initiated before development of the kidneys. Renal agenesis does not impair hepatic erythropoiesis and is not associated with anemia (37). The fetus makes erythropoietin independently of the mother (38). Fetal erythropoiesis is stimulated by hypoxia, androgens and thyroid hormone (34, 38) and is suppressed by antiserum to erythropoietin (39). Fetal erythropoietin production is not reduced by removal of the fetal kidneys but is reduced by partial hepatectomy (40). Taken together, these observations provide a basis for extrarenal erythropoietin production in the adult. In common with extramedullary erythropoiesis and fetal hemoglobin production, extrarenal erythropoietin production probably represents a reversion to fetal behavior when there is a severe and unsatisfied demand for red blood cells.

Until the recent purification of erythropoietin (3), there was no direct method for measuring the hormone in body fluids. Fortunately, mammalian erythropoietin is not species specific and a bioassay using rodents can be employed for its detection. Both in vivo and in vitro bioassays have been devised, each requiring a variety of manipulations in order to achieve an acceptable level of sensitivity and specificity. However, all the bioassays are cumbersome, insensitive and subject to artefact. In vivo bioassays of erythropoietin depend on techniques such as starvation (41), hypertransfusion (42), and hypoxia-induced polycythemia (43) which lower endogenous erythropoiesis in the test animal. The ability of test substances to stimulate erythropoiesis is monitored by the incorporation of ^{59}Fe into newly-formed red blood cells. The starved rat assay is the simplest but least sensitive bioassay (42). The hypertransfused mouse assay has the lowest threshold but is the most expensive and technically demanding. Although the exhypoxic polycythemic mouse has a higher level of endogenous erythropoiesis than the hypertransfused mouse, it is more responsive to erythropoietically-active test substances (44). Hypoxia is achieved by either placing the animals for 10 to 15 days in a low pressure tank (0.5 atm) or by exposing them to an atmosphere that contains only 10% oxygen at normal pressure or a low concentration of carbon monoxide (45). A low-cost alternative to the above methods is offered by animal cages that have been fitted with dimethyl silicone membranes (46, 47). Silicone rubber is more permeable for carbon dioxide than for oxygen and the oxygen tension inside the cage can therefore be adjusted by simply varying the number of animals living in a cage.

All strains of mice are not equally responsive to hypoxia (48). In addition, there is often a variation in the response to erythropoietin between mice from the same strain tested at different times (49). Consequently, a dose-response curve using a defined standard must be included in every assay to insure reasonable accuracy. The "Second International Reference Preparation of Erythropoietin" is distributed by the World Health Organization International Laboratory for Biological Standards, Holly Hill, London (50) for this purpose. Routinely, sheep plasma erythropoietin (Connaught Laboratories, Willowdale, Ontario, Canada) provides an adequate working standard. It is sometimes necessary to partially purify samples and reference preparations in order to remove endotoxin and other inhibitory contaminants which can cause nonparallel dose-response curves (51). Since erythropoietin is exquisitely sensitive to degradation by proteolytic and glycolytic enzymes, it is advisable to store samples under aseptic conditions at low temperatures. Bacterial growth in urine specimens can be suppressed by the addition of suitable antibiotics (penicillin and streptomycin) or 0.5% phenol. Finally, since plasma and urine may contain substances (androgens (17), prostaglandins (19), or cyclic nucleotides (20)) which can stimulate endogenous erythropoiesis in the test animal, bioassay results must be interpreted cautiously.

Even the most carefully performed in vivo erythropoietin bioassay is insensitive to concentrations of erythropoietin below 0.05 U/ml and thus fails to detect the presence of erythropoietin in unconcentrated samples of normal plasma or urine. Concentration of the urine to 1% of its original volume, however, permits detection of erythropoietin in normal individuals (52, 53). Recently, it has been demonstrated that by concentrating 200 ml plasma 40-fold, it is possible to detect 0.003 U erythropoietin per ml using the hypertransfused mouse bioassay (54).

In vitro bioassays for erythropoietin offer greater sensitivity than in vivo assays, facilitate testing of greater numbers of samples and produce results within a period of 24 to 48 hours. One type of in vitro assay measures the stimulatory effect of erythropoietin on the synthesis of heme by suspensions of freshly explanted marrow cells (55, 56, 57) or fetal liver cells (58). It detects erythropoietin at concentrations as low as 0.002 U/ml and it is highly specific since incorporation of ^{59}Fe into non-heme proteins is very small (55). Substitution of radioactive glucosamine or labeled amino acids for ^{59}Fe (59), is, however, not advisable since significant amounts of these compounds may be incorporated into nonerythroid cells, especially when crude erythropoietin is contaminated with substances such as granulocyte/macrophage colony stimulating factor (60). Samples and reference preparations must also be reasonably free of inhibitory and toxic contaminants which virtually precludes the direct assay of crude urinary erythropoietin. Even crude human serum may occasionally yield spurious results due to the presence of inhibitors and non-erythropoietin stimulators (62). All components of the culture medium, particularly the serum, have to be carefully tested in order to ensure optimum efficiency of the assay (57). Unlike the *in vivo* erythropoietin assays, *in vitro* assays also detect desialated erythropoietin (10).

The second type of *in vitro* bioassay for erythropoietin is based on clonal assays for erythroid progenitor cells developed during the past decade (4, 5, 6, 63). Erythroid progenitors are detected in viscous or semisolid media by their capacity to form colonies which contain morphologically recognizable members of the erythroid series. In mouse and human bone marrow, three classes of erythroid progenitor cells can be identified. One is a relatively mature member of the erythroid pathway (colony forming unit-erythroid or CFU-E), has a limited proliferative potential and gives rise to small, dense clusters consisting of up to 64 cells. Erythroid clusters originating from CFU-E are scored after 2 (mouse) or 7 (human) days in culture. Early erythroid progenitors (burst forming unit-erythroid or BFU-E) may be grouped into two subclasses, early and late BFU-E (64, 65). Late BFU-E form small multifocal colonies which are scored after 3-4 (mouse)or 10-12 (human) days in culture; early BFU-E form large multifocal colonies consisting of up to 10,000 cells which are scored after 8-10 (mouse) or 17-20 (human) days in culture. The number of colonies formed by the three types of progenitors is a function of the number of colony-forming cells plated, the concentration of erythropoietin, and in the case of BFU-E, the concentration of an additional growth factor called burst promoting activity (BPA; 66). Most mouse strains contain about 400 to 500 CFU-E per 10^5 nucleated bone marrow cells as opposed to only about 40-50 early and late BFU-E in the same number of marrow cells. CFU-E respond to erythropoietin concentrations as low as 0.01 U/ml, whereas BFU-E require at least 10 times higher concentrations. The lower threshold for CFU-E can be further reduced to about 0.002 U/ml if dimethyl sulfoxide is added to the culture medium (67). Colony formation by late erythroid progenitors thus provides a reasonably rapid, accurate and sensitive assay for erythropoietin.

Whether CFU-E are assayed in the plasma clot system of McLeod et al (4) or the methyl cellulose system described by Iscove et al (60) is largely a matter of personal preference. Plasma clot cultures consume less materials but due to the greater variability between individual clots more replicate cultures are usually required. They have to be fixed, squashed, and stained before they can be scored, but at the same time, this procedure provides a permanent record of the assay. Methylcellulose cultures offer the distinct advantage of employing fewer ill-defined medium components. Since these cultures are scored in situ by use of an inverted microscope, fixation and staining are usually not required, but a permanent record is not obtained. A distinction between erythroid and early granulocyte/macrophage colonies is not difficult and a contamination of the erythropoietin sample with granulocyte/macrophage colony stimulating factor thus does not interfere with the assay (60). Verification of the in situ analysis by standard histochemical techniques is easily achieved since methylcellulose is water soluble. It is, however, advisable to use neutral benzidine solutions for the identification of hemoglobinized cells since acidic benzidine solutions have been shown to stain nonerythroid cells as well. As with all in vitro bioassays, all components of the culture medium must be pretested and erythropoietin samples must be free of toxic and interfering contaminants. Identification of a suitable batch of fetal calf serum can be quite difficult. Replacement of fetal calf serum by a defined medium has recently been achieved (68). However, several components of this defined medium also require extensive screening. Connaught sheep plasma erythropoietin is usually acceptable as a working standard but additional purification may be necessary with certain lots (6). If urinary erythropoietin is to be measured by the in vitro colony assay, some purification and concentration is indispensable. Affinity chromatography on insolubilized phytohemagglutinin or wheat germ agglutinin is a simple way of directly and quantitatively extracting erythropoietin from crude urine in a form suitable for assay in tissue culture (8, 69).

To avoid the drawbacks inherent in bioassays, there has been much interest in developing a radioimmunoassay for erythropoietin. Schooley and Garcia (70) and Lange et al (71) were the first to describe the production of antibodies to erythropoietin; their results have been confirmed by other investigators (72, 73). Rabbits and goats have been found to be more suitable than guinea pigs and sheep for immunization (74) and both IgM and IgG neutralizing antibodies have been described (75, 76). Lange and co-workers (77) have described a hemmagglutination inhibition assay using a nonneutralizing erythropoietin antibody. A commercial kit based on this technique is available but results obtained with it by several investigators have not correlated well with the standard bioassay (78, 79).

Recently, Sherwood and Goldwasser (80) and Garcia et al (81) have developed radioimmunoassays employing pure erythropoietin as reference antigen. The results correlate well with the standard bioassay. The presence of asialoerythropoietin could cause discrepancies between the radioimmunoassay and the bioassay since desialated erythropoietin retains its immunological reactivity (80) but has a reduced biological activity in vivo (10). This is probably more a problem in the laboratory than the clinic since desialated glycoproteins are rapidly cleared from the circulation if liver function and blood flow are normal.

Under normal circumstances, only minute amounts of erythropoietin are present in plasma and urine. Calculations from bioassay data (82) and direct measurements with the newly developed radioimmunoassay (80) indicate that the concentration of erythropoietin in normal plasma is 0.02 U/mg. Based on an estimated specific activity of 70,000 U/mg protein for pure erythropoietin (3) each ml. of plasma contains 0.28 ng or 0.008 pM of hormone. A half-life of approximately 25 hours has been calculated for plasma erythropoietin (83) but owing to the insensitivity of the bioassay, a determination by radioimmunoassay will be required to establish an accurate value.

The liver is probably the major site of hormone degradation (10). Less than 7 units (0.1 μg) of erythropoietin are excreted in the urine each day (52, 53). Hormone excretion is greater in males than females under normal circumstances and during anemia (84). There is no correlation between urine erythropoietin levels and the degree of marrow cellularity (82). Whether erythropoietin in the urine represents hormone cleared from the plasma by glomerular filtration, hormone secreted directly into the urine or a combination of these is unknown. Probably only a small fraction of the erythropoietin present in the plasma appears in the urine (84) under normal conditions. Nevertheless, curves correlating urinary or serum erythropoietin concentrations with the hematocrit have the same slope (82) implying a close relationship between the hormone in serum and urine.

In spite of its insensitivity, the _in vivo_ bioassay for erythropoietin has been used widely for measuring erythropoietin levels in serum and urine in patients with disorders of erythropoiesis. Since the fundamental question of how much erythropoietin is enough remains unanswered, erythropoietin bioassay results, especially if negative, must be interpreted with caution. Nevertheless, much useful information concerning erythropoietin production has been obtained. An important relationship established by the bioassay is that serum and urine erythropoietin levels increase in a linear and logarithmic fashion with decreases in hematocrit (85). In this regard, it is of interest that a similar relationship exists between the P_{50} of hemoglobin and the hematocrit (86). Since under normal circumstances, the red cell mass varies directly with the arterial oxygen saturation but not with the arterial oxygen tension (87), it is evident that tissue oxygen delivery is the fundamental stimulus for erythropoietin production. This relationship provides an explanation for the disproportionately low levels of erythropoietin in serum or urine observed in certain anemias.

In both animals (88) and humans who are hypothyroid (89), erythropoietin titers are inappropriately reduced with respect to the degree of anemia. In patients with abnormal hemoglobins manifesting a low affinity for oxygen, erythropoietin excretion is also reduced below expectation for the level of the hematocrit (90). In each instance, however, tissue oxygen delivery is appropriate to tissue oxygen needs. In hypothyroidism, basal metabolism and consequently oxygen consumption are diminished and the demand for red cells is reduced. Hemoglobins which possess a high P_{50} release oxygen to the tissues more readily than does normal hemoglobin and thus less hemoglobin is required to satisfy tissue oxygen needs (86). Therefore, in evaluating the reason for a low hematocrit or a given level of erythropoietin production, it is always important to consider the role of tissue oxygenation.

Erythropoietin production is, of course, affected by factors other than tissue oxygenation. As mentioned above, androgenic steroids and thyroid hormone enhance erythropoietin production; protein deprivation reduces it. Thus castration, hypothyroidism and starvation are associated with low erythropoietin levels. Erythropoietin levels are also often low in relation to the hematocrit in patients with chronic infections, inflammatory or neoplastic diseases which do not impinge on the marrow (91, 92, 93). It must be emphasized, however, that the reduction in hormone concentration is relative, since the levels are elevated when compared to normal. Thus, anemia in these clinical situations is more likely to be the result of other factors such as hemolysis, inanition (94) or humoral factors (95) including but not limited to interferon (96) and endotoxin (15, 51) which can suppress erythroid progenitor cell proliferation.

Patients with a compensated hemolytic anemia defy the dictum that the rate of erythropoiesis reflects the balance between tissue oxygen demands and tissue oxygen supply. These patients maintain a normal hematocrit in the presence of a reduced red blood cell life span by increasing marrow erythropoiesis. However, the stimulus for increased erythropoiesis when the hematocrit is normal is a conundrum that to date defies solution. Hemoglobin oxygen affinity is normal in these patients and erythropoietin levels are not elevated by bioassay (97).

Although injection of red cell hemolysates or hemoglobin stimulates erythropoiesis in certain species (98), it fails to do so in others (99, 100). Furthermore, intravenous injection of red cell hemolysates or hemoglobin does not mimic the extravascular destruction of red blood cells which occurs in these patients.

In vitro studies of erythroid progenitor cells reveal that there is an age spectrum amongst these cells (64, 65). Erythropoietin appears to act only on the most mature progenitor cells (66) while earlier precursors may be under the control of regulatory factors secreted by lymphocytes (101) or monocytes (102). It is possible, therefore, that in a compensated hemolytic anemia, amplification of erythropoiesis is occurring at a level preceding erythropoietin-responsive progenitor cells and by mechanisms not involving erythropoietin.

Since erythropoietin is produced mainly in the kidneys, renal disease has a profound influence on erythropoiesis. Renal failure is a complex state and many factors contribute to anemia in this situation. In acute renal failure, the underlying disorder (vasculitis, septicemia, intravascular coagulation, or immune mediated hemolysis) is usually responsible for anemia. In chronic renal failure, complications due to the renal failure itself or its treatment (iron or folic acid deficiency, infection, toxin exposure during dialysis, hypersplenism, secondary hyperparathyroidism and disordered red cell metabolism) often produce anemia. The extent to which erythropoietin deficiency, in the absence of other complications, is responsible for the anemia of end stage renal disease is an unsettled question. In general, as renal excretory function declines, there is usually a reduction in erythropoietin production. This relationship is not absolute however. For example, after renal transplantation, erythropoietin production and renal excretory function appear to behave independently of each other (103) and in polycystic kidney disease, the hematocrit is higher than in chronic glomerulonephritis for the same level of urea nitrogen (104). Detectable levels of erythropoietin are found in most patients with chronic renal failure and even some anephric patients by both bioassay (33) and radioimmunoassay (80). For comparable degrees of anemia, however, the levels are much lower than would be expected in the absence of renal disease. Both anephric and uremic patients with their kidneys in situ respond to androgen therapy with an increase in erythropoietin production (105). In the anephric patients, however, the response is insufficient to eliminate the need for transfusions (106). Several anephric patients have been described in whom erythropoietin titers were quite high (35, 107) and in one instance, there was no reduction in erythropoietin levels after hypertransfusion (35).

A role for uremic toxins in the anemia of renal disease has been proposed by a number of investigators. Certainly, uremic patients undergoing intensive dialysis improve their rate of erythropoiesis (108) and may even demonstrate feedback inhibition by overtransfusion (109). Experimental data supporting a role for uremic toxins is, however, difficult to interpret since most studies have employed xenogenic assays to demonstrate the toxic effects of uremic serum (110, 111). In such assays, it is often difficult to distinguish nonspecific toxicity due to species differences, from the effects of a uremic toxin. Marrow cells from uremic patients respond normally to erythropoietin (112), indicating that target cell unresponsiveness is not a major component of the anemia of renal disease. Erythropoietin is stable in uremic serum (112) and administration of the hormone to uremic rats corrects their anemia (113). A patient with polycythemia vera, severe iron deficiency and end stage renal disease has been described, who was able to raise his hematocrit from 0.18 to 0.45 merely with iron replacement (114). Finally, a number of patients with chronic renal insufficiency developed transient erythrocytosis during the progression of their renal disease (115, 116). Taken together, these observations suggest that lack of erythropoietin is the major factor in the anemia of chronic renal disease. Reports of high erythropoietin levels in anephric patients with persistent anemia (107) suggest, however, that in some instances other factors have a role as well.

Although under-production of erythropoietin occurs as a result of renal disease or certain other acquired disorders, no convincing example of failure of erythropoietin production on a genetic basis has been described. Furthermore, immune-mediated impairment of erythropoietin activity also appears to be rare, if indeed it occurs at all. Lack of erythropoietin activity should result in pure red cell aplasia with an otherwise cellular marrow containing a normal complement of myeloid and megakaryocyte progenitor cells. Most patients with pure red cell aplasia have high levels of erythropoietin in their plasma and in many patients, antibodies cytotoxic to erythroblasts have been identified (117). In two patients with pure red cell aplasia, an inhibitor of erythropoietin was identified (117, 119). In one instance, subsequent studies indicated that the inhibitory factor was directed against erythroblasts and not erythropoietin (120); the other report requires confirmation.

An increase in the red cell mass is either due to excessive erythropoietin production or an intrinsic abnormality of erythroid progenitor cell proliferation. Tissue hypoxia is the commonest cause of excessive erythropoietin production. Of the many causes of tissue hypoxia, the most important clinically are chronic carbon monoxide intoxication, disorders of respiratory function and vascular abnormalities producing a venous admixture effect. Less commonly, erythropoietin production is elevated in the absence of tissue hypoxia in association with certain diseases of the kidney, with a variety of benign and malignant neoplasms, or after administration of androgenic steroids.

Careful measurements of erythropoietin levels in the serum have been helpful in distinguishing most patients with erythrocytosis due to polycythemia vera from patients with erythrocytosis due to other causes (54, 78, 121). However, even with the most sensitive radioimmunoassay, a definite distinction cannot be made in all cases (121). This appears to be due to the fundamental mechanisms for erythropoietin production.

Studies on rodents have demonstrated that transfusion-induced erythrocytosis does not completely suppress erythropoietin production (122). Furthermore, while hypoxemia initially produced a marked elevation of urinary and serum erythropoietin levels, in both rodents and humans the concentration of hormone declined, often to the extent that it was undetectable by bioassay, even though the hypoxemia persisted (11, 12). Indeed, patients with chronic pulmonary disease or high oxygen-affinity hemoglobins and erythrocytosis may manifest no increase in urinary erythropoietin excretion (85, 123), and thus behave like patients with a compensated hemolytic anemia. Consequently, in the patient with erythrocytosis, the absence of detectable levels of erythropoietin does not exclude the possibility of tissue hypoxia, nor does a low but detectable level of erythropoietin exclude the presence of polycythemia vera. It is obvious that an elevated level of erythropoietin in serum or urine is required for this distinction but in at least 10% of patients with secondary erythrocytosis, erythropoietin levels were not elevated to the extent required (121).

An explanation of the mechanism responsible for the low levels of erythropoietin observed in some plethoric patients with hypoxemia as well as those with polycythemia vera is provided by Adamson's studies of urine erythropoietin excretion in such patients after phlebotomy (85). In patients with erythrocytosis due to pulmonary disease in whom urinary erythropoietin excretion was normal, phlebotomy increased erythropoietin excretion several fold and hormone excretion was greater than in normal persons at the same hematocrit level (85). In two patients with high oxygen-affinity hemoglobins and erythrocytosis, similar observations were made (123). It appears that in these patients, the threshold of sensitivity of the renal oxygen sensor is increased. This is in keeping with the observation that patients with obstructive airway diseases have a more marked increase in red cell mass than normal persons for a given reduction in arterial oxygen saturation (87).

By contrast, in polycythemia vera where urinary erythropoietin excretion is low or absent, postphlebotomy erythropoietin excretion is reduced compared to normal individuals at the same hematocrit (85). In polycythemia vera, the sensitivity of the renal sensor for erythropoietin production appears to be reduced. Support for this was derived from experiments with rodents transfused with methemoglobin-containing red cells (124). In these animals, erythrocytosis suppressed erythropoiesis even though oxygen transport was not improved. This suggests that erythrocytosis by itself, rather than a surfeit of oxygen, can influence the renal mechanism for production of erythropoietin.

Studies of individuals with impaired tissue oxygenation due to chronic pulmonary disease or high oxygen-affinity hemoglobins, suggest that neither erythrocytosis nor maintenance of a normal resting venous oxygen saturation are invariable consequences of hypoxemia. Infection, chronic inflammation or inanition can be expected to prevent an appropriate increase in erythropoietin production in some patients with chronic pulmonary disease. In others, an alteration in hemoglobin-oxygen affinity, regional changes in blood flow or an elevated cardiac output could improve oxygenation sufficiently to obviate the need for an increase in red cell mass. Finally, in some instances it appears that patients adapt to a state of chronic tissue hypoxia. This has been observed in patients with high oxygen-affinity hemoglobins who maintain a low venous oxygen saturation without evident compensation either by an increase in cardiac output or the expected elevation in red cell mass (125, 126).

Although impaired erythropoietin production and anemia are the usual consequences of renal disease, inappropriate production of erythropoietin and erythrocytosis also occur. Structural lesions causing erythrocytosis include renal artery stenosis (127, 128), renal cysts (129) and obstructive hydronephrosis (130). It is noteworthy that renal artery stenosis causing erythrocytosis may involve vessels too small to be detectable by arteriography (128). In polycystic kidney disease, the hematocrit is often inappropriately high for the degree of renal failure (104) but true erythrocytosis is usually only observed with solitary renal cysts (131). The development of erythrocytosis does not correlate with the presence or absence of erythropoietin in the cyst fluid (132). Erythropoietin production is most likely due to local hypoxia which occurs as the cysts expand, compress adjacent renal tissue and disturb blood flow (132). It should be emphasized that erythrocytosis due to renal cysts, renal artery stenosis or hydronephrosis is uncommon and occurs predominantly in men (132). Furthermore, in several instances, polycythemia vera has been identified as the cause of erythrocytosis initially attributed to a renal cyst (133).

Erythrocytosis has also been observed in Bartter's syndrome (134) and paradoxically in patients with parenchymal renal disease, most notably in association with glomerular involvement and nephrosis (115, 116). In some but not all patients, the renal disease preceded the erythrocytosis. Eventually, anemia ensued but the erythrocytosis was sufficient to require periodic phlebotomies in several patients (115). Erythrocytosis associated with renal parenchymal disease is also more common in men.

Erythrocytosis is an unusual complication of renal transplantation but not necessarily a sign of graft rejection (135, 136). Erythrocytosis usually develops several months after transplantation and appears to occur more frequently when cadaver kidneys are employed (137). Although the mechanism for post-transplantation erythrocytosis is unresolved, a recent study has implicated the recipient's own kidneys as the site of uncontrolled erythropoietin production (138). This is not always the case since post-transplantation erythrocytosis has been observed in anephric recipients (103, 139). It should also be noted that denervation does not prevent the kidney from producing erythropoietin in response to hypoxia (103).

Erythrocytosis is a rare manifestation of benign and malignant neoplasms. Thorling's monograph (132) published in 1972 continues to be the definitive study of this subject. With the exception of tumors of the female reproductive tract, the majority of patients with tumor-associated erythrocytosis are men even when the particular tumor has no sexual predilection. Furthermore, women who develop inappropriate erythrocytosis do so at an older age than men. Distinguishing tumor-induced erythrocytosis from polycythemia vera is a major consideration since the age of onset of both is often similar. Although erythrocytosis has been associated with many different tumors, careful analysis of the published data has failed to substantiate many of these claims (132). Reliance on the hematocrit as an indicator of the red cell mass is unacceptable. In many instances, an elevated hematocrit merely reflects a reduction in plasma volume; occasionally, as in the case of hepatomas, an elevated plasma volume will mask an absolute increase in red cell mass (132). The best evidence for tumor-associated erythrocytosis is remission of the erythrocytosis with removal of the tumor but with certain tumors such as the hepatoma, this criterion is usually not applicable. Based on the published reports, erythrocytosis has been established as a paraneoplastic manifestation of the following tumors; renal tumors (hypernephroma, Wilms' tumor, adenoma and undifferentiated carcinoma), liver tumors (hepatoma and hamartoma), cerebellar hemangioblastoma, uterine fibromyoma, pheochromocytoma and adrenal adenoma. Hypernephroma, cerebellar hemangioblastoma and pheochromocytoma and adrenal adenoma are all observed in the von Hippel-Lindau syndrome suggesting that erythrocytosis associated with these tumors has a genetic predilection and does not occur by chance.

The mechanisms by which various tumors induce erythrocytosis have not been established. In several patients with tumor-associated erythrocytosis, urinary erythropoietin levels did not change with phlebotomy even when not elevated initially (85), suggesting both autonomous production of the hormone and possibly suppression of erythropoietin production by the kidney. Whether particular tumors produce erythropoietin, another molecule with similar activity or substance such as prostaglandins which stimulate renal erythropoietin production or potentiate the effect of erythropoietin (140) will require investigation with an antibody specific for the hormone. For certain tumors, such as virilizing ovarian or adrenal carcinomas, it is likely that erythrocytosis is due to production of androgenic steroids (141).

The incidence of erythrocytosis due to tumors is probably less than 1% (142); renal tumors are most often responsible (142, 143). Erythrocytosis occurs in approximately 3% of renal tumors, most commonly with the hypernephroma (143). An important clue to the presence of a tumor underlying the erythrocytosis is elevation of the erythrocyte sedimentation rate which is usually low in polycythemia vera (132). Removal of the tumor abolishes the erythrocytosis; persistence of erythrocytosis or its recurrence is associated with the presence of metastases (132). In most patients, Wilms' tumor does not produce erythrocytosis, but many of these patients, as well as non-polycythemic patients with renal tumors, have elevated levels of erythropoietin as measured by bioassay (144, 145). The meaning and significance of these observations require further evaluation. There is no correlation between the presence or absence of erythrocytosis and prognosis.

Approximately 3% of patients with hepatomas have erythrocytosis based on hemoglobin determinations (146). The incidence might well be higher if red cell mass determinations were employed, since the plasma volume in these patients is often elevated. The hemoglobin level can increase rapidly in the hepatoma patient and decline with equal rapidity (146). In patients with hemochromatosis, erythrocytosis can be an important clue to the development of a hepatoma (147). In one patient, chemotherapy and partial hepatectomy were associated with remission of the erythrocytosis but whether this was the result of drug-induced marrow damage as opposed to suppression of tumor growth or hormone production is unclear (148). It is worth emphasizing, however, that while hepatoma is a complication of cirrhosis, erythrocytosis can occur with cirrhosis in the absence of this neoplasm (149).

Erythrocytosis occurs in approximately 18% of patients with a cerebellar hemangioblastoma (150). These tumors usually occur in patients below age 50 and erythrocytosis is more common in men (150). Erythropoietin has been identified in fluid taken from these tumors and removal of the tumor is associated with remission of the erythrocytosis (151). It is unlikely that the erythrocytosis is due to compromise of respiratory function since it does not occur with other cerebellar tumors and is associated only with certain histologic types of hemangioblastoma (152).

Erythrocytosis has been occasionally described in association with uterine fibromyomas. A characteristic feature of these tumors is their immense size; the largest reported tumor weighed 14 kg (153). Because of their size, these tumors could cause erythrocytosis by interfering with renal blood flow or respiratory function (132). Erythropoietic activity which is neutralized by an antierythropoietin antibody has been extracted from uterine fibromyomas (154) but similar activity could not always be identified in plasma or urine by bioassay. However, the association of erythrocytosis with leiomyomas of the esophagus (155) and skin (156) supports the contention that erythrocytosis in patients with uterine fibromyomas is due to ectopic erythropoietin production.

Polycythemia vera is a clonal disorder of the hematopoietic stem cell (157) which is fully manifest as a panmyelopathy involving myeloid cells and megakaryocytes as well as erythrocytes. In a significant number of patients, however, the sole manifestation of the disorder initially is erythrocytosis. The disease is most common in patients over the age of 50 in whom a modest venous admixture effect or other cardiopulmonary abnormality is usually present (158). While arterial oxygen tension may be reduced in such individuals, arterial oxygen saturation is virtually never below 90% (158) and this permits distinction between autonomous erythrocytosis and that induced by tissue hypoxia. The disease has a predilection for Ashkenazic Jews (159) and familial occurrence has been documented (160). The only definitive method for identifying polycythemia vera as the cause of erythrocytosis is demonstration of clonality (157). Unfortunately, at present such a demonstration is technically limited to individuals heterozygous for the red cell enzyme glucose-6-phosphate dehydrogenase. However, since phlebotomy is the treatment of choice for erythrocytosis not associated with a correctable lesion, no harm ensues from not establishing a diagnosis of polycythemia vera early in the course of the disease.

The role of erythropoietin in the pathogenesis of polycythemia vera is an unsettled issue. The renal sensor for erythropoietin production is responsive to induced hypoxemia (85, 161), although its sensitivity is diminished. Erythropoiesis is stimulated by phlebotomy (85), but paradoxically is not suppressed by hyperoxia (162, 163). This suggests that the defect is in the target cell population and not in the kidney. In short term *in vitro* liquid cultures, marrow cells from patients with polycythemia vera are unresponsive to erythropoietin unless remission has been induced by chemotherapy (164). In long term *in vitro* liquid cultures, however, polycythemia vera marrow cells are erythropoietin-responsive (165). An explanation for these observations is provided by the elegant demonstration by Adamson and his colleagues of two populations of hematopoietic progenitor cells in the marrow in polycythemia vera, a normal population and one representing the abnormal clone (157). The latter population has a survival advantage since only its mature progeny circulate in the blood (157); as the disease progresses the abnormal clone probably becomes the dominant one in the marrow (166).

The use of *in vitro* clonal assay systems to study the response to erythropoietin in polycythemia vera has produced conflicting results. Erythroid colony formation by marrow cells from patients with polycythemia vera in contrast to normal marrow cells, occurs in the absence of added erythropoietin (167). From statistical considerations in studies employing glucose-6-phosphate dehydrogenase isoenzymes as markers of normal and abnormal erythroid colonies, it has been argued that the abnormal clone is erythropoietin-responsive (168). Studies employing antierythropoietin antibodies support this contention (169). Evidence has also been presented that the abnormal clone is exquisitely sensitive to erythropoietin (166, 170). However, the findings could also be interpreted as indicating that the abnormal clone is erythropoietin-independent. In this regard, an anephric patient with end stage polycythemia vera and myelofibrosis has been described who maintained a hematocrit of 0.37 (116). Taken together, the findings suggest that responsiveness to erythropoietin is maintained in polycythemia vera but the hormone may not be required to maintain proliferation of the abnormal clone. Further studies employing pure erythropoietin, monospecific antibodies to the hormone and the individual erythroid cell populations will be required to settle this issue.

An intriguing group of patients has been described with erythrocytosis occurring at an early age unassociated with an identifiable cause or evidence for polycythemia vera (171, 172, 173). In several instances, the disorder was familial, recessive, and associated with elevated levels of serum and urinary erythropoietin (171, 172). In one family, phlebotomy did not influence erythropoietin production (171). In another, however, neither serum nor urinary erythropoietin levels were elevated by bioassay but did increase after phlebotomy (174). One patient with erythrocytosis and excessive erythropoietin production has been followed for 14 years without evidence of any underlying disease (175) and our experience in a young patient with erythrocytosis has been similar. These patients serve to emphasize that phlebotomy is the only therapy which should be employed in treating erythrocytosis in patients in whom a correctable lesion is not found. There is no place for chemotherapeutic agents if a diagnosis of polycythemia vera cannot be established and a recent report suggests that chemotherapeutic agents are not warranted even in that disorder (176). The extent of phlebotomy should be dictated by the patient's symptoms when erythrocytosis is secondary to hypoxemia (126), but regardless of the cause of erythrocytosis, all patients are at risk of thromboembolic events unless the red cell mass is reduced. In polycythemia vera, phlebotomy will be most successful if the hematocrit is reduced below 0.45 (177) and a state of iron deficiency is induced.

Thirty-one years have passed since Reissmann demonstrated humoral regulation of erythropoiesis (178). Progress in erythropoietin research has been greatly hampered by lack of a sensitive and specific assay for the hormone and lack of pure erythropoietin for study. Yet, in spite of these difficulties, a substantial quantity of useful information about the physiology of erythropoietin and erythropoiesis has been obtained. The recent purification of the hormone (3) and the development of a highly sensitive and accurate radioimmunoassay (80, 81) together with the new clonal assays for hematopoietic progenitor cells hold great promise for the future. Obtaining an adequate supply of erythropoietin-rich urine for purification is the only remaining obstacle to widespread use of the hormone for research and therapeutic purposes. Isolation and cloning of the gene coding for erythropoietin would of course provide the most satisfactory solution to this problem.

Acknowledgements

Supported in part by grant AM 16702 from the National Institutes of Health. J. L. Spivak is a recipient of a Research Career Development Award from the National Heart Lung and Blood Institute. F. Sieber is a Hubert E. and Anne E. Rogers Scholar in Academic Medicine.

References

1. Jacobson, L.O., Goldwasser, E., Fried, W., Plzak, L.: Role of the kidney in erythropoiesis. Nature 179, 633-634 (1957).

2. Fried, W.: The liver as a source of extrarenal erythropoietin production. Blood 40, 671-677 (1972).

3. Miyake, T., Kung, C.K-H., Goldwasser, E.: Purification of human erythropoietin. J. biol.Chem. 252, 5558-5564 (1977).

4. McLeod, D.L., Shreeve, M.M., Axelrad, A.A.: Improved plasma culture system for production of erythrocytic colonies in vitro: quantitative assay method for CFU-E. Blood 44, 517-534 (1974).

5. Heath, D.S., Axelrad, A.A., McLeod, D.L., Shreeve, M.M.: Separation of the erythropoietin-responsive progenitors BFU-E and CFU-E in mouse bone marrow by unit gravity sedimentation. Blood 47, 777-792 (1976).

6. Iscove, N.N., Sieber, F.: Erythroid progenitors in mouse bone marrow detected by macroscopic colony formation in culture. Exp. Hemat. 3, 32-43 (1975).

7. Shelton, R.N., Ichiki, A.T., Lange, R.D.: Physicochemical properties of erythropoietin: isoelectric focusing and molecular weight studies. Biochem. Med. 12, 45-54 (1975).

8. Spivak, J.L., Small, D., Shaper, J.H., Hollenberg, M.D.: Use of immobilized lectins and other ligands for the partial purification of erythropoietin. Blood 52, 1178-1188 (1978).

9. Espada, J., Brandan, N.C., Dorado, M.: Effect of chemical and enzymatic agents in the biological activity of erythropoietin. Acta physiol. lat.-amer. 23, 193-201 (1973).

10. Goldwasser, E., Kung, C.K-H., Eliason, J.: On the mechanism of erythropoietin-induced differentiation. The role of sialic acid in erythropoietin action. J. biol. Chem. 249, 4202-4206 (1974).

11. Faura, J., Ramos, J., Reynafarje, C., English, E., Finne, P., Finch, C.A.: Effect of altitude on erythropoiesis. Blood 33, 668-676 (1969).

12. Abbrecht, P.H., Littell, J.K.: Plasma erythropoietin in men and mice during acclimatization to different altitudes. J. appl. Physiol. 32, 54-58 (1972).

13. Miller, M.E., Rorth, M., Parving, H.H., Howard, D., Keddington, I., Valeri, C.R., Stohlman, F., Jr.: pH Effect on erythropoietin response to hypoxia. New Engl. J. Med. 288, 706-710 (1974).

14. Schooley, J.C., Mahlmann, L-J.: Hypoxia and the initiation of erythropoietin production. Blood Cells 1, 429-448 (1975).

15. Schade, S.G., Fried, W.: Suppressive effect of endotoxin in erythropoietin-responsive cells in mice. Amer. J. Physiol. 231, 73-76 (1976).

16. Reissmann, K.R.: Protein metabolism and erythropoiesis. Erythropoietin formation and erythroid responsiveness in protein-deprived rats. Blood 23, 146-153 (1964).

17. Fried, W., Gurney, C.W.: Erythropoietic effect of plasma from mice receiving testosterone. Nature 206, 1160-1161 (1965).

18. Peschle, C.E., Zanjani, E.D., Gidari, A.S., McLaurin, W.D., Gordon, A.S.: Mechanism of thyroxin action on erythropoiesis. Endocrinology 89, 609-612 (1971).

19. Schooley, J.C., Mahlman, L-J.: Stimulation of erythropoiesis in plethoric mice by prostaglandins and its inhibition by antierythropoietin. Proc. Soc. exp. Biol. Med. 138, 523-524 (1971).

20. Schooley, J.C., Mahlman, L-J.: Stimulation of erythropoiesis in the plethoric mouse by cyclic-AMP and its inhibition by antierythropoietin. Proc. Soc. exp. Biol. Med. 137, 1289-1292 (1971).

21. Mirand, E.C., Gordon, A.S.: Mechanism of estrogen action in erythropoiesis. Endocrinology 78, 325-332 (1966).

22. Jepson, J.H., Lowenstein, L.: Effect of prolactin on erythropoiesis in the mouse. Blood 24, 726-738 (1964).

23. Kennedy, B.J., Gilbertsen, A.S.: Increased erythropoiesis induced by androgenic-hormone therapy. New Engl. J. Med. 256, 719-726 (1957).

24. Erslev, A.J.: In vitro production of erythropoietin by kidneys perfused with a serum-free solution. Blood 44, 77-85 (1974).

25. Libbin, R.M., Person, P., Gordon, A.S.: Renal lysozomes: role in biogenesis of erythropoietin. Science 185, 1174-1176 (1974).

26. Peschle, C., Condorelli, M.: Biogenesis of erythropoietin: evidence for proerythropoietin in a subcellular fraction of kidney. Science 190, 910-912 (1975).

27. Contrera, J.F., Camiscoli, J.F., Weintraub, A.H., Gordon,A.S.: Extraction of erythropoietin from kidneys of hypoxic and phenylhydrazine-treated rats. Blood 25, 809-815 (1965).

28. Sherwood, J.B., Goldwasser, E.: Extraction of erythropoietin from normal kidneys. Endocrinology 103, 866-870 (1978).

29. Schooley, J.C., Mahlman, L-J.: Evidence for de novo synthesis of erythropoietin in hypoxic rats. Blood 40, 662-670 (1972).

30. Naughton, B.A., Kaplan, S.M., Roy, M., Burdowski, A.J., Gordon, A.S., Piliero, S.J.: Hepatic regeneration and erythropoietin production in the rat. Science 196, 301-302 (1977)

31. Fried, W., Kilbridge, T., Krantz, S., McDonald, T.P., Lange, R.D.: Studies on extrarenal erythropoietin. J. Lab. clin. Med. 73, 244-241 (1969).

32. Nathan, D.G., Schupak, E., Stohlman, F., Jr., Merrill, J.P.: Erythropoiesis in anephric man. J. clin. Invest. 43, 2158-2165 (1964).

33. Caro, J., Brown, S., Miller, O., Murray, T., Erslev, A.J.: Erythropoietin levels in uremic and anephric patients. J. Lab. clin. Med. 93, 449-458 (1979).

34. Zanjani, E.D., Banisadre, M.: Hormonal stimulation of erythropoietin production and erythropoiesis in anephric sheep fetuses. J. clin. Invest. 64, 1181-1187 (1979).

35. Erslev, A.J., McKenna, P.J., Capelli, J.P., Hamburger, R.J., Cohn, H.E., Clark, J.E.: Rate of red cell production in two nephrectomized patients. Arch intern. Med. 122, 230-235 (1968)

36. Wang, F., Fried, W.: Renal and extrarenal erythropoietin production in male and female rats of various ages. J. Lab. clin. Med. 79, 181-186 (1972).

37. Finne, P.H., Halvorsen, S.: Regulation of erythropoiesis in the fetus and newborn. Arch. Dis. Childh. 47, 683-687 (1972).

38. Zanjani, E.D., Peterson, E.N., Gordon, A.S., Wasserman, L.R.: Erythropoietin production in the fetus: role of the kidney and maternal anemia. J. Lab. clin. Med. 83, 281-287 (1974).

39. Zanjani, E.D., Mann, L.I., Burlington, H., Gordon, A.S., Wasserman, L.R.: Evidence for a physiologic role of erythropoietin in fetal erythropoiesis. Blood 44, 285-290 (1974).

40. Zanjani, E.D., Poster, J., Burlington, H., Mann, L.I., Wasserman, L.R.: Liver as the primary site of erythropoietin formation in the fetus. J. Lab. clin. Med. 89, 640-644 (1977).

41. Fried, W., Plzak, L., Jacobson, L.O.: Studies on erythropoiesis. III. Factors controlling erythropoietin production. Proc. Soc. exp. Biol. Med. 94, 237-241 (1957).

42. DeGowin, R.L., Hofstra, D., Gurney, C.W.: A comparison of erythropoietin bioassays. Proc. Soc. exp. Biol. Med. 110, 48-51 (1962).

43. Cotes, P.M., Bangham, D.R.: Bio-assay of erythropoietin in mice made polycythaemic by exposure to air at a reduced pressure. Nature 191, 1065-1067 (1961).

44. O'Kunewick, J.P., Fulton, D.: Comparison of erythropoietin response in mice following polycythemia induced by transfusion or hypoxia. Blood 36, 239-245 (1970).

45. Fogh, J.: A sensitive erythropoietin assay on mice exposed to CO-hypoxia. Scand. J. clin. Lab. Invest. 18, 33-44 (1966).

46. Lange, R.D., Simmons, M.L., Dibelius, N.: A new technique. Polycythemic mice produced by hypoxia. Proc. Soc. exp. Biol. Med. 122, 761-764 (1966).

47. Spivak, J.L., Connor, E.C.: A simple hypoxic chamber. J. Lab. clin. Med. 89, 1375-1378 (1977).

48. Shadduck, R., Howard, D., Stohlman, F., Jr.: A difference in erythropoietin production between anemic and hypoxic mice. Proc. Soc. exp. Biol. Med. 128, 132-136 (1968).

49. Ichiki, A.T., Lange, R.D.: A method for the concentration of erythropoietin from human urine. Biochem. Med. 10, 50-60 (1974).

50. Annable, L., Cotes, P.M., Mussett, M.V.: The second international reference preparation of erythropoietin for bioassay. Bull. Wld Hlth Org. 47, 99-112 (1972).

51. Zuckerman, K.S., Quesenberry, P.J., Levin, J., Sullivan, R.: Contamination of erythropoietin by endotoxin: in vivo and in vitro effects on murine erythropoiesis. Blood 54, 146-158 (1979).

52. Adamson, J.W., Alexanian, R., Martinez, C., Finch, C.A.: Erythropoietin excretion in normal man. Blood 28, 354-364 (1966).

53. Alexanian, R.: Urinary excretion of erythropoietin in normal men and women. Blood 28, 344-353 (1966).

54. Erslev, A.J., Caro, J., Kansu, E., Miller, O., Cobbs, E.: Plasma erythropoietin in polycythemia. Amer. J. Med. 66, 243-247 (1979).

55. Gallien-Lartigue, O., Goldwasser, E.: Hemoglobin synthesis in marrow cell culture: the effect of rat plasma on rat cells. Science 145, 277-279 (1964).

56. Goldwasser, E., Eliason, J.F., Sikkema, D.: An assay for erythropoietin in vitro at the milliunit level. Endocrinology 97, 315-323 (1975).

57. Krystal, G., Eaves, A.C., Eaves, C.J.: A quantitative bioassay for erythropoietin, using mouse bone marrow. J. Lab. clin. Med. 97, 144-157 (1981).

58. Dunn, C.D.R., Lange, R.D.: Erythropoietin regulatory factors: correlation of detectable titers in vivo and in vitro. Blood 52, 1238-1242 (1978).

59. Dukes, P.P., Takaku, F., Goldwasser, E.: In vitro studies on the effect of erythropoietin on glucosamine-1-^{14}C incorporation into rat bone marrow cells. Endocrinology 74, 960-967 (1964).

60. Iscove, N.N., Sieber, F., Winterhalter, K.H.: Erythroid colony formation in cultures of mouse and human bone marrow: analysis of the requirement for erythropoietin by gel filtration and affinity chromatography on Agarose-Concanavalin A. J. cell. comp. Physiol. 83, 309-320 (1974).

61. Krystal, G., Eaves, A.C., Eaves, C.J.: Determination of normal human serum erythropoietin levels, using mouse bone marrow. J. Lab. clin. Med. 97, 158-169 (1981).

62. DeKlerk, R., Von Dem Borne, A.E.G. Kr., Goudsmit, R.: The nature of toxicity of human serum in the bioassay of erythropoietin using mouse fetal liver cells. Exp. Hematol. 6, 193-200 (1978).

63. Tepperman, A.D., Curtis, J.E., McCulloch, E.A.: Erythropoietic colonies in cultures of human marrow. Blood 44, 659-669 (1974).

64. Gregory, C.J.: Erythropoietin sensitivity as a differentiation marker in the hemopoietic system. J. cell. comp. Physiol. 89, 289-302 (1976).

65. Gregory, C.J., Eaves, A.C.: Human marrow cells capable of erythropoietic differentiation in vitro: definition of three erythroid colony responses. Blood 49, 855-864 (1977).

66. Iscove, N.N.: Erythropoietin-independent stimulation of early erythropoiesis in adult marrow cultures by conditioned media from lectin-stimulated mouse spleen cells. In: "Hematopoietic Cell Differentiation", Eds. Cline, M.J., Golde, D., Metcalf, D., Fox, C.F., Academic Press, New York, pp. 37-52 (1978).

67. Sieber, F.: Erythroid colony growth in culture: effects of desialated erythropoietin, neuraminidase, dimethyl sulfoxide, and Amphotericin B. In: "Progress in Differentiation Research", Ed. Müller-Bérat, N., North-Holland, Amsterdam, pp. 521-528 (1976).

68. Iscove, N.N., Guilbert, L.J., Weyman, C.: Complete replacement of serum in primary cultures of erythropoietin-dependent red cell precursors by albumin, transferrin, iron, unsaturated fatty acid, lecithin and cholesterol. Exp. Cell Res. 126, 121-126 (1980).

69. Sieber, F.: Chromatography of human urinary erythropoietin and granulocyte colony-stimulating factor on insolubilized phytohaemagglutinin. Biochim. biophys. Acta 496, 146-154 (1977).

70. Schooley, J.C., Garcia, S.F.: Immunochemical studies of human urinary erythropoietin. Proc. Soc. exp. Biol. Med. 109, 325-328 (1962).

71. Lange, R.D., Gardner, E. Jr., Wright, C.S., Gallagher, N.I.: Neutralization of the biological activity of erythropoietin by immune sera. Brit. J. Haematol. 10, 69-74 (1964).

72. Krugers Dagneaux, P.G.L.C., Goudsmit, R., Krijnen, H.W.: Investigations on an immunoassay of erythropoietin. Ann. N.Y. Acad. Sci. 149, 294-297 (1968).

73. Rioux, E., Erslev, A.J.: Immunologic studies of a partially purified sheep erythropoietin. J. Immunol. 101, 6-11 (1968).

74. Lange, R.D., O'Grady, L.F., Lewis, J.P., Trobaugh, F.E. Jr.: Application of erythropoietin antisera to studies of erythropoiesis. Ann. N.Y. Acad. Sci. 149, 281-291 (1968).

75. Lange, R.D., McDonald, T.P., Jordan, T.: Antisera to erythropoietin: partial characterization of two different antibodies. J. Lab. clin. Med. 73, 78-90 (1969).

76. Lange, R.D., Jordan, T.A., McDonald, T.P.: Partial characterization of an antiserum to erythropoietin. Israel J. med. Sci. 7, 877-884 (1971).

77. McKee, L.C., Johnson, L.E., Lange, R.D.: Circadian variation in reticulocyte counts and immuno-detectable erythropoietin. Proc. Soc. exp. Biol. Med. 145, 1284-1287 (1974).

78. Kolk-Vegter, A.J., Kolk, A.H.J., Napier, J.A.F., Dunn, C.D.R.: Some problems concerning the assay of erythropoietin using the haemagglutination inhibition kit. Brit. J. Haematol. 30, 371-372 (1975).

79. Erslev, A.J., Caro, J., Miller, O., Silver, R.: Plasma erythropoietin in health and disease. Ann. Clin. Lab. Sci. 10, 250-257 (1980).

80. Sherwood, J.B., Goldwasser, E.: A radioimmunoassay for erythropoietin. Blood 54, 885-893 (1979).

81. Garcia, J.F., Sherwood, J., Goldwasser, E.: Radioimmunoassay of erythropoietin. Blood Cells 5, 405-419 (1979).

82. Alexanian, R.: Erythropoietin excretion in bone marrow failure and hemolytic anemia. J. Lab. clin. Med. 82, 438-445 (1973).

83. Rosse, W.F., Waldman, T.A.: The metabolism of erythropoietin in patients with anemia due to deficient erythropoiesis. J. clin. Invest. 43, 1348-1354 (1964).

84. Alexanian, R.: Correlations between erythropoietin production and excretion. J. Lab. clin. Med. 74, 614-622 (1969).

85. Adamson, J.W.: The erythropoietin/hematocrit relationship in normal and polycythemic man: implications of marrow regulation. Blood 32, 597-609 (1965).

86. Huehns, E.R., Bellingham, A.J.: Diseases of function and stability of haemoglobin. Brit. J. Haematol. 17, 1-10 (1969).

87. Weil, J.V., Jamieson, G., Brown, D.W., Grover, R.F.: The red cell mass-arterial oxygen relationship in normal man. J. clin. Invest. 47, 1627-1639 (1968).

88. Donati, R.M., Fletcher, J.W., Warnecke, M.A., Gallagher, N.I.: Erythropoiesis in hypothyroidism. Proc. Soc. exp. Biol. Med. 144, 78-82 (1973).

89. Das, K.C., Mukherjee, M., Sarkar, T.K., Dash, R.J., Rastogi, G.K.: Erythropoiesis and erythropoietin in hypo- and hyperthyroidism. J. clin. Endocrinol. Metab. 40, 211-220 (1975).

90. Adamson, J.W.: Oxygen delivery by abnormal hemoglobins: effects on erythropoietin production. In: "Hematopoietic Cellular Proliferation", Ed. Stohlman, F., Grune and Stratton, New York, pp. 112-121 (1970).

91. Ward, H.P., Kurnick, J.E., Pisarczyk, M.J.: Serum level of erythropoietin in anemias associated with chronic infection, malignancy, and primary hematopoietic disease. J. clin. Invest. 50, 332-335 (1971).

92. Zucker, S., Friedman, S., Lysik, R.M.: Bone marrow erythropoiesis in the anemia of infection, inflammation and malignancy. J. clin. Invest. 53, 1132-1138 (1974).

93. Douglas, S.W., Adamson, J.W.: The anemia of chronic disorders: studies of marrow regulation and iron metabolism. Blood 45, 55-65 (1975).

94. DeGowin, R.L., Gibson, D.P.: Erythropoietin and the anemia of mice bearing extramedullary tumor. J. Lab. clin. Med. 94, 303-311 (1979).

95. Reissmann, K.R., Udupa, K.R.: Effect of inflammation on erythroid precursors in bone marrow and spleen of mice. J. Lab. clin. Med. 92, 22-29 (1978).

96. Lutton, J.D., Levere, R.D.: Suppressive effect of human interferons on erythroid colony growth in disorders of erythropoiesis. J. Lab. clin. Med. 96, 328-333 (1980).

97. Fernandez, L.A., Erslev, A.J.: Oxygen affinity and compensated hemolysis in hereditary spherocytosis. J. Lab. clin. Med. 80, 780-785 (1972).

98. Labardini, J., Sanchez-Medal, L., Arriaga, L., Lopez, D., Smyth, J.F.: Hemolysis and erythropoiesis. Effect of hemolysates on the erythropoiesis of normal, starved and polycythemic rats. J. Lab. clin. Med. 72, 419-428 (1968).

99. Okamura, H., Udupa, K.B., Reissmann, K.R.: On the mechanism of erythropoietic action of hemoglobin and its derivatives. Proc. Soc. exp. Biol. Med. 136, 794-797 (1971).

100. Erslev, A.J.: The effect of hemolysates on red cell production and erythropoietin release. J. Lab. clin. Med. 78, 1-7 (1971).

101. Nathan, D.G., Chess, L., Hillman, D.G., Clarke, B., Breard, J., Merler, E., Housman, D.E.: Human erythroid burst-forming cell. T cell requirement for proliferation in vitro. J. exp. Med. 147, 324-339 (1978).

102. Aye, M.T.: Erythroid colony formation in cultures of human marrow: effect of leukocyte conditioned medium. J. cell. comp. Physiol. 91, 69-77 (1977).

103. Denny, W.F., Flanigan, W.J., Zukoski, C.F.: Serial erythropoietin studies in patients undergoing renal homotransplantation. J. Lab. clin. Med. 67, 386-397 (1966).

104. Friend, D.G., Hoskins, R.G., Kirkin, M.W.: Relative erythrocytemia and polycystic kidney disease with uremia. New Engl. J. Med. 264, 17-19 (1961).

105. Eschbach, J.W., Adamson, J.W.: Improvement in the anemia of chronic renal failure with fluoxymesterone. Ann. intern. Med. 78, 527-532 (1973).

106. Hendler, E.D., Goffinet, I.A., Ross, S., Longnecker, R.E., Bakovic, V.: Controlled study of androgen therapy in anemia of patients on maintenance hemodialysis. New Engl. J. Med. 291, 1046-1051 (1974).

107. Ortega, J.A., Malekzadeh, M.H., Dukes, P.P., Ma, A., Pennisi, A.V., Fine, R.N., Shore, N.A.: Exceptionally high serum erythropoietin activity in an anephric patient with severe anemia. Amer. J. Hematol. 2, 299-306 (1977).

108. Kurtides, E.S., Rambach, W.A., Alt, H.L., Del Greco, F.: Effect of hemodialysis on erythrokinetics in anemia of uremia. J. Lab. clin. Med. 63, 469-479 (1964).

109. Eschbach, J.W., Adamson, J.W., Cook, J.D.: Disorders of red blood cell production in uremia. Arch. intern. Med. 126, 812-815 (1970).

110. Wallner, S.F., Vautrin, R.M., Kurnick, J.E., Ward, H.P.: The effect of serum from patients with chronic renal failure on erythroid colony growth in vitro. J. Lab. clin. Med. 92, 370-375 (1978).

111. Ohno, Y., Rege, A.B., Risher, J.W., Barona, J.: Inhibitors of erythroid colony-forming cells in sera of azotemic patients with anemia of renal disease. J. Lab. clin. Med. 92, 916-923 (1978).

112. Zucker, S., Lysik, R.M., Mohammad, G.: Erythropoiesis in chronic renal disease. J. Lab. clin. Med. 88, 528-535 (1976).

113. Anagnostou, A., Barone, J., Kedo, A., Fried, W.: Effect of erythropoietin therapy on the red cell volume of uraemic and non-uraemic rats. Brit. J. Haematol. 37, 85-91 (1977).

114. Spivak, J.L., Cooke, C.R.: Polycythemia vera in an anephric man. Amer. J. med. Sci. 272, 339-344 (1976).

115. Basu, T.K., Stein, R.M.: Erythrocytosis associated with chronic renal disease. Arch. intern. Med. 133, 442-447 (1974).

116. Sonneborn, R., Perez, G.O., Epstein, M., Martelo, O., Pardo, V.: Erythrocytosis associated with the nephrotic syndrome. Arch. intern. Med. 137, 1068-1072 (1977).

117. Krantz, S.B.: Diagnosis and treatment of pure red cell aplasia. Med. Clin. N. Amer. 60, 945-958 (1976).

118. Jepson, J.H., Lowenstein, L.: Inhibition of erythropoiesis by a factor present in the plasma of patients with erythroblastopenia. Blood 27, 425-434 (1966).

119. Peschle, C., Marmont, A.M., Marone, G., Genovese, A., Sasso, G.F., Condorelli, M.: Pure red cell aplasia studies on an IgG serum inhibitor neutralizing erythropoietin. Brit. J. Haematol. 30, 411-417 (1975).

120. Jepson, J.H., Vas, M.: Decreased in vivo and in vitro erythropoiesis induced by plasma of ten patients with thymoma, lymphosarcoma or idiopathic erythroblastopenia. Cancer Res. 34, 1325-1334 (1974).

121. Koeffler, H.P., Goldwasser, E.: Erythropoietin radioimmunoassay in evaluating patients with polycythemia. Ann. intern. Med. 94, 44-47 (1981).

122. Moccia, G., Miller, M.E., Garcia, J.F., Cronkite, E.P.: The effect of plethora on erythropoietin levels. Proc. Soc. exp. Biol. Med. 163, 36-38 (1980).

123. Adamson, J.W., Parer, J.T., Stamatoyannopoulos, G.: Erythrocytosis associated with hemoglobin Rainier: oxygen equilibria and marrow regulation. J. clin. Invest. 48, 1376-1386 (1969).

124. Kilbridge, T.M., Fried, W., Heller, P.: The mechanism by which plethora suppresses erythropoiesis. Blood 33, 104-113 (1979).

125. Woodson, R.D., Heywood, J.D., Lenfant, C.: Oxygen transport in hemoglobin Kohn. Arch. intern. Med. 134, 711-715 (1974).

126. Charache, S., Achuff, S., Winslow, R., Adamson, J., Chervenick, P.: Variability of the homeostatic response to altered P_{50}. Blood 52, 1156-1162 (1978).

127. Kisker, C.T., Kleinman, L.I.: Primary benign erythrocytosis and abnormal renal perfusion. Lancet 1, 1163-1165 (1971).

128. Maezawa, M., Takaku, F., Yoshimoto, M., Mizoguchi, H., Muira, Y.: A case of intrarenal artery stenosis associated with erythrocytosis. Scand. J. Haematol. 21, 278-282 (1978).

129. Rosse, W.F., Waldmann, T.A., Cohen, P.: Renal cysts, erythropoietin and polycythemia. Amer. J. Med. 34, 76-81 (1963).

130. Martt, J.M., Sayman, A., Neal, M.P.: Polycythemia and hydronephrosis. Ann. intern. Med. 54, 790-795 (1961).

131. Nixon, R.K., O'Rourke, W., Rupe, C.E., Korst, D.R.: Nephrogenic polycythemia. Arch. intern. Med. 106, 797-802 (1960).

132. Thorling, E.B.: Paraneoplastic erythrocytosis and inappropriate erythropoietin production. Scand. J. Haematol. 9, 13-14 (1972).

133. Koplan, J.P., Sprayregan, S., Lawrence Ossias, A., Zanjani, E.D.: Erythropoietin-producing renal cyst and polycythemia vera. Amer. J. Med. 54, 819-824 (1973).

134. Erkelens, D.W., Statius Van Eps, L.W.: Bartter's syndrome and erythrocytosis. Amer. J. Med. 55, 711-719 (1973).

135. Nies, B.A., Cohn, R., Schrier, S.L.: Erythemia after renal transplantation. New Engl. J. Med. 273, 785-788 (1965).

136. Swales, J.D., Evans, D.B.: Erythroemia in renal transplantation. Brit. med. J. 2, 80-83 (1969).

137. Wu, K. K-Y., Gibson, T., Freeman, R.M., Bonney, W.W., Fried, W., DeGowin, R.L.: Erythrocytosis after renal transplantation. Arch.intern. Med. 132, 898-902 (1973).

138. Dagher, F.J., Ramos, E., Erslev, A., Karmi, S., Alongi, S.V.: Erythrocytosis after renal allotransplantation: treatment by removal of the native kidneys. South. Med. J. 73, 940-942 (1980).

139. Westerman, M.P., Jenkins, J.L., Dekker, A., Kreutner, A. Jr., Fisher, B.: Significance of erythrocytosis and increased erythropoietin secretion after renal transplantation. Lancet 2, 755-757 (1967).

140. Hammond, D., Winnick, S.: Paraneoplastic erythrocytosis and ectopic erythropoietins. Ann. N.Y. Acad. Sci. 230, 219-226 (1974).

141. Muechler, E.K.: Testosterone-producing ovarian tumor associated with erythrocytosis, hyperuricemia and recurrent deep vein thrombosis. Amer. J. Obstet. Gynec. 129, 467-469 (1977).

142. Lawrence, J.H., Donald, W.G. Jr.: Polycythemia and hydronephrosis or renal tumors. Ann. intern. Med. 50, 959-969 (1959).

143. Damon, A., Holub, D.A., Melicow, M.M., Uson, A.C.: Polycythemia and renal carcinoma. Amer. J. Med. 25, 182-197 (1958).

144. Murphy, G.P., Mirand, E.A., Sinks, L.F., Allen, J.E., Staubitz, W.J.: Ectopic production of erythropoietin in Wilms tumor patients in relationship to clinical stage and disease activity. J. Urol. 113, 230-233 (1975).

145. Sufrin, G., Mirand, E.A., Moore, R.H., Murphy, G.P.: Hormones in renal carrier. J. Urol. 117, 433-438 (1977).

146. Brownstein, M.H., Ballard, H.S.: Hepatoma associated with erythrocytosis. Amer. J. Med. 40, 204-210 (1966).

147. Raphael, B., Cooperberg, A.A., Niloff, P.: The triad of hemachromatosis, hepatoma and erythrocytosis. Cancer 43, 690-694 (1979).

148. Okazaki, N., Ozaki, H., Arima, M., Hattou, N., Kimura, K.: Hepatocellular carcinoma associated with erythrocytosis. A nine year survival after successful chemotherapy and left lateral hepatectomy. Acta Hepatogastroenterol. 26, 248-252 (1979).

149. Hutchinson, D.C.S., Sapru, R.P., Sumerling, M.D., Donaldson, G.W.K., Richmond, J.: Cirrhosis, cyanosis and polycethemia: multiple pulmonary arteriovenous anastomose. Amer. J. Med. 45, 139-151 (1968).

150. Jeffreys, R.: Clinical and surgical aspects of posterior fossa haemangioblastoma. J. Neurol. Neurosurg. Psychiat. 38, 105-111 (1975).

151. Waldmann, T., Levin, E.H., Baldwin, M.: The association of polycythemia with a cerebellar hemangioblastoma. Amer. J. Med. 31, 318-324 (1961).

152. Jeffreys, R.: Pathological and haematological aspects of posterior fossa haemangioblastomata. J. Neurol. Neurosurg. Psychiat. 38, 112-119 (1975).

153. Naets, J.P., Wittek, M., Delwiche, F., Kram, I.: Polycythemia and erythropoietin producing uterine fibromyoma. Scand. J. Haematol. 19, 75-78 (1977).

154. Lawrence Ossias, A., Zanjani, E.D., Zalusky, R., Estren, S., Wasserman, L.R.: Case report: studies on the mechanism of erythrocytosis associated with uterine fibromyoma. Brit. J. Haematol. 25, 179-185 (1973).

155. Fried, W., Ward, H.P., Hopeman, A.R.: Leiomyoma and erythrocytosis: a tumor producing a factor which increases erythropoietin production. Blood 31, 813-816 (1968).

156. Eldor, A., Even-Paz, A., Polliack, A.: Erythrocytosis associated with multiple cutaneous lecomyomata. Scand. J. Haematol. 16, 245-249 (1976).

157. Adamson, J.W., Fialkow, P.J., Murphy, S., Prchal, J.F., Steinman, L.: Polycythemia vera: stem cell and probable clonal origin of the disease. New Engl. J. Med. 295, 913-916 (1976).

158. Murray, J.F.: Arterial studies in primary and secondary polycythemic disorders. Amer. Rev. resp. Dis. 92, 435-449 (1965).

159. Modan, B., Kallner, H., Zerner, D.: Increased risk of polycythemia vera in Jews. Blood 37, 172-176 (1971).

160. Ratnoff, W.D., Gress, R.E.: The familial occurrence of polycythemia vera. Blood 56, 233-236 (1980).

161. Bomchil, G., Carmena, A.O., Segade, A., Cavagnaro, F., DeTesta, N.G.: Studies on the response to hypoxia and relative hyperoxia in two polycythemia vera patients. J. med. Res. 55, 543-548 (1967).

162. Barach, A.L., McAlpin, K.R.: Negative results of oxygen therapy in polycythemia vera. Amer. J. med. Sci. 185, 178-181 (1933).

163. Lawrence, J.H., Elmlinger, P.J., Fulton, G.: Oxygen and the control of red cell production in primary and secondary polycythemia: effects on the iron turnover patterns with Fe^{59} as tracer. Cardiologia (Basel) 21, 337-346 (1952).

164. Krantz, S.B.: Response of polycythemia vera marrow to erythropoietin in vitro. J. Lab. clin. Med. 71, 999-1012 (1968).

165. Golde, D.W., Cline, M.J.: Erythropoietin-responsiveness in polycythemia vera. Brit. J. Haematol. 29, 567-573 (1975).

166. Eaves, C.J., Eaves, A.L.: Erythropoietin dose-response curves for three classes of erythroid progenitors in normal human marrow and in patients with polycythemia vera. Blood 52, 1196-1210 (1978).

167. Prchal, J.F., Axelrad, A.A.: Bone marrow response in polycythemia vera. New Engl. J. Med. 289, 1382 (1974).

168. Prchal, J.F., Adamson, J.W., Murphy, S., Steinmann, L., Fialkow, P.J.: Polycythemia vera. The in vitro response of normal and abnormal stem cell lines to erythropoietin. J. clin. Invest. 61, 1044-1047 (1978).

169. Zanjani, E.D., Lutton, J.D., Hoffman, R., Wasserman, L.R.: Erythroid colony formation by polycythemia vera bone marrow in vitro: dependence on erythropoietin. J. clin. Invest. 59, 841-848 (1977).

170. Golde, D.W., Bersch, N., Cline, M.J.: Polycythemia vera: hormonal modulation of erythropoiesis in vitro. Blood 49, 399-405 (1977).

171. Adamson, J.W., Stamatoyannopoulos, G., Kontras, S., Lascau, A., Detter, J.: Recessive familial erythrocytosis: aspects of marrow regulation in two families. Blood 41, 641-652 (1973).

172. Yonemitsu, H., Yamoguchi, K., Shigeta, H., Okuda, K., Takaku, F.: Two cases of familial erythrocytosis with increased erythropoietin activity in plasma and urine. Blood 42, 793-797 (1973).

173. Whitcomb, W.H., Peschle, C., Moore, M., Nitschke, R., Adamson, J.W.: Congenital erythrocytosis: a new form associated with an erythropoietin-dependent mechanism. Brit. J. Haematol. 44, 17-24 (1980).

174. Greenberg, B.R., Golde, D.W.: Erythropoiesis in familial erythrocytosis. New Engl. J. Med. 296, 1080-1084 (1977).

175. Dainiak, N., Hoffman, R., Lebowitz, A.I., Solomon, L., Maffei, L., Ritchey, K.: Erythropoietin-dependent primary pure erythrocytosis. Blood 53, 1076-1084 (1979).

176. Berk, P.D.: The Polycythemia Vera Study Group: Increased incidence of acute leukemia in polycythemia vera associated with chlorambucil therapy. New Engl. J. Med. 304, 441-447 (1981).

177. Thomas, D.J., Marshall, J., Ross Russell, R.W.: Cerebral blood-flow in polycythaemia. Lancet 2, 161-163 (1977).

178. Reissmann, K.R.: Studies on the mechanism of erythropoietic stimulation in parabiotic rats during hypoxia. Blood 5, 372-380 (1950).

THE ROLES OF RECEPTORS AND METABOLISM IN ANDROGEN ACTION : STUDIES IN CULTURED CELLS AND ISOLATED TISSUES FROM MALE PSEUDOHERMAPHRODITES

M. B. Hodgins
Department of Dermatology, University of Glasgow, Glasgow, Scotland, U.K.

In mammals, the testes control the embryonic differentiation of the male urogenital tract and external genitalia as well as reproductive function in the adult. Two secretions of the embryonic testes control development of the male phenotype. Anti-Mullerian hormone causes regression of the Mullerian ducts, the anlage of the female reproductive tract. Androgen stimulates the differentiation of the Wolffian ducts, urogenital sinus and external genitalia into the male reproductive tract, penis and scrotum. In the absence of testes, the Wolffian ducts regress and a female phenotype develops (1).

A male pseudohermaphrodite is a karyotypically normal male with an incompletely developed reproductive tract and external genitalia. This can be caused by either deficient androgen production or insensitivity of the tissues to androgens.

Much recent research into the mechanisms of androgen action has been concerned with the properties of specific hormone receptors and also with the conversion of testosterone, the major testicular androgen, into active metabolites, notably 5α-dihydrotestosterone (DHT). Investigations into the pathogenesis of male pseudohermaphroditism have provided important evidence about the properties of androgen receptors and the physiological roles of testosterone and DHT.

Recent reviews have covered male sexual differentiation (2), the mechanism of androgen action (3) and the clinical and endocrinological features of male pseudohermaphroditism (4-6).

Hormones in Normal and Abnormal Human Tissues, Vol. III

This review considers the contribution to our understanding of androgen action which may be made by studies of tissue biopsies and cultured cells from male pseudohermaphrodites.

Androgen Insensitivity - Hormone Receptor Defects

The initial step in androgen action appears to be the binding of the hormone to a cytoplasmic receptor protein, the hormone-receptor complex binding in turn to chromatin to influence gene expression (3). It is important to establish that the androgen binding proteins, detected in many tissues, are receptors by demonstrating a correlation between hormone binding and biological activity. One approach has been to search for mutations affecting hormone binding and tissue responsiveness.

Testicular feminization - complete androgen insensitivity

Testicular feminization (Tfm) is an X-linked recessive trait which confers insensitivity to androgens. In the Tfm/Y male mouse, specific binding of testosterone and DHT in androgen target organs is greatly reduced (7-10), possibly due to a structurally abnormal receptor (11). In man, affected males have elevated serum testosterone and LH levels but a female phenotype, except for the absence of Mullerian duct structures and pubic or axillary hair (4-6). Unresponsiveness to exogenously administered testosterone and DHT has been demonstrated (12).

Fibroblasts, grown from the skin of some patients with complete androgen insensitivity, contain undetectably low levels of saturable binding sites for DHT (13-16). Binding sites can readily be detected in normal foreskin fibroblasts, and are similar to the putative androgen receptors of other target tissues in affinity for DHT, specificity and sedimentation characteristics (13-18). Thus, it has been possible to correlate the presence of specific androgen binding molecules with the ability of tissues to respond to the hormone.

The concentration of specific DHT binding sites in normal genital fibroblasts varies from about 20 to 100 fmol/mg protein, leaving ample room for the detection of "receptor negative" androgen insensitivity. However, normal, non-genital fibroblasts frequently show very low levels of DHT binding so that it is important to use genital fibroblasts when searching for androgen receptor defects (16, 19-21). Evidence has been obtained which supports X-linkage of the gene for the androgen receptor (or of a gene controlling its expression). Fibroblast clones from a woman heterozygous for the testicular feminization trait could be divided into two populations. One contained saturable DHT binding sites, the other was deficient in DHT binding (22). Because of random X-chromosome inactivation in the female, this distribution would be expected if a gene controlling receptor activity were on the X-chromosome. However, this study used non-genital fibroblasts, cultures of which could contain a significant proportion of cells with undetectable DHT binding, even from normal persons. It will be important to confirm these results with genital fibroblasts. An attractive possibility may be to use autoradiography to screen for DHT binding in monolayer cultures (23).

Methods are being developed to detect specific androgen binding in extracts of skin biopsies. It is important to distinguish receptors from sex hormone binding globulin (SHBG), either by using synthetic ligands such as methyltrienolone (24, 25) or by separating the receptors from SHBG physically (26, 27). Analysis of binding in tissue extracts is quicker than cell culture for the simple detection of receptor deficiency. However, cell cultures provide an almost unlimited supply of material for more detailed work.

Partial androgen insensitivity

Several forms of male pseudohermaphroditism have been attributed to partial insensitivity to androgens. Familial incomplete male pseudohermaphroditism type-1, exemplified by the Reifenstein syndrome, shows X-linked inheritance. The characteristic patient is a man with gynaecomastia and perineal hypospadias, although there is considerable variation in the degree of feminization, even within one family (28). Incomplete testicular feminization is considered to be a distinct clinical entity by Madden et al. (29). The phenotype is female with clitoromegaly and posterior labial fusion. The mode of inheritance is unclear. Certain cases of infertility in otherwise normal men also appear to be due to partial insensitivity (30).

It has been possible to demonstrate reduced levels of DHT binding in genital skin fibroblasts of some patients with partial androgen insensitivity (30-32). However, there is no correlation between the level of DHT binding in intact fibroblasts at 37°C and the extent of feminization. Undetectable binding was reported in one case where a bifid scrotum and infertility were the only clinical abnormalities (30).

The latter finding has led to a search for abnormalities of DHT binding in fibroblasts of men with idiopathic gynaecomastia and also in hirsute women (33, 34). So far, the results have been negative. Deficient DHT binding was not demonstrated in a number of cases of pseudohermaphroditism of unexplained aetiology (35). DHT binding in foreskin cytosol has been measured in a group of patients with simple hypospadias. The majority showed no reduction in DHT binding but a few patients had levels below the range of normal controls (25). It would be of great interest to establish fibroblast cultures from some of these patients for more detailed characterization of their androgen receptors (vide infra).

The concentration of receptor sites cannot be the only factor determining tissue sensitivity to androgens. Partial receptor deficiency, expressed in cultured skin fibroblasts, may be only a faint reflection of the defect in different target tissues at different stages of development.

Recent work has been directed towards qualitative analysis of the properties of the androgen binding proteins in partial androgen insensitivity. Fibroblasts of patients with Reifenstein syndrome showed reduced concentrations of DHT binding sites, without any apparent abnormalities in affinity for the hormone or in receptor turnover. This suggested a decreased rate of receptor synthesis (31). Griffin (36) has studied the temperature stability of DHT binding in intact fibroblasts. Normal cells showed little change in binding between 37°C and 42°C. Temperature stability was normal in cells from patients with Reifenstein syndrome, but was markedly reduced in several patients with either incomplete or complete testicular feminization. In these patients, binding levels were normal at 25°C, reduced at 37°C and almost undetectable at 42°C. A family history compatible with X-linkage of the mutation was found in several cases. There appear to be a number of X-linked mutations affecting the androgen receptor such as mutations affecting the structure and stability of the receptor or causing reduced receptor synthesis. Whether or not the mutations are allelic is unknown.

Decreased affinity of the receptor for DHT has not yet been reported. It is possible that the methods used have not been sufficiently reproducible to detect small but physiologically significant changes in the equilibrium dissociation constant (Kd) of the DHT-receptor complex. Even a few-fold decrease in binding affinity may be important, but current estimates of Kd range from about 0.1 - 3.0 nmol/l. Some recent studies (37 and Kaufman, personal communication) indicate that the rate of dissociation of DHT from its receptor in fibroblasts may be measured more precisely than Kd derived by saturation analysis. Two patients with partial androgen insensitivity had an increased rate of dissociation of DHT from receptor sites. It is likely that this would be reflected in decreased binding of the hormone under equilibrium or steady state conditions, unless the increased rate of dissociation were balanced by an increased rate of association.

Receptor positive androgen insensitivity

In some cases of complete and of partial androgen insensitivity there is a normal concentration of DHT binding sites in fibroblasts (38-40). Present techniques may have failed to detect subtle changes in the interaction between hormone and receptor (36). However, defects in later stages of hormone action are possible, such as in binding of the hormone-receptor complex in the cell nucleus or in later steps (41-43).

The distribution of DHT-receptor complexes between cytoplasm and nucleus at 37°C is relatively constant over a wide range of total binding levels in fibroblasts of normal and androgen insensitive persons (38-40). However, present methods of assessing nuclear binding may not distinguish true acceptor sites, or specific acceptor binding regions of the receptor, from less specific nuclear binding.

Future work on androgen binding in fibroblasts

Detailed studies of hormone-receptor-nucleus interaction are hampered by the lack of methods suitable for isolating the unbound receptor from the cells; all analyses so far published have required incubation of the steroid with intact cells before isolation of receptor complexes.

A search for complementation between fibroblasts carrying different mutations causing androgen insensitivity should help to establish whether or not more than one X-linked gene is involved in normal expression of androgen receptor activity. This type of analysis is somewhat limited, especially in the case of "receptor positive defects", by the apparent lack of response of normal cultured fibroblasts to androgens. The cells in culture may lose their hormone responsiveness while continuing to synthesize receptors or their response may be very specific, involving only a few proteins. Alternatively androgens may be amplifiers of processes under multi-hormonal control so that in culture other influences override those of androgens. Androgens may antagonize the growth inhibition caused by glucocorticosteroids in human fibroblasts (44). A possible analogous situation has been reported for the rat uterus maintained *in vitro*; oestrogen stimulation of glucose-6-phosphate dehydrogenase could be demonstrated only after suppression of enzyme synthesis with dexamethasone (45).

Ultimately, the analysis of receptors purified from normal and androgen insensitive fibroblasts could lead to a detailed understanding of the mechanism of androgen binding and of receptor activation.

Metabolism of Testosterone : The Physiological Roles of Testosterone and DHT

DHT is the major androgen bound in cell nuclei of the adult male rat ventral prostate, seminal vesicles and epididymis (46, 47). Conversion of testosterone into DHT has been demonstrated in androgen sensitive tissues of many vertebrates from fish to mammals (48, 49). The NADPH dependent 5α-reductase, which catalyses the reaction, has been partially characterized in human foreskin (50) and rat ventral prostate (51). There is evidence that accumulation of DHT in the prostate glands of man and dog is the cause of benign hyperplasia (52-54). DHT is concentrated in human scrotal skin (55). These observations support the theory that testosterone is primarily a prehormone which is converted into DHT within target cells. However, some androgen sensitive tissues contain little or no 5α-reductase; examples are skeletal muscle (48) and bone marrow (56). The Wolffian ducts of the embryos of rat, rabbit and man contain little 5α-reductase during the period of male sexual differentiation while activity is high in the urogenital sinus and external genitalia (57, 58). This led to the proposal that testosterone is responsible for Wolffian duct differentiation, while DHT causes masculinization of the urogenital sinus and external genitalia.

If there are separate testosterone and DHT responsive tissues, there is little evidence of separate receptors for the two steroids. Early studies found that testosterone bound only weakly to the receptor in rat ventral prostate gland (59). More recent studies of a number of tissues (60-70) including human genital fibroblasts (71, 72) support the view that both steroids act through the same receptor. Testosterone may bind to and dissociate from receptors more rapidly than DHT (64, 72).

Attempts to elucidate the roles of testosterone and DHT by inhibiting 5α-reductase activity *in vivo* have provided equivocal results (73-75). Potent 5α-reductase inhibitors, such as progesterone and certain secosteroids, also inhibit the binding of androgens to receptors (69, 76). A recent report has suggested that 5α-reduction of testosterone may be more important in the control of LH secretion than for the stimulation of male accessory sex organ growth (77) yet treatment of rats with a potent 5α-reductase inhibitor failed to antagonize the effect of testosterone on plasma LH levels (75).

The syndrome of 5α-reductase deficiency

The characterization of this form of male pseudohermaphroditism has provided new insight into the physiological roles of testosterone and DHT.

5α-Reductase deficiency is known only in man. It was first recognised by Imperato-McGinley et al. (78, 79) and Walsh et al. (80). The clinical manifestation is pseudovaginal perineoscrotal hypospadias. Affected males appear superficially as normal females at birth but at puberty profound virilization occurs. Testes are clearly discernable in the labioscrotal folds, the clitoris grows considerably, epididymes and seminal vesicles develop and an ejaculate containing sperm can be produced; the prostate remains small. Although they have been brought up as girls, affected adult males who were not castrated prepubertally have a male gender identity (81). Thus 5α-reductase deficiency affects particularly the differentiation of the embryonic genitalia and the urogenital sinus, in accord with the hypothesis that these events would be DHT dependent (58). The disorder is inherited as an autosomal recessive trait, expressed clinically only in males. Recent studies of urinary steroid excretion patterns in one large pedigree have found that 5α-reduction of androgens, cortisol and progesterone is deficient (J. Imperato and R.E. Peterson, personal communication). Further cases of 5α-reductase deficiency have now been described (82-88).

Measurement of 5α-reductase activity in tissue biopsies

Normal human genital skin retains the high 5α-reductase activity characteristic of the embryonic external genitalia (58, 89). Walsh et al. (80) were first to demonstrate that 5α-reductase deficiency could be detected in genital skin biopsies. This has been confirmed in other patients (82-86 and Table 1). In patients of two families the enzyme deficiency has also been demonstrated in the epididymes (80, 85). This is important, as the epididymes are well developed in 5α-reductase deficiency, in spite of the fact that normal adult epididymes (in contrast to embryonic Wolffian ducts) contain high concentrations of the enzyme (85).

It is important to consider whether or not low 5α-reductase activity is found in skin biopsies from other forms of male pseudohermaphroditism. Earlier studies of patients with testicular feminization yielded conflicting results (89-92). However, more recent studies support the view that 5α-reductase activity of genital skin (labia, scrotum, prepuce) is not lowered significantly in complete or partial androgen insensitivity due to androgen receptor defects (29, 80). This indicates that low 5α-reductase activity in this tissue is not simply a consequence of androgen insensitivity nor of androgen deprivation. The enzyme activity is normal in genital skin of patients with simple hypospadias (93, 94). It has been reported that 5α-reductase activity of pubic skin is low in testicular feminization (95) and raised in women with hirsutism (96). Treatment of men with oestrogens lowered 5α-reductase activity in pubic skin (95). However, this apparent hormone dependence of the enzyme activity in pubic skin could result simply from the concentration of 5α-reductase in sebaceous glands (97, 98), which are greatly reduced in size after oestrogen treatment or in testicular feminization (99).

In conclusion, it appears that 5α-reductase activity in genital skin biopsies can provide evidence of 5α-reductase deficiency. It would be advantageous if non-genital skin could be

Table 1. Conversion of Testosterone into DHT by Skin Slices of Normal Donors and Two Patients with Clinical and Endocrinological evidence of 5α-Reductase Deficiency.

5α-Reduction of testosterone (f mol DHT formed/2h/100 mg tissue) was measured as described in ref. 82. Male genital skin: prepuce and scrotum, donor age 3-56 years. Male non-genital skin: upper back of young adults. Female genital skin: anterior labium majus, clitoral hood, glans clitoris, labium minus and posterior fourchette region of adults. Female non-genital skin: suprapubic and breast of adults with varying degrees of hirsutism. Results for normal donors are mean, ± S.D. with ranges in parentheses. Results for two patients are for single assays.

Donor and Body Site	5α-Reductase Activity
Normal male genital	2436 ± 822 (1128 - 4161) n = 22
Normal male non-genital	337 ± 66 (258 - 417) n = 7
Normal female genital	1089 ± 762 (247 - 2321) n = 14
Normal female non-genital	216 ± 98 (92 - 546) n = 35
Patient 1 genital	78, 70
Patient 1 non-genital	97, 113, 106
Patient 2 genital	78
Patient 2 non-genital	78, 66

used. With suitably sensitive enzyme assays, this might be possible in prepubertal patients where the problem of sex hormone dependence of enzyme activity might not arise. Better still may be to assay the enzyme in plucked hair roots. 5α-Reductase activity can be measured in a few roots and, when corrected for DNA content, does not seem to be markedly affected by hormonal status in normal persons (100).

Testosterone metabolism in cultured fibroblasts

Normal genital skin fibroblasts tend to retain the high 5α-reductase activity of genital skin (101-109). However, there is considerable interstrain variation in enzyme activity, making it doubtful that simple enzyme assays on cultured fibroblasts can provide definitive evidence of 5α-reductase deficiency (103-107). Clonal variability may underlie the differences between normal fibroblast strains (102). This could result either from variable differentiation of the cells in culture or from cellular heterogeneity in the original tissue biopsy. Nevertheless, all the reported strains of genital skin fibroblasts, from patients having clinical and endocrinological evidence of 5α-reductase deficiency, have had enzyme activities close to the lower limits of assay sensitivity (103-107). High 5α-reductase activity in genital skin fibroblasts may exclude a diagnosis of 5α-reductase deficiency while very low activity, especially if combined with normal levels of androgen receptors, may give a strong suspicion of 5α-reductase deficiency.

A report of sex differences in testosterone metabolism by human non-genital fibroblasts (110) has not been confirmed (111). It has been claimed that 5α-reductase deficiency could be detected in non-genital skin fibroblasts after extended incubation with testosterone (84). In extended incubations, it is important to recover possible 5α-reduced metabolites in case of further metabolism of DHT. This has not always been done, such key products as 5α-androstane-3,17-dione being omitted (84, 109).

Characterization of the fibroblast 5α-reductase

The 5α-reductase of normal genital skin fibroblasts is tightly bound to microsomal membranes, is NADPH dependent and has an apparent Michaelis constant (Km) for testosterone and progesterone of about 10^{-7} mol/l (104, 112). The Km for testosterone measured in intact cells (107) is similar to that in microsomes incubated at optimal pH with excess NADPH, suggesting that the availability of co-enzyme does not limit the reaction in normal fibroblasts. In normal genital fibroblast extracts there is a sharp peak of enzyme activity at pH 5.5-6.0, with a shoulder at pH 7-9. Moore and Wilson (112) found that normal non-genital fibroblasts lacked the peak activity at pH 5.5 and proposed that this peak represented a separate species of enzyme from the activity at more alkaline pH. We have found that the pH profile in normal non-genital fibroblasts can be identical to that in genital cells (unpublished results). It remains to be proved that the activities at acid and alkaline pH are due to separate enzymes. There is evidence that a single enzyme catalyses 5α-reduction of testosterone and cortisol in human epididymal microsomes (85) yet the maximum activity with cortisol as substrate is around pH 7 and the pH - activity profile for cortisol is much broader than that for testosterone.

Attempts have been made to characterize the residual enzyme activity in 5α-reductase deficient fibroblasts. Increased values of Km for testosterone have been reported in genital fibroblasts of patients from four different families (105, 107). It is still uncertain whether normal fibroblasts also contain this enzyme with apparently low affinity for testosterone. The apparent Km for testosterone in normal non-genital fibroblasts with low 5α-reductase activity was similar to that in genital cells (107).

There is evidence of genetic heterogeneity in 5α-reductase deficiency. Two patients studied by Leshin et al. (105) have a disorder affecting the binding of NADPH to the enzyme. Another patient (87) appears to have a defect intermediate between these patients and those with lowered affinity of the 5α-reductase for testosterone.

It will be necessary to solubilize and purify the 5α-reductase of the male reproductive organs before a detailed understanding of the various defects is possible. Recent studies of the 5α-reductase of rat liver indicate a complex reaction mechanism, involving initial transfer of hydrogen from NADPH to ubiquinone, by NADPH - cytochrome C reductase (113). However, the 5α-reductase of fibroblasts from the patients reported by Leshin et al. (105) had a greatly increased Km for NADPH, while NADPH - cytochrome C reductase activity in the cells was normal.

Function of 5α-reductase in androgen action

It can be concluded that, in man and possibly in other mammals, high 5α-reductase activity is essential for the normal differentiation of the prostate gland, urethra, penis and scrotum in the male embryo. The enzyme is not essential for normal Wolffian duct differentiation, nor for most of the androgen dependent events of puberty, including genital growth and feedback control of gonadotrophin secretion.

This apparently specific need for high 5α-reductase activity needs to be explained. In human fibroblasts there is a correlation between the amount of exogenous testosterone bound and the activity of 5α-reductase (108). Can small differences in the binding of testosterone and DHT to the androgen receptor account for the requirement of some tissues for DHT at a specific stage of development (72) ?

The requirement for high 5α-reductase activity is usually equated with a need for DHT. However, 5α-reductases are widely distributed and relatively non-specific enzymes. The 5α-reductase of human male reproductive tissues acts on cortisol, testosterone and progesterone, the last being the best substrate (85, 104). One possible explanation of the problem considers the hormonal environment to which the mammalian embryo is exposed during male sexual differentiation.

The development of the male sex organs is dependent upon androgens. However, in many mammals, especially in man, the maintenance of pregnancy requires high concentrations of progesterone, a relatively potent antiandrogen (114, 115). Progesterone in amniotic fluid could act directly on the external genitalia and urogenital sinus to inhibit the binding of testosterone to androgen receptors. This could be less serious for the Wolffian ducts, which might receive high concentrations of testosterone directly from the testis. It has been suggested that exogenous progestins may cause hypospadias (116). The concentration of progesterone in human amniotic fluid can exceed 10^{-7} mol/l in early mid-pregnancy (117, 118).

5α-Reduction converts progesterone into less active metabolites but with 5α-reductase deficient human fibroblasts these are less effective than progesterone in displacing testosterone from androgen receptors (119 and Fig. 1); DHT is less readily displaced than testosterone. Thus, simultaneous 5α-reduction of testosterone and progesterone may allow androgen action in the presence of high concentrations of the latter steroid.

This may not be the sole function of 5α-reductase in androgen action. In normal adult animals of some species, DHT is obviously the major androgen bound in certain target tissues. Possibly the slower dissociation of the DHT-receptor complex than the testosterone-receptor complex is important in some situations. In some tissues, the fact that DHT, unlike testosterone, cannot be converted into oestrogens may be significant.

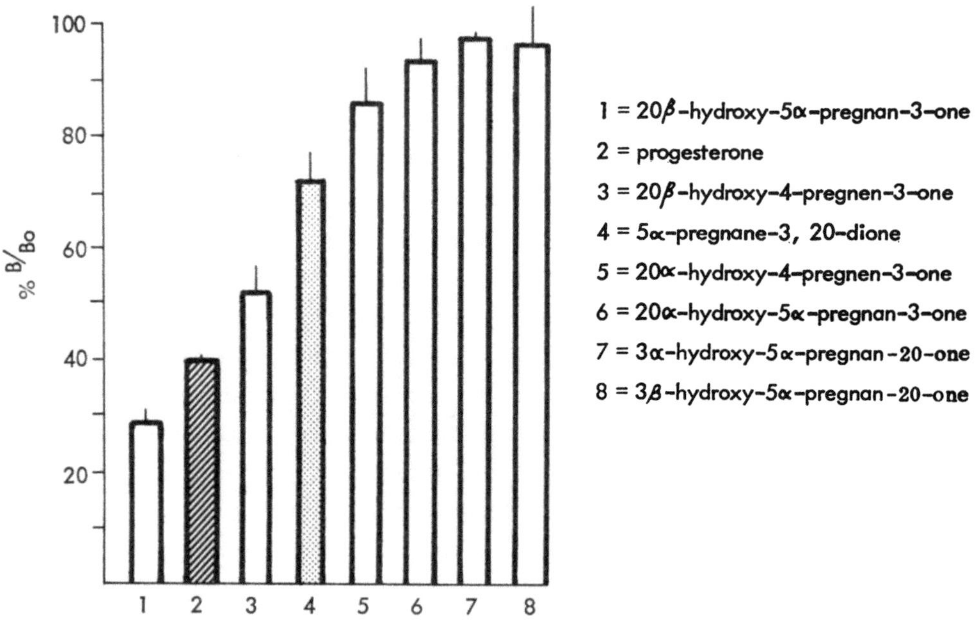

Fig. 1

Future work on 5α-reductase

Further studies of the mechanism of the 5α-reductase reaction are needed before the molecular basis of 5α-reductase deficiency can be understood. The possibility that there are several different 5α-reductases, especially in human tissues, needs to be reinvestigated.

An animal model of 5α-reductase deficiency is needed. More work on the inhibition of 5α-reductase *in vivo* may help. However, if deductions are to be made about the physiological importance of testosterone and DHT, it is essential to demonstrate that the 5α-reductase inhibitor does not also inhibit the binding of testosterone to the androgen receptor. Comparative studies of the embryonic development of testosterone metabolism should be extended, especially to marsupials, where male sexual differentiation takes place after the young have entered the pouch (120).

Acknowledgements

I thank J. E. Griffin, J. D. Wilson, M. Kaufman and L. Pinsky for stimulating discussions of the ideas presented in this review. I thank Una Syme for typing the manuscript.

References

1. Jost, A.: A new look at the mechanisms controlling sex differentiation in mammals. Johns Hopkins Med. J. 130, 38-53 (1972).
2. Wilson, J.D.: Sexual differentiation. A. Rev. Physiol. 40, 279-306 (1978).
3. Mainwaring, W.I.P.: The mechanism of action of androgens. In: "Monographs on Endocrinology", vol. 10, Springer Verlag, New York, Heidelberg, Berlin (1977).
4. Pinsky, L.: The nosology of male pseudohermaphroditism due to androgen insensitivity. Birth Defects: Original Article Ser. XIV (6C), 73-95 (1978).

5. Fichman, K.R., Migeon, B.R., Migeon, C.J.: Genetic disorders of male sexual differentiation. In: "Advances in Human Genetics - 10", Eds. Harris, H., Hirschhorn, K., Plenum Press, New York and London, pp. 333-377 (1980).

6. Griffin, J.E., Wilson, J.D.: The syndromes of androgen resistance. New Engl. J. Med. 302, 198-209 (1980).

7. Gehring, U., Tomkins, G.M., Ohno, S.: The effect of the androgen insensitivity mutation on a cytoplasmic receptor for dihydrotestosterone. Nature 232, 106-107 (1971).

8. Gehring, U., Tomkins, G.M.: Characterization of a hormone receptor defect in the androgen insensitivity mutant. Cell 3, 59-64 (1974).

9. Bullock, L.P., Bardin, C.W.: Androgen receptors in mouse kidney: A study of male, female and androgen insensitive (tfm/y) mice. Endocrinology 94, 746-756 (1974).

10. Verhoeven, G., Wilson, J.D.: Cytosol androgen binding in submandibular gland and kidney of the normal mouse and the mouse with testicular feminization. Endocrinology 99, 79-92 (1976).

11. Wieland, S.J., Fox, T.O.: Putative androgen receptors distinguished in wild-type and testicular feminized (Tfm) mice. Cell 17, 781-787 (1979).

12. Strickland, A.L., French, F.S.: Absence of response to dihydrotestosterone in the syndrome of testicular feminization. J. clin. Endocrinol. Metab. 29, 1284-1286 (1969).

13. Keenan, B.S., Meyer, W.J., Hadjian, A.J., Jones, H.W., Migeon, C.J.: Syndrome of androgen insensitivity in man: absence of 5α-dihydrotestosterone binding protein in skin fibroblasts. J. clin. Endocrinol. Metab. 38, 1143-1146 (1974).

14. Griffin, J.E., Punyashthiti, K., Wilson, J.D.: Dihydrotestosterone binding by cultured fibroblasts. Comparison of cells from control subjects and from patients with hereditary male pseudohermaphroditism due to androgen resistance. J. clin. Invest. 57, 1342-1351 (1976).

15. Kaufman, M., Straisfeld, C., Pinsky, L.: Specific 5α-dihydrotestosterone binding in labial skin fibroblasts cultured from patients with male pseudohermaphroditism. Clin. Genet. 9, 567-574 (1976).

16. Kaufman, M., Straisfeld, C., Pinsky, L.: Male pseudohermaphroditism presumably due to target organ unresponsiveness to androgens. Deficient 5α-dihydrotestosterone binding in cultured skin fibroblasts. J. clin. Invest. 58, 345-350 (1976).

17. Keenan, B.S., Meyer, W.J., Hadjian, A.J., Migeon, C.J.: Androgen receptor in human fibroblasts characterization of a specific 17β-hydroxy-5α-androstan-3-one protein complex in cell sonicates and nuclei. Steroids 25, 535-552 (1975).

18. Kaufman, M., Pinsky, L., Kubski, A., Straisfeld, C., Dobrenis, K., Shiroky, J., Chan, T., MacGibbon, B.: Some properties of the specific androgen binding activities in cultured human genital skin fibroblasts. J. clin. Endocrinol. Metab. 47, 738-745 (1978).

19. Kaufman, M., Straisfeld, C., Pinsky, L.: Expression of androgen responsive properties in human skin fibroblasts of genital and non-genital origin. Somat. Cell Genet. 3, 17-25 (1977).

20. De Wailly, D., Maes, M., Amrhein, J.A., Rothwell, S.W., Migeon, C.J.: Antibody method for measurement of dihydrotestosterone receptors in cultured human skin fibroblasts. J. Lab. clin. Med. 94, 106-113 (1979).

21. Herfert, J., Wienker, T.F., Ropers, H.H.: The presence of androgen binding receptors in genital and non-genital skin fibroblasts. Hum. Genet. 53, 271-273 (1980).

22. Meyer, W.J. III, Migeon, B.R., Migeon, C.J.: Locus on human X-chromosome for dihydrotestosterone receptor and androgen insensitivity. Proc. natn. Acad. Sci. U.S.A. 72, 1469-1472 (1975).

23. Ozasa, H., Tominaga, T., Nishimura, T., Takeda, T.: Radioautographic demonstration of dihydrotestosterone receptor in cultured human fibroblasts. Experientia 36, 1230-1231 (1980).

24. Menon, M., Tananis, C.E., Hicks, L.L., Hawkins, E.F., McLoughlin, M.G., Walsh, P.C.: Characterization of the binding of a potent synthetic androgen, methyltrienolone, to human tissues. J. clin. Invest. 61, 150-162 (1978).

25. Svensson, J., Snochowski, M.: Androgen receptor levels in preputial skin from boys with hypospadias. J. clin. Endocrinol. Metab. 49, 340-345 (1979).

26. Evain, D., Savage, M.O., Binet, E.: A specific and rapid determination of human skin dihydrotestosterone cytosol receptor. J. clin. Endocrinol. Metab. 45, 363-366 (1977).

27. Mowszowicz, I., Riahi, M., Wright, F., Bouchard, P., Kutten, F., Mauvais-Jarvis, P.: Androgen receptor in human skin cytosol. J. clin. Endocrinol. Metab. 52, 338-344 (1981).

28. Wilson, J.D., Harrod, M.J., Goldstein, J.L., Hemsell, D.L., MacDonald, P.C.: Familial incomplete male pseudohermaphroditism, type 1. Evidence for androgen resistance and variable clinical manifestations in a family with the Reifenstein syndrome. New Engl. J. Med. 290, 1097-1103 (1974).

29. Madden, J.D., Walsh, P.C., MacDonald, P.C., Wilson, J.D.: Clinical and endocrinologic characterization of a patient with the syndrome of incomplete testicular feminization. J. clin. Endocrinol. Metab. 41, 751-760 (1975).

30. Aiman, J., Griffin, J.E., Gazak, J.M., Wilson, J.D., MacDonald, P.C.: Androgen insensitivity as a cause of infertility in otherwise normal men. New Engl. J. Med. 300, 223-227 (1979).

31. Griffin, J.E., Wilson, J.D.: Studies on the pathogenesis of the incomplete forms of androgen resistance in man. J. clin. Endocrinol. Metab. 45, 1137-1143 (1977).

32. Amrhein, J.A., Klingensmith, G.J., Walsh, P.C., McKusick, V.A., Migeon, C.J.: Partial androgen insensitivity. The Reifenstein syndrome revisited. New Engl. J. Med. 297, 350-356 (1977).

33. Eil, C., Loriaux, D.L.: The androgen receptor in skin fibroblasts from men with idiopathic gynecomastia. Proceedings Endocrine Society 61st Annual Meeting, p. 259, Abs. no. 746 (1979).

34. Eil, C., Belman, A.B., Johnsonbaugh, R.E., Loriaux, D.L.: Fibroblasts androgen receptors in men with genito-urinary anomalies and in women with idiopathic hirsutism. Proceedings Endocrine Society 62nd Annual Meeting, p. 207, Abs. no. 529 (1980).

35. Amrhein, J.A., Meyer, W.J., III, Danish, R.K., Migeon, C.J.: Studies of androgen production and binding in 13 male pseudohermaphrodites and 13 males with micropenis. J. clin. Endocrinol. Metab. 45, 732-738 (1977).

36. Griffin, J.E.: Testicular feminization associated with a thermo-labile androgen receptor in cultured human fibroblasts. J. clin. Invest. 64, 1624-1631 (1979).

37. Pinsky, L., Kaufman, M., Feldstein, W., Nudo, J.: Androgen insensitivity (AI) due to a kinetically abnormal 5α-dihydrotestosterone receptor. Paediat. Res. 14, 483 (1980).

38. Amrhein, J.A., Meyer, W.J., III, Jones, H.W., Jr., Migeon, C.J.: Androgen insensitivity in man: evidence for genetic heterogeneity. Proc. natn. Acad. Sci. U.S.A. 73, 891-894 (1976).

39. Collier, M.E., Griffin, J.E., Wilson, J.D.: Intranuclear binding of [^{3}H] dihydrotestosterone by cultured human fibroblasts. Endocrinology 103, 1499-1505 (1978).

40. Kaufman, M., Pinsky, L., Bird, P.A., McGillivray, B.C.: Complete androgen insensitivity with a normal amount of 5α-dihydrotestosterone binding in labium majus skin fibroblasts. Am. J. Med. Genet. 4, 401-411 (1979).

41. Yamamoto, K.R., Gehring, U., Stampfer, M.R., Sibley, C.H.: Genetic approaches to steroid hormone action. Recent Progr. Hormone Res. 32, 3-32 (1976).

42. Thompson, E.B., Aviv, D., Lippman, M.E.: Variants of HTC cells with low tyrosine aminotransferase inducibility and apparently normal glucocorticoid receptors. Endocrinology 100, 406-418 (1977).

43. Bruchovsky, N., Rennie, P.S.: Classification of dependent and autonomous variants of Shionogi mammary carcinoma based on heterogeneous patterns of androgen binding. Cell 13, 273-280 (1978).

44. Harvey, W., Grahame, R., Panayi, G.S.: Effects of steroid hormones on human fibroblasts in vitro. II. Antagonism by androgens of cortisol induced inhibition. Ann. rheum. Dis. 35, 148-151 (1976).

45. Yen, P.T.K., Barker, K.L.: In vitro induction of synthesis and inhibition of degradation of glucose-6-phosphate dehydrogenase in the uterus by estradiol. Biol. Reprod. 20, (Suppl. 1), 12A (1979).

46. Bruchovsky, N., Wilson, J.D.: The intranuclear binding of testosterone and 5α-androstan-17β-ol-3-one by rat prostate. J. biol. Chem. 243, 5953-5960 (1968).

47. Baker, H.W.G., Bailey, D.J., Feil, P.D., Jefferson, L.S., Santen, R.J., Bardin, C.W.: Nuclear accumulation of androgens in perfused rat accessory sex organs and testes. Endocrinology 100, 709-721 (1977).

48. Wilson, J.D., Gloyna, R.E.: Intranuclear metabolism of testosterone in the accessory organs of reproduction. Recent Progr. Hormone Res. 26, 309-336 (1970).

49. Hay, J.B., Hodgins, M.B., Roberts, R.J.: Androgen metabolism in skin and skeletal muscle of the rainbow trout and in accessory sexual organs of the spur dogfish. Gen. comp. Endocrinol. 29, 402-413 (1976).

50. Voigt, W., Fernandez, E.P., Hsia, S.L.: Transformation of testosterone into 17β-hydroxy-5α-androstan-3-one by microsomal preparations of human skin. J. biol. Chem. 245, 5594-5599 (1970).

51. Frederiksen, D.W., Wilson, J.D.: Partial characterization of the nuclear reduced nicotinamide adenine dinucleotide phosphate: Δ^4-3-ketosteroid reductase of rat prostate. J. biol. Chem. 246, 2584-2593 (1971).

52. Siiteri, P.K., Wilson, J.D.: Dihydrotestosterone in prostatic hypertrophy. 1. The formation and content of dihydrotestosterone in the hypertrophic prostate of man. J. clin. Invest. 49, 1737-1745 (1970).

53. Hammond, G.L.: Endogenous steroid levels in the human prostate from birth to old age: a comparison of normal and diseased tissues. J. Endocrinol. 78, 7-19 (1978).

54. Moore, R.J., Gazak, J.M., Quebbeman, J.F., Wilson, J.D.: Concentration of dihydrotestosterone and 3α-androstanediol in naturally occurring and androgen induced prostatic hyperplasia in the dog. J. clin. Invest. 64, 1003-1010 (1979).

55. Deslypere, J.P., Sayed, A., Verdonck, L., Vermeulen, A.: Androgen concentration in sexual and non-sexual skin as well as in striated muscle in man. J. Steroid Biochem. 13, 1455-1458 (1980).

56. Minguell, J., Grant, J.K.: Rat bone marrow cells: androgen metabolism and actions at the molecular level. J. Steroid Biochem. 3, 803-805 (1972).

57. Wilson, J.D., Lasnitzki, I.: Dihydrotestosterone formation in fetal tissues of rabbit and rat. Endocrinology 89, 659-668 (1971).

58. Siiteri, P.K., Wilson, J.D.: Testosterone formation and metabolism during male sexual differentiation in the human embryo. J. clin. Endocrinol. Metab. 38, 113-125 (1974).

59. Liao, S., Liang, T., Fang, S., Casteneda, E., Shao, T.-C.: Steroid structure and androgenic activity. Specificities involved in the receptor binding and nuclear retention of various androgens. J. biol. Chem. 248, 6154-6162 (1973).

60. Schultz, F.M., Wilson, J.D.: Virilization of the Wolffian duct in the rat fetus by various androgens. Endocrinology 94, 979-986 (1974).

61. Shain, S.A., Boesel, R.W.: Saturation analysis of the binding of androgens, antiandrogens and estrogens by the cytoplasmic high affinity androgen receptor of the rat ventral prostate. J. Steroid Biochem. 6, 43-50 (1975).

62. Verhoeven, G., Heyns, W., De Moor, P.: Ammonium sulphate precipitation as a tool for the study of androgen receptor proteins in rat prostate and mouse kidney. Steroids 26, 149-169 (1975).

63. Heyns, W., Verhoeven, G., De Moor, P.: Androgen binding in rat uterus cytosol. J. Steroid Biochem. 7, 335-343 (1976).

64. Wilson, E.M., French, F.S.: Binding properties of androgen receptors: evidence for identical receptors in rat testis, epididymis and prostate. J. biol. Chem. 251, 5620-5629 (1976).

65. Krieg, M., Voigt, K.D.: Biochemical substrate of androgenic action at a cellular level in prostate, bulbocavernosus/ levator ani and in skeletal muscle. Acta Endocrinol. Suppl. 214, 43-89 (1977).

66. Norris, J.S., Kohler, P.O.: The co-existence of androgen and glucocorticoid receptors in the DDT.1 cloned cell line. Endocrinology 100, 613-618 (1977).

67. Morishige, W.K., Uetake, C.-A.: Receptors for androgen and estrogen in the rat lung. Endocrinology 102, 1827-1837 (1978).

68. Krieg, M., Smith, K., Bartsch, W.: Demonstration of a specific androgen receptor in rat heart muscle: relationship between binding, metabolism and tissue levels of androgens. Endocrinology 103, 1686-1694 (1978).

69. Kirchoff, J., Soffie, M., Rousseau, G.G.: Differences in the steroid binding site specificities of rat prostate androgen receptor and epididymal androgen binding protein. J. Steroid Biochem. 10, 487-497 (1979).

70. Nimrod, A., Rosenfield, R.L., Otto, P.: Relationship of androgen action to androgen metabolism in isolated rat granulosa cells. J. Steroid Biochem. 13, 1015-1019 (1980).

71. Hodgins, M.B.: Specific binding of testosterone and dihydrotestosterone in human fibroblasts. Biol. Reprod. 20, (Suppl. 1), 59 (1979).

72. Maes, M., Sultan, C., Zerhouni, N., Rothwell, S.J., Migeon, C.J.: Role of testosterone binding to the androgen receptor in male sexual differentiation of patients with 5α-reductase deficiency. J. Steroid Biochem. 11, 1385-1390 (1979).

73. Voigt, W., Hsia, S.L.: The antiandrogenic action of 4-androsten-3-one-17β-carboxylic acid and its methyl ester on hamster flank organ. Endocrinology 92, 1216-1228 (1973).

74. Voigt, W., Castro, A., Covey, D.F., Robinson, C.H.: Inhibition of testosterone 5α-reductase by and antiandrogenicity of allenic 3-keto-5,10-secosteroids. Acta Endocrinol. 87, 688-692 (1978).

75. Kao, L.W.L., Weisz, J.: Inhibition of steroid 5α-reductase in vivo: effect on suppression of luteinizing hormone and stimulation of accessory sex organs by testosterone in the orchidectomized rat. J. Endocrinol. 81, 209-220 (1979).

76. Zerhouni, N.A., Maes, M., Sultan, C., Rothwell, S., Migeon, C.J.: Selective inhibition by secosteroids of 5α-reductase activity in human sex skin fibroblasts. Steroids 33, 277-285 (1979).

77. Lotz, W.: Importance of 5α-reduction for the trophic effects of androgens on rat accessory sex organs and LH control. J. Steroid Biochem. 13, 1261-1264 (1980).

78. Imperato-McGinley, J., Guerrero, L., Gautier, T., Peterson, R.E.: Steroid 5α-reductase deficiency in man: an inherited form of male pseudohermaphroditism. Science 186, 1213-1215 (1974).

79. Peterson, R.E., Imperato-McGinley, J., Gautier, T., Sturla, E.: Male pseudohermaphroditism due to 5α-reductase deficiency. Am. J. Med. 62, 170-191 (1977).

80. Walsh, P.C., Madden, J.D., Harrod, M.J., Goldstein, J.L., MacDonald, P.C., Wilson, J.D.: Familial incomplete male pseudohermaphroditism, type 2. Decreased dihydrotestosterone formation in pseudovaginal perineoscrotal hypospadias. New Engl. J. Med. 291, 944-949 (1974).

81. Imperato-McGinley, J., Peterson, R.E., Gautier, T., Sturla, E.: Androgens and the evolution of male gender identity among male pseudohermaphrodites with 5α-reductase deficiency. New Engl. J. Med. 300, 1233-1237 (1979).

82. Hodgins, M.B., Clayton, R.N., London, D.R.: Androgen metabolism and binding in skin and fibroblasts from a case of incomplete male pseudohermaphroditism. J. Endocrinol. 75, 24P (1977).

83. Greene, S.A., Symes, E., Brook, C.G.D.: 5α-Reductase deficiency causing male pseudohermaphroditism. Arch. Dis. Childh. 53, 751-753 (1978).

84. Saenger, P., Goldman, A.S., Levine, L.S., Korthschutz, S., Muecke, E.C., Katsumata, M., Doberne, Y., New, M.I.: Prepubertal diagnosis of steroid 5α-reductase deficiency. J. clin. Endocrinol. Metab. 46, 627-634 (1978).

85. Fisher, L.K., Kogut, M.D., Moore, R.J., Goebelsmann, U., Weitzman, J.J., Isaacs, H. Jr., Griffin, J.E., Wilson, J.D.: Clinical endocrinological and enzymatic characterization of two patients with 5α-reductase deficiency: evidence that a single enzyme is responsible for the 5α-reduction of cortisol and testosterone. J. clin. Endocrinol. Metab. 47, 653-664 (1978).

86. Kutten, F., Mowszowicz, I., Wright, F., Baudot, N., Jaffiol, C., Robin, M., Mauvais-Jarvis, P.: Male pseudohermaphroditism: a comparative study of one patient with 5α-reductase deficiency and three patients with the complete form of testicular feminization. J. clin. Endocrinol. Metab. 49, 861-865 (1979).

87. Imperato-McGinley, J., Peterson, R.E., Leshin, M., Griffin, J.E., Cooper, G., Draghi, S., Berenyi, M., Wilson, J.D.: Steroid 5α-reductase deficiency in a 65 year-old male pseudohermaphrodite: the natural history, ultrastructure of the testes, and evidence for inherited enzyme heterogeneity. J. clin. Endocrinol. Metab. 50, 15-22 (1980).

88. Savage, M.O., Preece, M.A., Jeffcoate, S.L., Ransley, P.G., Rumsby, G., Mansfield, M.D., Williams, D.I.: Familial male pseudohermaphroditism due to deficiency of 5α-reductase. Clin. Endocr. 12, 397-406 (1980).

89. Wilson, J.D., Walker, J.D.: Conversion of testosterone to dihydrotestosterone by skin slices of man. J. clin. Invest. 48, 371-379 (1969).

90. Northcutt, R.C., Island, D.P., Liddle, G.W.: An explanation for the target organ unresponsiveness to testosterone in the testicular feminization syndrome. J. clin. Endocrinol. Metab. 29, 422-425 (1969).

91. Jenkins, J.S., Ash, S.: The metabolism of testosterone by skin in normal subjects and in testicular feminization. J. Endocrinol. 49, 515-520 (1971).

92. Rosenfield, R.L., Lawrence, A.M., Liao, S., Landau, R.L.: Androgens and androgen responsiveness in the feminizing testis syndrome. Comparison of complete and incomplete forms. J. clin. Endocrinol. Metab. 32, 625-632 (1971).

93. Svensson, J., Eneroth, P., Gustafsson, J.A., Ritzen, M., Stenberg, A.: Metabolism of androstenedione in skin and serum levels of gonadotrophins and androgens in prepubertal boys with hypospadias. J. Endocrinol. 76, 399-409 (1978).

94. Svensson, J., Eneroth, P., Gustafsson, J.A., Ritzen, M., Stenberg, A.: Reduction of androstenedione by skin in vitro and serum levels of gonadotrophins and androgens in men with hypospadias. J. Endocrinol. 82, 395-401 (1979).

95. Kutten, F., Mauvais-Jarvis, P.: Testosterone 5α-reduction in the skin of normal subjects and of patients with abnormal sex development. Acta Endocrinol. 79, 164-176 (1975).

96. Kutten, F., Mowszowicz, I., Schaison, G., Mauvais-Jarvis, P.: Androgen production and skin metabolism in hirsutism. J. Endocrinol. 75, 83-91 (1977).

97. Hay, J.B., Hodgins, M.B.: Distribution of androgen metabolizing enzymes in isolated tissues of human forehead and axillary skin. J. Endocrinol. 79, 29-39 (1978).

98. Takayasu, S., Wakimoto, H., Itami, S., Sano, S.: Activity of testosterone 5α-reductase in various tissues of human skin. J. invest. Dermatol. 74, 187-191 (1980).

99. Strauss, J.S., Pochi, P.E.: Recent advances in androgen metabolism and their relation to the skin. Arch. Dermatol. 100, 621-636 (1969).

100. Schweikert, H.U., Wilson, J.D.: Regulation of human hair growth by steroid hormones. I. Testosterone metabolism in isolated hairs. J. clin. Endocrinol. Metab. 38, 811-819 (1974).

101. Pinsky, L., Finkelberg, R., Straisfeld, C., Zilahi, B., Kaufman, M., Hall, G.: Testosterone metabolism by serially subcultured fibroblasts from genital and non-genital skin of individual human donors. Biochem. biophys. Res. Commun. 46, 364-369 (1972).

102. Kaufman, M., Pinsky, L., Straisfeld, C., Shanfield, B., Zilahi, B.: Qualitative differences in testosterone metabolism as an indication of cellular heterogeneity in fibroblast monolayers derived from human preputial skin. Exp. Cell Res. 96, 31-36 (1975).

103. Wilson, J.D.: Dihydrotestosterone formation in cultured human fibroblasts. Comparison of cells from normal subjects and patients with familial incomplete pseudohermaphroditism type-2. J. biol. Chem. 250, 3498-3504 (1975).

104. Moore, R.J., Griffin, J.E., Wilson, J.D.: Diminished 5α-reductase activity in extracts of fibroblasts cultured from patients with familial incomplete male pseudohermaphroditism, type 2. J. biol. Chem. 250, 7168-7172 (1975).

105. Leshin, M.E., Griffin, J.E., Wilson, J.D.: Hereditary male pseudohermaphroditism associated with an unstable form of 5α-reductase. J. clin. Invest. 62, 685-691 (1978).

106. Pinsky, L., Kaufman, M., Straisfeld, C., Zilahi, B., St. G. Hall, C.: 5α-reductase activity of genital and non-genital skin fibroblasts from patients with 5α-reductase deficiency, androgen insensitivity, or unknown forms of male pseudohermaphroditism. Am. J. Med. Genet. 1, 407-416 (1978).

107. Hodgins, M.B.: Further studies of testosterone 5α-reductase deficiency in human fibroblasts. J. Endocrinol. 83, 31P-32P (1979).

108. Lamberigts, G., Dierickx, P., De Moor, P., Verhoeven, G.: Comparison of the metabolism and receptor binding of testosterone and 17β-hydroxy-5α-androstan-3-one in normal skin fibroblast cultures. J. clin. Endocrinol. Metab. 48, 924-930 (1979).

109. Mowszowicz, I., Kirchhoffer, M.-O., Kutten, F., Mauvais-Jarvis, P.: Testosterone 5α-reductase activity of skin fibroblasts increase with serial subcultures. Mol. Cell. Endocrinol. 17, 41-50 (1980).

110. Shanies, D.D., Hirschhorn, K., New, M.I.: Metabolism of testosterone-^{14}C by cultured human cells. J. clin. Invest. 51, 1459-1468 (1972).

111. Pinsky, L., Kaufman, M., Straisfeld, C., Shanfield, B.: Lack of difference in testosterone metabolism between cultured skin fibroblasts of human adult males and females. J. clin. Endocrinol. Metab. 39, 395-398 (1974).

112. Moore, R.J., Wilson, J.D.: Steroid 5α-reductase in cultured human fibroblasts. Biochemical and genetic evidence for two distinct enzyme activities. J. biol. Chem. 251, 5895-5900 (1976).

113. Golf, S.W., Graef, V.: Reconstitution of NADPH: 4-ene-3-oxosteroid-5α-reductase from solubilized components of rat liver microsomes. J. Steroid Biochem. 9, 1087-1092 (1978).

114. Dorfman, R.I., Dorfman, A.S.: A test for antiandrogens. Acta Endocrinol. 33, 308-316 (1960).

115. Dorfman, R.I.: The antioestrogenic and antiandrogenic activities of progesterone in defense of a normal fetus. Anat. Rec. 157, 547-557 (1967).

116. Aarskog, D.: Maternal progestins as a possible cause of hypospadias. New Engl. J. Med. 300, 75-78 (1979).

117. Johansson, L.E., Johansson, G.D.B.: Progesterone levels in amniotic fluid and plasma from women. Acta obstet. gynec. scand. 50, 339-343 (1971).

118. Wu, C.H., Mennuti, M.T., Mikhail, G.: Free and protein bound steroids in amniotic fluid of mid pregnancy. Am. J. Obstet. Gynec. 133, 666-672 (1979).

119. Hodgins, M.B.: The function of 5α-reductase in androgen action. Proc. Soc. Endocrinol. Proceedings 161st Meeting Abstract no. 19 (1980).

120. Burns, R.K. Jr.: The differentiation of the phallus in the opossum and its reactions to sex hormones. Publications of the Carnegie Institute of Washington, No. 557. Contrib. Embryol. XXXI (205), 147-162 (1945).

MASS SPECTROMETRIC DETERMINATION OF STEROID HORMONES AND RELATED COMPOUNDS IN HUMAN ENDOCRINE TISSUES

S. J. Gaskell
Tenovus Institute for Cancer Research, Welsh National School of Medicine, Heath, Cardiff CF4 4XX, U.K.

Introduction

The importance of analyses of normal and diseased endocrine tissues for steroid hormones may be summarised as follows:

(i) In the study of the mechanism of hormone action, a knowledge of the intracellular distribution of steroid hormones is required.

(ii) Quantitative analyses provide an indication of *in vivo* metabolism in terms of both direction and extent at the target level.

(iii) A knowledge of the molar proportions of hormone and receptor is important in assessing the biochemical and clinical relevance of receptor determinations.

(iv) An assessment of the hormonal milieu of tumour tissue, as an alternative to receptor determinations, may indicate the likelihood of success of endocrine therapy.

(v) In the evaluation of synthetic hormones and anti-hormones, a knowledge of the tissue concentrations of both drugs and endogenous hormones is essential to guide therapy and elucidate the mechanism of action of the synthetic compounds.

The reliable quantitative determination of steroids in tissue extracts represents a complex analytical problem. Clearly, for routine applications, immunoassays are the present methods of choice on the grounds of speed, simplicity and low cost. Doubts concerning the specificity of such methods, however, indicate the need for very highly specific procedures

Hormones in Normal and Abnormal Human Tissues, Vol. III

to provide reference data for initial research purposes and to enable the assessment of routine assays. Techniques based on gas chromatography-mass spectrometry (GC-MS) have recently assumed importance as reference procedures for the analysis of steroid hormones in blood (1, 2, 3). It is the purpose of this chapter to describe the principles upon which such procedures are based and to review applications to the analysis of steroids and related compounds in endocrine tissues.

Principles of Mass Spectrometry Analysis

A typical analytical procedure incorporating GC-MS includes the following stages.

(i) Solvent extraction of a tissue homogenate or sub-cellular fraction, to which internal standard (see below) has been added.
(ii) Fractionation of the total extract using, for example, gel chromatography on ion-exchange columns.
(iii) Chemical derivatisation to optimise gas chromatographic and mass spectrometric properties. Thus, oxosteroids are frequently converted to substituted oximes and hydroxyl groups to alkylsilyl ethers.
(iv) Combined gas chromatography-mass spectrometry to effect further separation of the derivatised mixture and achieve selective detection of the chosen analyte.

It should be emphasised that the characterisation of the analyte is generally dependent on several stages of the procedure. Thus, for example, isolation of an oestrogen fraction by chromatography on an anion exchange derivative of Lipidex 5000 (4, 5) complements the highly selective mass spectrometric detection. Similarly, gas chromatographic separation of isomeric compounds is frequently essential to identify individual steroids.

Specificity of mass spectrometric detection

In tandem GC-MS, the mass spectrometer may be considered to function as a highly specific GC detector. When complex mixtures are analysed and chromatographic resolution is incomplete, use of the mass spectrometer in the selected ion monitoring (SIM) mode improves the selectivity of detection and maximises sensitivity. While it is the specificity of this technique which is frequently emphasised, it should be recognised that the procedure necessarily ignores the majority of mass spectrometric information derived from the analyte. Thus, confidence in the characterisation of the analyte (and hence in the accuracy of the quantitative determination) is limited. GC-MS/SIM analyses most commonly employ low mass spectrometric resolution, so that all ions of a given nominal mass, corresponding to a possibly large number of elemental compositions, are detected.

In the field of steroid hormone analysis, two approaches have been adopted to further improve the specificity of GC-MS/SIM analyses. Both techniques employ a double-focusing mass spectrometer, a schematic diagram of which is shown in Figure 1. (An instrument of Mattauch-Herzog geometry is shown here since the applications described below were carried out on an instrument of this type. The same principles, however, apply to instruments of the more common Nier-Johnson geometry). The double-focusing instrument is required to achieve high resolution of the ion beam and hence separate ions of the same nominal mass but different exact mass. In single-focusing magnetic sector instruments, resolution is limited by the energy dispersion of the ions formed in the ion source and by the angular divergence of the ion beam. In a double-focusing instrument, initial velocity dispersion of isobaric ions in traversing a radial electric field (the electric sector) is followed by compensating deflections in the magnetic field. Isobaric ions of slightly differing energies thus converge at a focal point after emergence from the magnetic field.

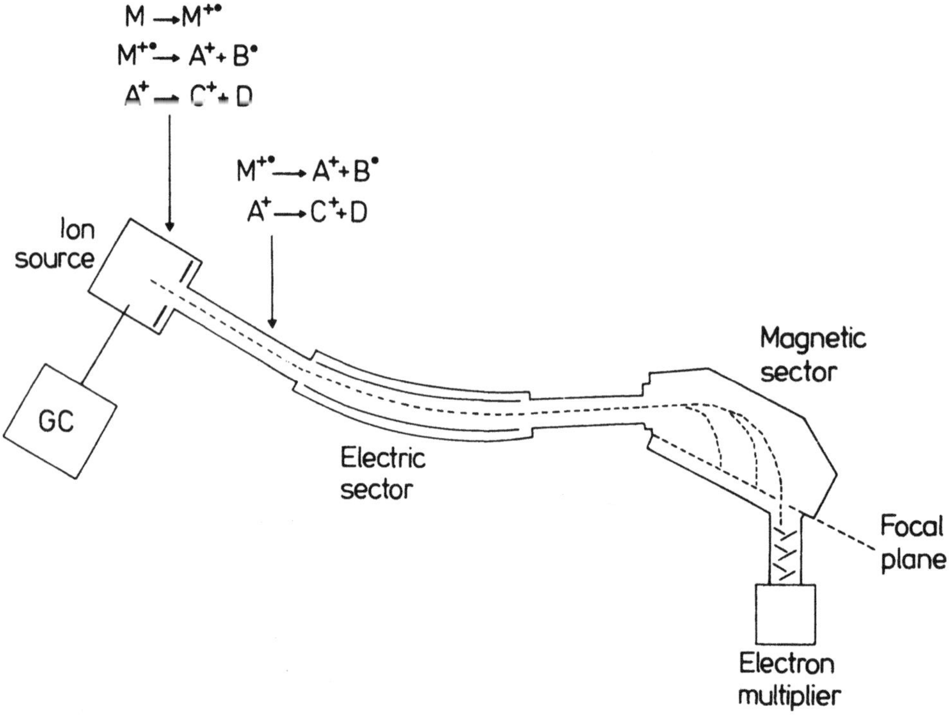

Fig. 1. Schematic diagram of double-focusing mass spectrometer of Mattauch-Herzog geometry.

The properties of double-focusing mass spectrometers have two major implications for SIM analyses. In the first place, the capacity for high resolution permits the selective detection of ions of a chosen exact mass (corresponding to a single or few elemental compositions) with a consequent increase in the specificity of detection. Secondly, the energy focusing properties permit the selective detection of ions, of reduced energy, formed in the field-free region immediately following the ion source (Fig. 1). Such ions, the products of "metastable" transitions, may be focussed by synchronised adjustment of magnetic and electric sector fields or of accelerating voltage and electric sector field. In contrast with the focusing of ions formed in the ion source, focusing conditions of ions formed in the field-free region are dependent not only on the mass-to-charge ratio of the ions detected but also on that of the "parent" ions. Specificity of analysis is accordingly enhanced during metastable peak monitoring.

The importance of mass spectrometric detection of enhanced specificity has been demonstrated in the analysis of testosterone in prostatic tissue from the golden hamster (6). In this instance, quantification was not possible using conventional low resolution selected ion monitoring due to the detection of interfering constituents. Both high resolution selected ion monitoring and metastable peak monitoring, however, permitted quantitative analyses and afforded data in good agreement.

A further example of the benefit of the high resolution technique is provided by the analysis of oestradiol-17β in human breast tumour homogenates. Figure 2 compares the GC-MS analyses of a fraction derived from a tumour extract using selected ion monitoring at low and high resolution. The determination of oestradiol-17β at low resolution is confused by the detection of other constituents eluting from the gas chromatographic column. A clearer trace is obtained by high resolution selected ion monitoring (Fig. 2). It is particularly noteworthy that, despite the decrease in signal intensity which accompanies the increase in mass spectrometric resolution, useful sensitivity, expressed as the signal/noise ratio, is actually enhanced at high resolution due to the reduction in "chemical noise".

Applications to the Analysis of Human Endocrine Tissues

Early applications of GC-MS to the study of steroids in human tissues included analyses of foetal adrenal (7) and testicular (8) tissue. While quantitative data were approximate, the value of the technique in elucidating metabolic pathways was clearly

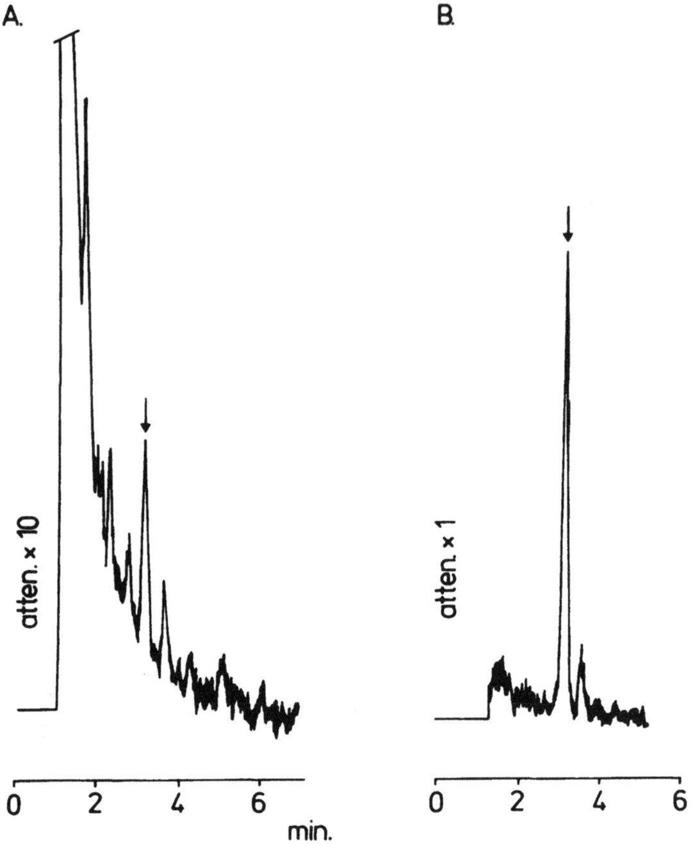

Fig. 2. GC-MS analyses of an extract of human breast tumour tissue for oestradiol-17β after conversion to the trimethylsilyl (TMS) ether. A. Selected monitoring of m/z 416 at low mass spectrometric resolution (1000). B. Analysis of a similar aliquot with selected monitoring of m/z 416.2566 (the molecular ion for oestradiol-17β bis-TMS ether) at a mass spectrometric resolution of 8000. The oestradiol-17β TMS peak is indicated; the concentration was approximately 1 ng/g wet weight of tissue.

established. The use of selected ion monitoring extends this application by improving sensitivity and selectivity of detection. Thus, ovarian steroidogenesis in the human and sheep has been studied in vitro by Phillipou and coworkers (9) who applied GC-MS/SIM to the analysis of culture media for a number of C-18, C-19 and C-21 steroids. The benefits of the high resolution SIM technique were emphasised by Millington et al. (10) in their studies of in vitro steroid synthesis by a feminising adrenocortical carcinoma. The advantages of the method, compared with radioimmunoassay, were particularly evident in oestradiol assays where cross-reaction with oestrone, present at relatively high concentrations, reduced the accuracy of the immunoassay data.

The steroid hormone content of human prostatic tissue has attracted much interest in attempts to understand the aetiology of benign and malignant disease. The majority of such studies (c.f. Vihko et al., 11) have used radioimmunoassay (RIA) though Millington et al. (12) demonstrated the effectiveness of GC-high resolution MS/SIM in the detection of the major androgens in benign prostatic hypertrophic tissue. The value of GC-MS/SIM as a reference technique, however, has yet to be exploited in this area.

Determination of steroid hormones in human breast tissue

Early work by Millington et al. (13, 14) established approximate concentrations for several steroids (dehydroepiandrosterone, testosterone, androsterone, epiandrosterone, oestrone, oestradiol-17β, estriol) in human breast tumour tissue. GC-high resolution MS/SIM was employed, the specificity of the mass spectrometric detection allowing the use of simple work-up procedures. Later work, using internal standards, has permitted the acquisition of more accurate and precise data. Table 1 details mass spectrometric studies of three steroid hormones in human breast tissue. Maynard et al. (15-17) used structurally related steroids as internal standards in their determinations of dehydroepiandrosterone and 5-androstene-3β,17β-diol.

Table 1. Mass spectrometric quantification (using internal standards) of steroid hormones in human breast tissue.

Steroid	Technique	Internal Standard	Tissue Type*	Concentration	Reference
dehydroepiandrosterone	GC-high resolution MS/SIM	3α-hydroxy-5-androsten-17-one	tumours	2.5-466 ng/g tissue wet weight	15,16
			fibroadenomata	245-1000 ng/g tissue wet weight	17
5-androstene-3β,17β-diol	GC-high resolution MS/SIM	5α-androstane-3α,17α-diol	tumours	<1-40 ng/g tissue wet weight	15,16
			fibroadenomata	42-130 ng/g tissue wet weight	17
oestradiol-17β	high resolution GC-low resolution MS/SIM	$|16,16,17-{}^{2}H_3|$-oestradiol-17β	tumours: ER+	15.9+7.0 pg/mg protein	18
			ER-	5.5 $\pm$5.6 pg/mg protein	

*ER+ : oestrogen receptor positive; ER- : oestrogen receptor negative.

The recent work of Edery et al. (18) incorporated the more rigorous approach of using a stable-isotopically labelled analogue as internal standard in the analysis of oestradiol. The latter study established three important points. (i) The molar concentrations of oestradiol, relative to receptor protein, were generally insufficient to create a significant risk of false negative receptor assays due to the presence of the hormone. This confirmed similar conclusions drawn previously from studies using RIA for oestradiol determinations (16, 19, 20).

(ii) Oestrogen receptor positive tumour tissue contained significantly higher levels of oestradiol than receptor negative tissue, again in accord with data obtained earlier by workers using RIA (16, 19, 20). (iii) Satisfactory agreement between RIA and GC-MS determinations of oestradiol were obtained except where the concentration was less than 2.8 pg/mg protein. This was attributed to the high imprecision of RIA at these levels, associated with blank contributions and the presence of cross-reacting substances.

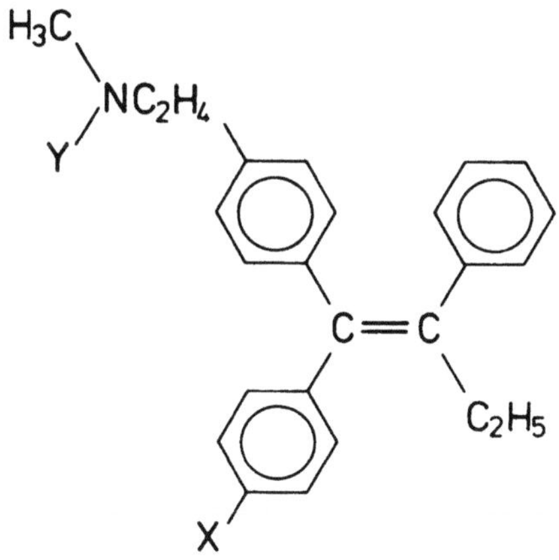

		X	Y
I	tamoxifen	H	CH_3
II	N-desmethyl tamoxifen	H	H
III	tamoxifen 'metabolite B'	OH	CH_3
IV	N-desmethyl tamoxifen, N-heptafluorobutyryl	H	C_3F_7CO
V	tamoxifen 'metabolite B' trimethylsilyl ether	$OSi(CH_3)_3$	CH_3

Fig. 3. Structures of tamoxifen and major metabolites, with the derivatives employed for GC-MS analyses.

Determination of tamoxifen and metabolites in breast tumour tissue.

The antioestrogen tamoxifen (Fig. 3; I) is now widely used in the treatment of breast cancer and is principally effective against those tumours in which a specific intracellular receptor for oestradiol can be detected. The mechanism of action of the drug may be considered in terms of three related processes (21); (i) reduction in the concentration of the nuclear oestrogen-receptor complex through competition for receptor binding with endogenous oestrogen, (ii) substitution of the tamoxifen-receptor complex which fails to elicit a full oestrogenic response and (iii) reduction in the concentration of available oestrogen receptor sites at high concentrations of the drug. The evaluation of these hypotheses clearly requires the determination of tamoxifen and its major metabolites in tumour tissue. Furthermore, comparisons of drug concentrations achieved in tumour tissue from subjects who do and do not respond to treatment may permit the assessment of factors affecting the success of therapy.

Procedures for the determination of tamoxifen and its metabolites in blood plasma have been reported, using thin layer chromatography with densitometry (22) and high pressure liquid chromatography with fluorimetric detection (23, 24), as well as GC-high resolution MS (25, 26). Only the latter technique has so far been applied to the determination of tamoxifen in tumour tissue (27).

In brief, the GC-MS procedure consists of the addition of internal standards (the pentene analogues of analyte I-III, Fig. 3) to tissue homogenates or sub-cellular fractions, solvent extraction and partition between diethyl ether and aqueous ammonia. Further purification is achieved on micro-columns of the cation exchange gel sulphoethyl Sephadex LH-20 (28). For GC-MS analysis, the monohydroxylated metabolite (metabolite B, Fig. 3) is converted to the trimethylsilyl ether (V) and the N-desmethyl metabolite to the N-heptafluorobutyryl derivative (IV). Quantitative analyses employ GC-high resolution MS in the selected ion monitoring mode, with selective detection of ions with exact mass corresponding to the molecular ions of the analytes.

Table 2 lists representative data from the study of Daniel et al. (27). Tamoxifen was detected in blood plasma at concentrations at least 1000-fold higher than the concentration

Table 2. Concentrations of tamoxifen, metabolites and oestradiol-17β in blood plasma and breast tumour tissue homogenates from tamoxifen-treated patients[a].

Patient	Length of treatment (days)	Plasma Concentration[b] (ng/ml)				Tissue Concentration[b] (ng/mg protein)			
		tam	N-des	B	E_2^c	tam	N-des	B	E_2^c
QB	21	160	356	4.5	0.14	18.7	24	0.37	$<1.3 \times 10^{-4}$
ESt	26	410	534		0.10	42.5	21.1	0.29	$<2.6 \times 10^{-4}$
FS	34	146	299	6.0	0.14	13.8	25.0		
FS	60	248	396	5.4	0.14	18.4	35.6		
JC	75	149	416	5.8	0.18	5.4	92.3	1.13	4.7×10^{-4}

a. Data taken from Daniel *et al.* (27)
b. tam : tamoxifen (I; Fig. 3); N-des : N-desmethyl tamoxifen (II); B : tamoxifen metabolite B (III); E_2 : oestradiol-17β. Where no concentration is quoted, no result was available.
c. Determined by radioimmunoassay.

of oestradiol-17β and the concentration of tamoxifen relative to oestradiol-17β was somewhat greater in tumour tissue. The data are therefore consistent with effective competition for binding to the oestradiol receptor (29). The high concentrations of the N-desmethyl compound and significant levels of the monohydroxylated drug suggest supportive roles for these metabolites. Further studies have indicated that the tamoxifen content of tumour samples is concentrated in a crude nuclear fraction (27).

Conclusions

The importance of mass spectrometric procedures for the quantification of steroid hormones and related compounds in tissues parallels their value in biological fluid analysis. The principal advantages of techniques based on GC-MS are (i) high sensitivity, (ii) wide applicability and (iii) rapid method development. Thus, such techniques will find increasing applications in establishing the identity of hormonal constituents of tissues and in providing quantitative data which may be used to assess more routine methods.

Acknowledgements

Research in the author's laboratory is generously supported by the Tenovus Organisation. The collaboration of Drs. C.P. Daniel and R.I. Nicholson in analyses of human breast tumour tissue is gratefully acknowledged.

References

1. Siekmann, L.: Isotope dilution-mass spectrometry of steroid hormones - a definitive method in clinical chemistry. In: "Quantitative Mass Spectrometry in Life Sciences", Vol. 2 Eds. De Leenheer, A.P., Roncucci, R.R., Van Peteghem, C., Elsevier, Amsterdam, pp. 3-16 (1978).

2. Bjorkhem, I., Blomstrand, R., Lantto, O., Svensson, L., Ohmann, G.: Toward absolute methods in clinical chemistry : application of mass fragmentography to high-accuracy analyses. Clin. Chem. 22, 1789-1801 (1976).

3. Finlay, E.M.H., Gaskell, S.J.: Determination of testosterone in plasma from men by gas chromatography/mass spectrometry, with high-resolution selected-ion monitoring and metastable peak monitoring. Clin. Chem. 27, 1165-1170 (1981).

4. Axelson, M., Sjovall, J.: Analysis of unconjugated steroids in plasma by liquid-gel chromatography and glass capillary GC-MS. J. Steroid Biochem. 8, 683-692 (1977).

5. Gaskell, S.J., Finlay, E.M.H., Pike, A.W.: Analyses of steroids in saliva using highly selective mass spectrometric techniques. Biomed. Mass Spectrom. 7, 500-504 (1980).

6. Gaskell, S.J., Finney, R.W., Harper, M.E.: The determination of testosterone in hamster prostate by gas chromatography - mass spectrometry with selected metastable peak monitoring. Biomed. Mass Spectrom. 6, 113-116 (1979).

7. Huhtaniemi, I., Luukkainen, T., Vihko, R.: Identification and determination of neutral steroid sulphates in human foetal adrenal and liver tissue. Acta Endocrinol. 64, 273-286 (1970).

8. Huhtaniemi, I., Ikonen, M., Vihko, R.: Presence of testosterone and other neutral steroids in human fetal tissues. Biochem. biophys. Res. Commun. 38, 715-720 (1970).

9. Seamark, R.F., Phillipou, G., McIntosh, J.E.A.: Ovarian steroidogenesis studied by mass fragmentography. J. Steroid Biochem. 8, 885-891 (1977).

10. Millington, D.S., Golder, M.P., Cowley, T., London, D., Roberts, H., Butt, W.R., Griffiths, K.: In vitro synthesis of steroids by a feminising adrenocortical carcinoma : effect of prolactin and other protein hormones. Acta Endocrinol. 82, 561-571 (1976).

11. Vihko, R., Bolton, N., Hammond, G.L., Lahtonen, R.: Steroids in normal and diseased human prostatic tissue. In: "Hormones in Normal and Abnormal Human Tissues", Vol. 1, Eds. Fotherby, K., Pal, S.B., Walter de Gruyter, Berlin, pp. 523-539 (1981).

12. Millington, D.S., Buoy, M.E., Brooks, G., Harper, M.E., Griffiths, K.: Thin-layer chromatography and high resolution selected ion monitoring for the analysis of C_{19} steroids in human hyperplastic prostate tissue. Biomed. Mass Spectrom. 2, 219-224 (1975).

13. Millington, D.S., Jenner, D.A., Jones, T., Griffiths, K.: Endogenous steroid concentrations in human breast tumours determined by high-resolution mass fragmentography. Biochem. J. 139, 473-475 (1974).

14. Millington, D.S.: Determination of hormonal steroid concentrations in biological extracts by high resolution mass fragmentography. J. Steroid Biochem. 6, 239-245 (1975).

15. Maynard, P.V., Bird, M., Basu, P.K., Shields, R., Griffiths, K.: Dehydroepiandrosterone and androstenediol in human primary breast tumours. Europ. J. Cancer 14, 549-553 (1978).

16. Maynard, P.V., Griffiths, K.: Clinical, pathological and biochemical aspects of the oestrogen receptor in primary human breast cancer. In: "Steroid Receptor Assays in Human Breast Tumours", Ed. King, R.J.B., Alpha Omega Publishing, Cardiff, pp. 86-99 (1979).

17. Maynard, P.V., Pike, A.W., Weston, A., Griffiths, K.: Analysis of dehydroepiandrosterone and androstenediol in human breast tissue using high resolution gas chromatography-mass spectrometry. Europ. J. Cancer 13, 971-975 (1977).

18. Edery, M., Goussard, J., Dehennin, L., Scholler, R., Reiffsteck, J., Drosdowsky, M.A.: Endogenous oestradiol-17β concentrations in breast tumours determined by mass fragmentography and by radioimmunoassay : relationship to receptor content. Europ. J. Cancer 17, 115-120 (1981).

19. Fishman, J., Nisselbaum, J.S., Mendez-Botet, C.J., Schwartz, M.K.: Estrone and estradiol content in human breast tumours: relationship to estradiol receptors. J. Steroid Biochem. 8, 893-896 (1977).

20. Abul-Hajj, Y.J.: Relationship between estrogen receptors, 17β-hydroxysteroid dehydrogenase and estrogen content in human breast cancer. Steroids 34, 217-225 (1979).

21. Nicholson, R.I., Daniel, C.P., Gaskell, S.J., Syne, J.S., Davies, P., Griffiths, K.: The biochemistry of tamoxifen therapy of breast cancer. In: "Antihormones", Ed. Agarwal, M.K., Elsevier/North Holland, Amsterdam, pp. 253-267 (1979).

22. Adam, H.K., Douglas, E.J., Kemp, J.V.: The metabolism of tamoxifen in humans. Biochem. Pharmacol. 27, 145-147 (1979).

23. Mendenhall, D.W., Kobayashi, H., Shih, F.M.L., Sternson, L.A., Higuchi, T., Fabian, C.: Clinical analysis of tamoxifen, an anti-neoplastic agent, in plasma. Clin. Chem. 24, 1518-1524 (1978).

24. Golander, Y., Sternson, L.A.: Paired-ion chromatographic analysis of tamoxifen and two major metabolites in plasma. J. Chromatog. 181, 41-49 (1980).

25. Gaskell, S.J., Daniel, C.P., Nicholson, R.I.: Determination of tamoxifen in rat plasma by gas chromatography - mass spectrometry. J. Endocrinol. 78, 293-294 (1978).

26. Daniel, C.P., Gaskell, S.J., Bishop, H., Nicholson, R.I.: Determination of tamoxifen and an hydroxylated metabolite in plasma from patients with advanced breast cancer using gas chromatography-mass spectrometry. J. Endocrinol. 83, 401-408 (1979).

27. Daniel, C.P., Gaskell, S.J., Bishop, H., Campbell, C., Nicholson, R.I.: Determination of tamoxifen and biologically active metabolites in human breast tumours and plasma. Europ. J. Cancer 17, 1183-1189 (1981).

28. Setchell, K.D.R., Almé, B., Axelson, M., Sjövall, J.: The multi-component analysis of neutral steroids in urine by lipophilic ion exchange chromatography and computerised gas chromatography-mass spectrometry. J. Steroid Biochem. 7, 615-629 (1976).

29. Nicholson, R.I., Syne, J.S., Daniel, C.P., Griffiths, K.: The binding of tamoxifen to oestrogen receptors under equilibrium and non-equilibrium conditions. Europ. J. Cancer 15, 315-329 (1979).

PROSTAGLANDINS IN HUMAN TISSUES : THEIR IMPLICATION IN CANCER, HYPERCALCEMIA AND CELLULAR REGULATION

L. M. Pelus and M. A. S. Moore
Laboratories of Developmental Hematopoiesis, Sloan-Kettering Institute, 1250 First Avenue, New York, New York 10021, U.S.A.

Introduction

The prostaglandins form a family of natural twenty carbon oxygenated unsaturated fatty acids detected in or associated with most mammalian tissues. These compounds have been attributed with an ever increasing number of pharmacological and physiological activities. In addition to the primary prostaglandins, the recent discovery of more short-lived intermediates in the formation of prostaglandins, the prostaglandin endoperoxides, and other extremely biologically active substances, the thromboxanes, prostacyclin and the non-cyclized leukotrienes, all formed during the metabolism of prostaglandin precursors, has added a new dimension to prostaglandin research and already expanded the bewildering array of biological effects attributable to members of the prostaglandin family.

Biosynthesized in cell membranes, particularly microsomes, from simple fatty acids, the prostaglandins are perhaps the most short-lived, ubiquitous and biologically active substances found in mammalian tissues. The magnitude and multiplicity of prostaglandin effects are beyond the scope of this chapter (see reviews 1-4), however, to illustrate the biological diversity of their effects one may cite their implication in hormonal regulation, modulation of intracellular metabolism, muscle contraction, lipolysis, inflammation, immunity,

Hormones in Normal and Abnormal Human Tissues, Vol. III

digestion, respiration, pain, blood flow, fertility, renal function, parturition, hemodynamics and hematopoiesis.

The diversity of prostaglandin action has given rise to much speculation and some insight into mechanisms of action. There is general consensus that the site of action of the prostaglandins is the plasma membrane, and a number of studies have demonstrated specific cell surface receptors or binding sites (5-7). It is likewise held that many of the effects of prostaglandins are mediated via interactions with membrane bound adenyl and guanyl cyclase enzymes. An opposition between elevation of cyclic 3' - 5' - adenosine monophosphate levels by the E series prostaglandins and endoperoxides, and cyclic 3' - 5' - guanosine monophosphate levels by the F series prostaglandins has been suggested as an explanation for the complex regulation of cellular function by the prostaglandins (8). Studies of calcium ion changes at the membrane level by prostaglandin has led to an alternate hypothesis suggesting that prostaglandin effects could be transmitted via alterations in the transmembrane distribution of calcium ions (9). While it is most likely a combination of effects, the precise mechanism of prostaglandin action remains unclear. The interpretation of their effect is further complicated by the fact that different prostaglandins and/or different concentrations of the same prostaglandin can have opposing effects on the same or different systems. Thus one must finally consider the balance of effects between target system, which members of the prostaglandin pathway are present, and at what concentration.

The realization that prostaglandins are important in the control of many cellular mechanisms has stimulated intense research on their significance in cancer, spread of metastases and cell proliferation in general, control of immune cell function and regulation of hematopoietic cells. This chapter will deal primarily with the roles ascribed to prostaglandins in these areas and with mechanisms which bear on the pathophysiology associated with the abnormal state.

Prostaglandins and Cancer

The capacity of malignant tumours to progressively grow and ultimately to metastise is perhaps one of their most important properties. While factors such as site, size and morphology have long been a starting point for appraisal of tumour growth and metastatic potential, a shift towards characterization of tumour-derived products, as a mechanism associated with uncontrolled growth, has recently occurred. In this same context, one must also consider tumour-associated products as it is likely that many "tumour factors" are generated partly or wholly from host elements such as fibrovascular stroma, inflammatory cells and immune cells. This category is justified since these factors are a direct response to the presence of the neoplastic cells and may indeed be evoked by the neoplasm or result from an interaction between host and tumour.

In the past fifteen years, a great deal of effort has been directed towards understanding the role of prostaglandins, whether tumour-derived or tumour-associated, in the physiology of tumour growth. The studies performed to date have concentrated on four major areas; 1) Prostaglandin synthesis by normal and neoplastic tissue; 2) Prostaglandins as humoral mediators of the symptoms associated with some neoplasm; 3) Bone resorption and hypercalcaemia in neoplastic disease; and 4) Prostaglandins in the regulation of immune cell function.

The first evidence that prostaglandins may be associated with tumour growth was suggested by Williams et al. who described the association of diarrhoea with medullary carcinoma of the thyroid (11). Analysis of tumour tissue revealed substantial quantities of prostaglandins E_2 and $F_{2\alpha}$, and in two patients raised plasma concentration of these two prostaglandins were demonstrated, with particularly high levels noted in veins draining the tumour (12). These studies suggested that the clinical symptoms of diarrhoea associated with medullary carcinoma of the thyroid may result from excessive tumour prostaglandin production. This concept was strengthened by studies (13) which demonstrated that monolayer cultures of medullary carcinoma of the thyroid continuously synthesized large quantities of prostaglandin E_2 and F_2 and by radioimmunoassay measurements which demonstrated increased circulating prostaglandin E_2 levels in most patients with carcinoid syndrome, pheochromocytomas and neuroblastoma (14, 15). Tumour tissue and plasma from patients with Kaposi's sarcoma contained large quantities of prostaglandins of both the E and F series (16). Furthermore, prostaglandin concentrations correlated with the degree of vasomotor complaints such as pain, itching, edema and sweating associated with this neoplastic disease. Based upon these studies it appears that, regardless of source of origin, some clinical symptoms associated with certain neoplastic lesions correlate with the demonstrable presence of elevated tissue or plasma prostaglandin levels. These studies also support the concept that prostaglandins play a role in the physiology of tumour growth.

Early studies of prostaglandins associated with neoplasia subsequently stimulated a large number of investigations aimed at measurement of the synthesis of prostaglandins by tumours and neoplastic cell lines and the determination of serum and plasma prostaglandin concentrations. A number of human neoplastic cell lines and primary tumour cell cultures are capable of producing large quantities of prostaglandins in vitro (Table 1). It was not possible to categorize these studies quantitatively but, qualitatively, it appears that most cell lines and primary cultures are capable of producing prostaglandins of both the E and F series, and in most cases, prostaglandin E (primarily prostaglandin E_2) is the major synthetic product. These studies are important in that they unequivocally demonstrate the production of prostaglandin by several pure cell populations (neoplastic cell lines) in an environment most likely free of contaminating host cells and host environmental influences.

Table 1

Human Neoplastic Cell Lines and Primary Cell Cultures Shown to Produce Prostaglandins

Tumor Type	Major Prostaglandin Products	Reference
Urinary Bladder Carcinoma	PGE	(17)
Renal Cell Carcinoma	PGE, PGF_2	(18) (19) (20)
Acute Lymphoblastic Leukemia	PGE_2, PGF_2	(22)
Neuroblastoma	PGE_2, PGF_2	(23)
Breast Carcinoma	PGE_2, PGF_2	(24)
Medullary Carcinoma of Thyroid	PGE_2, PGF_2	(13)

Table 2

Human Tumors Associated with Elevated Plasma or Urinary Levels of Prostaglandin

Tumor Type	Prostaglandin Level	Reference
Medullary Carcinoma of Thyroid	3ng/ml, PGE	(12) (14)
	1-2.4 (0.4)[1] ng/ml, PGE	
Carcinoid Tumor Neuro Blastoma	1-3.3 (0.4) ng/ml, PGE	(14)
Neuro Blastoma	> 10 (0.4) ng/ml, PGE	
Renal Cell Carcinoma	1-1.5 (.04-24) ng/ml, PGE	(25)
	0.5 (.04-.24) ng/ml, PGE	(26)
Transititional Cell Carcinoma of Bladder	14 μg/day (6-8) (urine) PGE	(27)
Bronchial Carcinoid Tumor	120 (4.5) ng/L., PGE_2	(28)
	86 (7.5) ng/L., $PGE_{2\alpha}$	
Melanoma	168-521 (25-100) pg/ml, PGE	(29)
Carcinoma of Lung	714 (25-100) pg/ml, PGE	
Ovarian Carcinoma	5292 (25-100) pg/ml, PGE	
Breast Carcinoma	114-398 (25-100) pg/ml, PGE	
Hepatoma	561 (25-100) pg/ml, PGE	
Esophageal Carcinoma	500 (40-240) pg/ml, PGE	(18)
Adeno Carcinoma-Lung	301 (40-240) pg/ml, PGE	
Parotid Carcinoma	272 (40-240) pg/ml, PGE	

1. Normal values simultaneously reported by these authors are within parenthesis.

Elevated plasma or urinary prostaglandin levels were found to be associated with the presence of neoplastic disease in many cases (Table 2). In general good agreement could be found among reported studies and prostaglandin E levels (3×10^{-9}M to 1.5×10^{-8}M) were approximately 2.5 to 25 times higher than those found in normal subjects (approximately 3×10^{-10}M to 1×10^{-9}M). Inherent in the measurement of serum or plasma prostaglandin levels are sampling errors due to rapid metabolism of circulating prostaglandins which leads to an underestimate of actual levels particularly locally, within the tumour environment and platelet damage and clotting which leads to an overestimate of prostaglandin levels as a result of the contribution of platelet prostaglandin production.

Substantial evidence now supports prostaglandin production by a variety of human neoplastic tissues (Table 3). These compounds seem to be involved in carcinomas of the mammary gland, the colon and rectum, renal cell, thyroid and in bronchial malignancies. In most cases, sampling of histologically normal adjacent tissue taken at the time of tumour excision clearly demonstrates a significant elevation of prostaglandin levels in the tumour tissue. As demonstrated earlier, the most prevalent prostaglandin produced is prostaglandin of the E series, primarily prostaglandin E_2.

One major criticism of studies on prostaglandin production by excised tumour tissue is that of cellular origin of the prostaglandin measured. Since most neoplastic lesions are also inflammatory lesions, they are highly infiltrated with host cells, many of which are capable of significant prostaglandin synthesis (40-42).

In Hodgkin's disease, prostaglandin production by host monocytes has been documented and may play a role in defective cell mediated immunity associated with this disease. Enhanced immune responsiveness of lymphocytes from patients with Hodgkin's disease has been observed following the addition of indomethacin <u>in vitro</u> (43). This phenomenon does not appear to result from direct tumour derived prostaglandin production and provides

Table 3.

Direct Measurements of Prostaglandins in Human Tumors

Tumor Type	Prostaglandin Detected[1]	Reference
Malignant Breast Carcinoma	1 7-62 (0-1.4)[2] ng PGE_2/g tissue	(30)
Benign Breast Tumor	0 2.5 (0-1.4) ng PGE_2/g tissue	
Breast Carcinoma	0 76.4 ng PGE_2/g tissue	(31)
Breast Carcinoma	5 9-101.5 ng PGE_2/g tissue	(32)
Benign Breast Tumor	2 7-22.8 ng PGE_2/g tissue	
Malignant Breast Carcinoma	5 34 (0-1.7) ng PGE_2/g tissue	(33)
Benign Breast Tumor	0 29 (0-1.7) ng PGE_2/g tissue	
Breast Carcinoma		
Schirrhous Adenocarcinoma	11-66 (< 2.0) ng PGE/g tissue	(34)
Medullary Carcinoma	18-64 (< 2.0) ng PGE/g tissue	
Intraduct carcinoma	18-41 (< 2.0) ng PGE/g tissue	
Breast Carcinoma	25 98 ng PGE/g tissue	(35)
Renal Carcinoma	74 ± 34 (5.2 ± 1) ng PGE/g tissue	(34)
Renal Cortical Carcinoma	73 ± 9.6 (8.4 ± 4.2) ng PGE/g tissue	(36)
Renal Cell Carcinoma (Liver Metastasis)	13.6 ± 1.8 (2.0 ± 0.1) ng PGE/g tissue	(20)
Adenocarcinomas of the Rectum Caccum and Colon	37-125 (11-37) ng PGE/g tissue	(21) (37)
Carcinomas of descending colon and rectum	89-304 (42-196) ng PGE/g tissue	(30)
Colon Carcinoma	65-140 ng PGE/g tissue	(35)
Neural Crest Tumors	7-52 ng PGE/g tissue	(35)
	12.4-297 ng PGE_2/g tissue	(39)
Lung Carcinoma	4000 ng PGE/g tissue	(35)
Bronchial Carcinoid	32 ng PGE_2/g tissue	(39)
Carcinoma of Bronchus	25-110 ng PGE_2/g tissue	
Kaposi's Sarcoma	18-237 ng PGE_2/g tissue	(16)

1. Basal Tissue Levels

2. Normal values simultaneously reported by these authors.

clear evidence of host-derived or tumour-associated prostaglandin production and its implications in the pathophysiology of tumour growth.

Whether the prostaglandin produced is a natural tumour-derived product or is generated in response to the tumour, it is clear that elevated levels of prostaglandins are associated with certain neoplastic tissues. This leaves us with the question of what role this elevated concentration plays.

In answer to this question, recent work has focussed upon two relevant areas. Prostaglandin synthesis has been implicated in many physiological and pathological processes that influence the progression of tumour growth in patients with breast cancer. Some human tumours, including carcinoma of the breast, release or are associated with the release of osteolytic substances which cause bone degradation. This process can often be inhibited by prostaglandin synthesis inhibitors. It is believed that excessive tumour prostaglandin production may be responsible for certain cases of hypercalcaemia associated with certain neoplastic diseases, often more life threatening than the neoplasm itself, and may contribute to the development of bone metastases. A second area of interest has focussed upon tumour derived or tumour associated prostaglandin production as a mechanism against immune destruction and possibly responsible, in part, for generilised immune depression. Since both of these concepts bear directly on the role of prostaglandins in tumour growth and progression, they will be discussed in greater detail.

Hypercalcaemia, Osteolysis and Metastatic Spread

The pathophysiology of hypercalcaemia frequently associated with certain solid tumours is poorly understood, but is believed to be caused by humoral mediators. Animal models using the murine $HSDM_1$ cell line (44-46) and the VX_2 tumour model in rabbits (47) clearly indicate that tumour-derived prostaglandin can mediate osteolysis of bone in culture. In the $HSDM_1$ model, bone resorbing activity could be blocked by indomethacin and restored by the exogenous addition of prostaglandin E_2. In addition, mice bearing the transplantable tumour displayed elevated serum calcium and prostaglandin E levels which returned to normal after indomethacin treatment _in vivo_. Additional studies using the Walker mammary tumour demonstrated hypercalcaemia and osteolytic bone metastases in tumour-bearing rats (48). Again, after indomethacin administration serum calcium levels returned to normal and the animals displayed a decreased incidence of bony metastases.

Although prostaglandin E_2 appears to be the cause of hypercalcaemia and bone degradation in these animal models, the results in humans are less convincing. Morphological studies have identified two osteolytic processes, initial bony degradation by osteoclasts alone and direct bone destruction by tumour cells. A large body of experimental and clinical evidence suggests that the osteoclast-mediated phase of bone resorption is stimulated by tumour associated products, one of which is prostaglandin. The prostaglandins have been implicated most extensively in carcinomas of the breast (30, 33, 34, 49, 50), to a lesser extent in carcinoma of the colon (21) and renal cell carcinoma (19, 34) and have been demonstrated in patients with a variety of cancers (51, 52). The experimental evidence is based upon the demonstration of bone resorbing activity produced by tumour tissue *in vitro*, identification of prostaglandin, notably prostaglandin E, in the tumour medium and the abolition of bone resorbing activity by addition of prostaglandin synthesis inhibitors. In addition, clinical evidence indicates that inhibition of prostaglandin synthesis *in vivo*, has beneficial effects on serum calcium levels in some patients (26, 52). Further evidence is provided by experimental studies demonstrating osteoclast activation by soluble factors from tumours enclosed in millipore chambers (53).

Prostaglandins are also likely to be involved in mediating local effects of tumour metastases on bone, possibly as a mechanism for creation of "bone space". An increased incidence of bone metastases in patients whose tumours produced large quantities of prostaglandin *in vitro* was observed in comparison to patients whose tumours produced only relatively small quantities (54). Similarly, concentrations of prostaglandin-like material were higher and the ability to convert substrate to prostaglandin product greater in malignant breast tumours than in normal tissue or benign breast tumours (30). In addition, survival time after surgery of patients with mammary carcinoma correlated inversely with the quantity of prostaglandin (55).

A second level of involvement of prostaglandins in metastatic bone disease is their association with lymphocyte-derived osteolytic activity and macrophage collagenase secretion. The release of osteoclast activating factor from simulated lymphocytes (55, 57) and collagenase secretion by monocytes and macrophages (58) appear to be dependent upon prostaglandin production. This evidence indicates that prostaglandins can resorb bone directly as well as indirectly via host derived mediators.

Many aspects of this subject are still unclear, most notably the sources of prostaglandin under different situations. Most bone lesions contain tumour cells, inflammatory cells and bone itself. Raised levels of prostaglandin are commonly found in situations of subacute or chronic inflammation associated with bone resorption (59, 60). Macrophages in particular appear to be centrally involved (40, 61, 62). While a strong association between prostaglandins, hypercalcaemia and bone metastases can be demonstrated for certain patients with breast and renal cell carcinomas, some negative results have been reported. Most recently, in a double blind clinical study, prostaglandin synthesis inhibitors were found to be of little value in diminishing bone metastases in patients with breast cancer although significant relief from pain was reported (63). However, although circulating prostaglandin levels were decreased, it was unknown if levels of synthesis inhibitors were sufficient to inhibit localized prostaglandin synthesis.

Prostaglandins and Immune Response

A great deal of early evidence documented that prostaglandins, notably prostaglandin E_1 and E_2, were capable of inhibiting most types of immunological reactions in vitro (1, 64). However, in most of these studies, pharmacological concentrations (10^{-6}M - 10^{-4}M) were required to demonstrate the inhibitory effect. These concentrations of prostaglandins were well beyond the levels which could be demonstrated *in vivo*, even under conditions of inflammation and neoplastic disease (10^{-8}M), and cast doubt as to the potential *in vivo* role of prostaglandins in immune function. However, recent studies using more sensitive assay systems and concentrations of prostaglandin in the range of 10^{-8}M - 10^{-10}M, clearly indicate that prostaglandins can indeed mediate immune cell inhibition and in many cases may play a role in homeostatic immune cell function. The realization of the importance of macrophages in regulation of immunity (65) and the demonstration that macrophages are the major immunological source of prostaglandins (40, 41, 43, 61) have strengthened this hypothesis. It is now believed that prostaglandins play a regulatory role in cytolytic T-cell responses, antibody formation, natural and antibody-dependent cytotoxicity, lymphokine production and inflammatory and delayed type hypersensitivity reactions (1, 64).

Immunological responsiveness, both tumour specific immunity and overall immune competence, is often depressed in tumour bearing mice and patients with neoplastic disease. Early studies which demonstrated increased immunological function after surgical resection of the tumour (66, 67) suggested that depressed immune responsiveness may be mediated by tumour factors, and naturally stimulated interest in tumour-derived prostaglandins as mediators of immunosuppression. Murine studies provided initial evidence that the immunosuppression caused by certain tumours *in vitro* could be reversed by the addition of prostaglandin synthesis inhibitors (68) and that tumour growth *in vivo* could be slowed by administration of indomethacin (69). These studies suggested that tumour-derived prostaglandins were responsible for host immune suppression. However, analysis of the immunological responsiveness of mice bearing a number of different tumours indicated that in vivo treatment of mice bearing both prostaglandin E-producing and non-producing tumours with indomethacin, enhanced immunological responsiveness (70). Furthermore, direct addition of prostaglandin synthesis inhibitors to spleen cell cultures from these mice likewise enhanced both B- and T-cell immune response, while having little effect on normals (70). Since all the tumour types studies were non-metastatic, these studies suggested that the immune suppressive effect observed was host-mediated.

Host-mediated immunosuppression in mice and man is now well documented and can be mediated by a variety of cell types. While prostaglandin does not appear to be involved in all cases of host-mediated suppression associated with neoplastic disease, when its involvement is demonstrated, the host source of the prostaglandin appears to be cells of monocytic lineage (43, 64, 71, 72). Prostaglandin effects can be both directly upon the effector immune cells or indirectly mediated through the generation of other immune cell derived inhibitory substances (73). Macrophages isolated from spleen and peritoneal cavity of mice bearing progressively growing non-metastasizing tumours possessed a markedly enhanced capacity for synthesis and release of prostaglandin E much greater than the tumour itself. In this system it appears that enhanced substrate conversion and cyclooxygenase production could represent a unique tumour-induced macrophage (host) activity resulting in prostaglandin mediated immunosuppression (40).

At present, little evidence exists to demonstrate an effect of systemic prostaglandin concentrations on immune responses in patients with neoplastic disease. However, in any circumstance where prostaglandin levels rise, associated with, or derived from, the tumour, either locally or systemically, their inhibitory effects on immune responses must be suspected. Administration of indomethacin to patients with depressed cellular immunity has been reported to enhance hypersensitivity (64) and can boost secondary antibody response in normal subjects (74). Enhanced immune responsiveness _in vitro_, after inhibition of prostaglandin synthesis, was observed in patients with Hodgkin's disease, supporting a role for prostaglandins in the pathophysiology of the disease (43). This is supported by the demonstration of four-fold elevations in prostaglandin production by monocytes from these patients (43). A beneficial effect of in vivo prostaglandin synthesis inhibition on immunological responsiveness in these patients remains to be evaluated.

Prostaglandins and Hematopoiesis

The implications of prostaglandins, whether synthesized by the tumour itself or by the host cells in response to the tumour, in the alteration of immunological effector responses is of primary importance as a mechanism associated with progressive tumour growth. Of equal importance, are the effects of prostaglandins on the differentiation and expansion of immune cell populations. Studies have been described which indicate that prostaglandins can suppress the proliferation of mature lymphoid cell populations. Prostaglandins have also been shown to play a central regulatory role in the formation of granulocytes and macrophages (74, 75), cells which are involved in inflammatory lesions and which contribute greatly to locally elevated prostaglandin levels (40, 61, 62).

In vitro, a class of committed hematopoietic progenitor cells, termed GM-CFC or CFU-C, restricted solely to granulocyte/monocyte-macrophage differentiation, will proliferate in soft agar giving rise to colonies of up to several thousand cells. This clonal expansion requires the obligatory presence of regulatory macromolecules termed granulocyte macrophage colony stimulating factors (GM-CSF). These glycoproteins are present in biological fluids from most mammalian tissues and situations which exert a demand on myelopoiesis are characterized by high serum and tissue levels. Monocytes and macrophages are the dominant hematopoietic cell types which produce these factors, and their detection in most tissues may represent the presence of these cells. The demonstration that prostaglandins, which can inhibit cellular proliferation, are likewise major monocytic cell products suggested that they might serve to counterbalance GM-CSF induced proliferation and thus regulate myelopoiesis. A significant role for prostaglandin E has now been shown in

Table 4

Selective In Vitro Inhibition of
Hemopoietic and Lymphoid CFU by Prostaglandin E

Progenitor Cells Detected by In Vitro Clonal Techniques	Concentration of PGE Producing 50% Inhibition of Cloning	
	Murine	Human
Macrophage CFU-c	$6x10^{-9}M$	$5x10^{-9}M$
Macrophage-Neutrophil CFU-c	$3x10^{-5}M$	$7x10^{-6}M$
Neutrophil CFU-c	$>10^{-5}M$	$>10^{-5}M$
Eosinophil CFU-c	$>10^{-5}M$	$>10^{-5}M$
Megakaryocyte CFU-c	$>10^{-5}M$	ND
Erythroid BFU-e, CFU-e	$>10^{-5}M$	$>10^{-5}M$
B-Lymphocyte CFU	$3x10^{-9}M$	ND
T-Lymphocyte CFU	ND	$3x10^{-8}M$

the regulation of both murine and human progenitor cell expansion (75, 76) (Table 4). Its effect appears to be selective for cells committed solely to monocyte differentiation and bipotentially committed to mixed monocytic-granulocytic differentiation where it probably reflects an effect on the monocytic component of these colonies. The ability to clonally expand is a characteristic of mature lymphoid cells, thus the effect of prostaglandin E on B and T lymphocyte colony formation is a measure of mature cell function and does not represent an effect at the stem cell level.

In the neoplastic state, two mechanisms for myelopoietic suppression can be postulated. Elevated tumour prostaglandin production could suppress monocyte-macrophage proliferation within the local tumour environment and thus comprise the first line of host defence. Secondly, sustained elevation in systemic prostaglandins could have an effect on monocytopoiesis and lead to a monocytopenic condition and alteration of immune functions dependent upon monocytic cell interaction. The situation is somewhat different in myeloid leukemia, where the neoplastic cell is a monocyte. In these conditions, a lack of responsiveness to the effects of prostaglandin E at the stem cell level appears to be a defect intrinsic to the leukemic stem cell (77). Little evidence exists at present concerning prostaglandin production by leukemic monocytoid cells and its role in affecting immunological and hematopoietic function.

Summary

In spite of the large amount of experimental information available concerning the potential physiological effects of the prostaglandins, their precise role in neoplastic growth and the syndromes associated with it remains primarily one of implication. At present, firm evidence is available only for a role in hypercalcaemia associated with some solid tumours. Clearly, in vitro studies document the ability of prostaglandins to alter and control many cellular events, i.e. bone degradation and immune and myeloid cell suppression. Likewise, radioimmuno- and biological assays have documented both host and neoplastic cell production of prostaglandins and measured concentrations, both locally and systemic, sufficient to mediate the effects observed in vitro. Future directions in these fields would now benefit from a redirection of effects towards the development of meaningful in vivo models and clinical studies designed to define the physiological and pathophysiological roles of the prostaglandins and to explore methods by which their effects can be manipulated

Acknowledgements

This work was supported by Grant CA-28512 from the National Cancer Institute, D.H.E.W. and the Gar Reichman Foundation.

L.M. Pelus is a Special Fellow of the Leukemia Society of America, Inc.

References

1. Pelus, L.M., Strausser, H.R.: Prostaglandins and the immune response. Life Sci. 20, 903-914 (1977).

2. Karmali, R.A.: Prostaglandins and Cancer. Prostaglandins and Medicine 5, 11-28 (1980).

3. Horrobin, D.F.: In: "Prostaglandins : Physiology, Pharmacology and Clinical Significance", Eden Press Inc., Montreal (1978).

4. Ramwell, P.W., Foegh, M., Loeb, R., Leovey, E.M.: Synthesis and metabolism of prostaglandins, prostacyclin and thromboxanes. Seminars in Perinatology 4, 1-38 (1980).

5. Smigel, M., Fleisher, S.: Characterization of Triton-X-solubilized prostaglandin E binding protein of rat liver plasma membranes. J. biol. Chem. 252, 3689-3696 (1977).

6. Cooper, B., Gregerman, R.I.: Hormone Sensitive fat cell adenylate cyclase in the rat. J. clin. Invest. 57, 161-168 (1976).

7. Humes, J.L., Oien, H.G., Kuehl, F.A.Jr.: Prostaglandin receptors in adipose tissue. In: "Methods in Receptor Research", Ed. Bleecher, M., Marcell Dekker Inc., New York, pp. 599-614 (1976).

8. Kuehl, F.A.Jr.: Prostaglandins cyclic nucleotides and cell function.Prostaglandins 5, 325-340 (1974).

9. Baum, H., Kirtland, S.J., Corvetti, F., Carafoli, E.: Prostaglandin E_1 anti-inflammatory agents and calcium : Interactions at the mitochondrial membrane. In: "Mechanisms in Bioenergetics", Ed. Azzone, G.G., Academic Press, New York, pp. 365-374 (1973).

10. Kirtland, S.J., Baum, H.: Prostaglandin E_1 may act as a "Calcium Ionophore". Nature, New Biol. 236, 47-49 (1972).

11. Williams, E.D.: Diarrhoea and Thyroid Carcinoma. Proc. roy. Soc. Med. 59, 602-604 (1966).

12. Williams, E.D., Karim, S.M.M., Sandler, M.: Prostaglandin Secretion by Medullary Carcinoma of the Thyroid.Lancet I, 22-23 (1968).

13. Grimley, P.M., Deftos, L.J., Weeks, J.R., Robson, A.S.: Growth in vitro and ultrastructure of cells from medullary carcinoma of the human thyroid gland. J. nat. Cancer Inst. 42, 663-666 (1969).

14. Jaffe, B.M., Behrman, H.R., Parker, C.W.: Radioimmunoassay measurements of prostaglandins E, A and F in human plasma. J. clin. Invest. 52, 398-405 (1973).

15. Kaplan, E.L., Sizemore, G.W., Peskin, G.W., Jaffee, B.M.: Humoral Similarities of carcinoid tumors and medullary carcinomas of the thyroid. Surgery 74, 21-29 (1973).

16. Bhana, D., Hillier, K., Karim, S.M.M.: Vasoactive Substances in Kaposi's Sarcoma. Cancer 27, 233-237 (1971).

17. Droller, M.J., Lindgren, J.A., Claesson, H.E., Perlmann,P.: Production of prostaglandin E_2 by bladder tumor cells in tissue culture and a possible mechanism of lymphocyte inhibition. Cell. Immunol. 47, 261-273 (1979).

18. Cummings, K.B., Whellis, R.F., Robertson, R.P.: Prostaglandin: Increased production by renal cell carcinoma. Surg. Forum 26, 572-574 (1975).

19. Atkins, D., Ibbotson, K.J., Hillier, K., Hunt, N.H., Hammonds, J.C., Martin, T.J.: Secretion of prostaglandins as bone-resorbing agents by renal cortical carcinoma in culture. Br. J. Cancer 36, 601-607 (1977).

20. Cummings, K.B., Robertson, R.P.: Prostaglandin: Increased production by renal cell carcinoma. J. Urol. 118, 720-723 (1977).

21. Bennett, A., Deltacca, M., Stamford, I.F., Zebro, T.: Prostaglandins from tumors of human large bowel. Br. J. Cancer 35, 881-884 (1977).

22. Carpentieri, U., Brouhard, B.H., LaGrove, L., Lockhart, L.H.: Observations on prostaglandins in normal and leukemic lymphocytes. Prostaglandins 20, 1117-1129 (1980).

23. Tansik, R.L., White, H.L.: Prostaglandin Synthesis in homogenates of cultured neuroblastoma cells. Prostaglandins and Medicine 2, 225-234 (1979).

24. Dowsett, M., Easty, G.C., Powles, T.J., Easty, D.M., Neville, A.M.: Human breast tumour-induced osteolysis and prostaglandins. Prostaglandins 11, 447-460 (1976).

25. Robertson, R.P., Baylink, D.J., Marini, J.J., Adkinson, H.W.: Elevated prostaglandins and suppressed parathyroid hormone associated with hypercalcemia and renal cell carcinoma. J. clin. Endocrinol. Metab. 41, 164-167 (1975).

26. Robertson, R.P., Baylink, D.J., Metz, S.A., Cummings, K.B.: Plasma prostaglandin E in patients with cancer with and without hypercalcemia. J. clin. Endocrinol. Metab. 43, 1330-1335 (1976).

27. McKay, H.A., Garren, G.J., Meehan, W.L., Kaplan, R.A., LeBlanc, G.A.: Prostaglandin-mediated hypercalcemia in transitional cell carcinoma of the bladder. J. Urol. 119, 689-692 (1978).

28. Delmont, J., Rampal, P.: Prostaglandins and carcinoid tumors. Br. med. J. 4, 165 (1977).

29. Demers, L.M., Allegra, J.C., Harvey, H.A., Lipton, A., Luderer, J.R., Mortel, R., Brenner, D.E.: Plasma prostaglandins in hypercalcemic patients with neoplastic disease. Cancer 39, 1559-1562 (1977).

30. Bennett, A., McDonald, A.M., Simpson, J.S., Stamford, I.F.: Breast Cancer, Prostaglandins and Bone Metastases. Lancet I, 1218-1220 (1975).

31. Kibbey, W.E., Bronn, D.G., Minton, J.P.: Prostaglandin synthetase and prostaglandin E_2 levels in human breast carcinoma. Prostaglandins and Medicine 2, 133-139 (1979).

32. Feller, N., Malachi, T., Halbrecht, I.:Prostaglandin E_2 and Cyclic AMP levels in human breast tumors. Cancer Res. Clin. Oncol. 93, 275-280 (1979).

33. Bennett, A., McDonald, A.M., Stamford, I.F., Charlier, E.M., Simpson, J.S., Zebro, T.: Prostaglandins and breast cancer. Lancet I, 624-626 (1977).

34. Greaves, M., Ibbotson, K.J., Atkins, D., Martin, T.J.: Prostaglandins as mediators of bone resorption in renal and breast tumors. Clin. Sci. 58, 201-210 (1980).

35. Husby, G., Strickland, R.G., Rigler, G.L., Peake, G.T., Williams, R.C.: Direct immunochemical detection of prostaglandin E and cyclic nucleotides in human malignant tumors. Cancer 40, 1629-1642 (1977).

36. Greaves, M., Martin, T.J., Gyde, O.H.B., Harris, B.R.: Renal cortical carcinoma, erythropoietin and prostaglandin E. Proc. Soc. Endocrinol. 21P (1977).

37. Bennett, A., Deltacca, M.: Prostaglandins in human colonic carcinoma. Gut 16, 409 (1975).

38. Papanicolaou, N., Mountoralakis, T., Teherdakoff, P., Bariety, J., Milliez, P.: Prostaglandins in neural crest tumours. Prostaglandins 10, 405-411 (1975).

39. Sandler, M., Karim, S.M.M., Williams, E.D.: Prostaglandins in amine-peptide-secreting tumours. Lancet 2, 1053-1055 (1968).

40. Pelus, L.M., Bockman, R.S.: Increased prostaglandin synthesis by macrophages from tumor-bearing mice. J. Immunol. 123, 2118-2125 (1979).

41. Kurland, J.I., Broxmeyer, H.E., Pelus, L.M., Bockman, R.S., Moore, M.A.S.: Role for monocyte-macrophage-derived colony-stimulating factor and prostaglandin E in the positive and negative feedback control of myeloid stem cell proliferation. Blood 52, 388-407 (1978).

42. Weissman, G., Korchak, H.M., Perez, H.D., Smolen, J.E., Goldstein, I.M., Hoffstein, S.T.: Leukocytes as secretory organs of inflammation. In: "Advances in Inflammation Research" vol. 1, Eds.Weissman, G., Samuelsson, B., Paoletti, R., Raven Press, New York, pp. 95-112 (1979).

43. Goodwin, J.S., Messner, R.P., Bankhurst, A.D., Peake, G.T., Saiki, J.H., Williams, R.C.Jr.: Prostaglandin producing suppressor cells in Hodgkin's Disease. New Engl. J. Med. 297, 963-972 (1977).

44. Levine, L., Hinkle, P.M., Voelkel, E.F., Tashjian, A.H.Jr.: Prostaglandin production by mouse fibrosarcoma cells in culture. Biochem. biophys. Res. Commun. 47, 888-894 (1972).

45. Tashjian, A.J.Jr., Voelkel, E.F., Goldhaber, P., Levine, L.: Successful treatment of hypercalcemia by indomethacin in mice bearing a prostaglandin producing fibrosarcoma. Prostaglandins 3, 515-524 (1973).

46. Tashjian, A.H., Voelkel, E.F., Levine, L., Goldhaber, P.: Evidence that the bone resorption stimulating factor produced by mouse fibrosarcoma cells is prostaglandin E_2. J. exp. Med. 136, 1329-1343 (1972).

47. Voelkel, E.F., Tashjian, A.H.Jr., Franklin, R.B., Wasserman, E., Levine, L.: Hypercalcemia and tumor prostaglandins. Metabolism 24, 973-986 (1975).

48. Powles, T.J., Clark, S.A., Easty, D.M., Easty, G.C., Neville, A.M.: The inhibition by aspirin and indomethacin of osteolytic tumor deposits and hypercalcemia in rats with Walker Tumors. Br. J. Cancer 28, 316-321 (1973).

49. Powles, T.J., Dowsett, M., Easty, D.M., Easty, G.C., Neville, A.M.: Breast cancer, osteolysis, bone metastases and antiosteolytic effects of aspirin. Lancet I, 608-610 (1976).

50. Bennett, A., Charlier, E.M., McDonald, A.M., Simpson, J.S., Stamford, I.F.: Bone destruction by breast tumours. Prostaglandins 11, 461-463 (1976).

51. Powell, D., Singer, F.R., Murray, T.M., Minrin, C., Potts, T.J.Jr.: Non parathyroid humoral hypercalcemia in patients with neoplastic disease. New Engl. J. Med. 289, 176-181 (1973).

52. Seyberth, H.W., Segre, G.V., Morgan, J.L., Sweetman, B.J., Potts, T.J., Oates, J.A.: Prostaglandinsas mediators of hypercalcemia associated with certain types of cancer. New Engl. J. Med. 293, 1278-1283 (1975).

53. Calesko, C.S.B., Bennett, A.: Relationship of bone destruction in skeletal metastases to osteoclast activation and prostaglandins. Nature 263, 508-509 (1976).

54. Powles, T.J., Alexander, P., Miller, J.L.: Enhancement of anti-cancer activity of cytotoxic chemotherapy with protection of normal tissues by inhibition of prostaglandin synthesis. Biochem. Pharmacol. 27, 1389-1394 (1978).

55. Bennett, A., Berstock, D.A., Stamford, I.F.: Survival time after surgery is inversely related to the amounts of prostaglandins extracted from human breast cancers. Proc. Br. Pharmacol. Soc. 451P (1979).

56. Yoneda, T., Mundy, G.R.: Prostaglandins are necessary for osteoclast activating factor production by activated peripheral blood leukocytes. J. exp. Med. 149, 279-283 (1979).

57. Yoneda, T., Mundy, G.R.: Monocytes regulate osteoclast-activating factor production by releasing prostaglandins. J. exp. Med. 150, 338-350 (1979).

58. Wahl, L., Olsen, C.E., Sandberg, A.L., Mergenhagen, S.E.: Prostaglandin regulation of macrophage collagenase production. Proc. natn. Acad. Sci. U.S.A. 74, 4955-4958 (1977).

59. Harris, M., Jenkins, M.V., Bennett, A., Hird, V.M., Wills, M.R.: Leukocytes, bone resorption and prostaglandins. Lancet I, 265 (1974).

60. Robinson, D.R., Tashjian, A.H., Levine, L.: Prostaglandin stimulated bone resorption by rheumatoid synovia. J. clin. Invest. 56, 1181-1188 (1975).

61. Humes, J.L., Bonney, R.J., Pelus, L.M., Dahlgren, M.E., Sadowski, S.J., Kuehl, F.A., Davies, P.: Macrophages synthesize and release prostaglandins in response to inflammatory stimuli. Nature 269, 149-150 (1977).

62. Davies, P., Allisson, A.C.: Secretion of macrophage enzymes in relation to the pathogenesis of chronic inflammation. In: "Immunobiology of the Macrophage", Ed. Nelson, D.S., Academic Press, New York, pp. 427-461 (1976).

63. Powles, T.J., Dady, P.J., Williams, J., Easty, G.C., Coombes, R.C.: Use of inhibitors of P.G. synthesis in patients with breast cancer. In: "Advances in Prostaglandin and Thromboxane Research", vol. 6, Eds. Samuelsson, B., Ramwell, P., Paoletti, R., Raven Press, New York, pp. 511-516 (1980).

64. Goodwin, J.S., Webb, D.R.: Regulation of the immune response by prostaglandins. Clin. Immunol. Immunopathol. 15, 106-122 (1980).

65. Unanue, E.R., Rosenthal, A.S.: Eds. "Macrophage Regulation of Immunity", Academic Press, New York (1980).

66. Gillette, R.W., Boone, C.W.: Changes in mitogen response of lymphoid cells with progressive tumor growth. Cancer Res. 35, 3774-3779 (1975).

67. Whitney, R.B., Levy, J.G., Smith, A.G.: Influence of tumor size and surgical resection on cell mediated immunity in mice. J. natn. Cancer Inst. 53, 111-116 (1974).

68. Plescia, O.J., Smith, A.H., Gvinwick, R.: Subversion of immune system by tumor cells and the role of prostaglandins. Proc. natn. Acad. Sci. U.S.A. 72, 1848-1851 (1975).

69. Humes, J.L., Cupo, J.J., Strausser, H.R.: Effects of indomethacin on moloney sarcoma virus-induced tumors. Prostaglandins 6, 463-473 (1974).

70. Pelus, L.M., Strausser, H.R.: Indomethacin enhancement of spleen cell responsiveness to mitogen stimulation in tumorous mice. Int. J. Cancer 18, 653-660 (1976).

71. Rice, L., Laughter, A.H., Twomey, J.J.: Three suppressor systems in human blood that modulate lymphoproliferation. J. Immunol. 122, 991-996 (1979).

72. Laughter, A.H., Twomey, J.J.: Suppression of lymphoproliferation by high concentrations of human mononuclear leukocytes. J. Immunol. 119, 173-178 (1977).

73. Webb, D.R., Nowowiejski, I.: Mitogen induced changes in lymphocyte prostaglandin levels. Cell Immunol. 41, 72-85 (1978).

74. Goodwin, J.S., Selinger, D.S., Messner, R.P.: Immunity in Humans. Infect. Immun. 19, 400-433 (1978).

75. Pelus, L.M. Broxmeyer, H.E., Kurland, J.I., Moore, M.A.S.: Regulation of macrophage and granulocyte proliferation. J. exp. Med. 150, 277-292 (1979).

76. Pelus, L.M., Broxmeyer, H.E., Moore, M.A.S.: Regulation of human myelopoiesis by prostaglandin E and lactoferrin. Cell Tissue Kinet. 14, 515-526 (1981).

77. Pelus, L.M., Broxmeyer, H.E., Clarkson, B.D., Moore, M.A.S.: Abnormal responsiveness of granulocyte-macrophage committed colony-forming cells from patients with chronic myeloid leukemia to inhibition by prostaglandin E. Cancer Res. 40, 2512-2515 (1980).

BIOSYNTHESIS OF CORTICOSTEROID SULPHATES BY HUMAN FOETAL ADRENALS

P. C. Ghosh
Sheffield and Region Endocrine Investigation Centre, Jessop Hospital for Women, Sheffield S3 7RE, England

Concerted studies of the metabolism of steroid hormones during human pregnancy brought about the concept of the term "foeto-placental unit". Sulpho-conjugated neutral steroids are possibly the most significant form of metabolites produced during foetal steroid metabolism (1). Cortisol, cortisone and corticosterone are excreted by the human newborn during the first few days of life in the form of ester sulphates (2, 3) and the secretion rates of cortisol and corticosterone sulphates are considerably higher in the newborn than in the adult (4). The most likely source of these compounds in the foetus is maternal progesterone suitably hydroxylated to form corticosteroids (5, 6). Progesterone in the incubation medium stimulates the 11β- and 21-hydroxylase enzyme activities of the foetal adrenal, an essential requirement for the synthesis of corticosteroids. This is probably due to stabilization of pre-existing enzyme molecules rather than the synthesis of neoteric ones (7); a condition exists during pregnancy where the foetal adrenals are exposed to large amounts of progesterone elaborated by the maternal placenta (8).

Progesterone Synthesis

Placental tissue extensively converts endogenous cholesterol to pregnenolone which is further converted to progesterone (9).

Hormones in Normal and Abnormal Human Tissues, Vol. III

A large proportion entering the foetal compartment (10) is utilized by the foetal adrenal in the biosynthesis of corticosteroids with 4-en-3-one configuration (11). Autoradiography of the whole body after perfusion of the foetus with radioactive progesterone showed that the highest accumulation of radioactivity was in the adrenal cortex (12). A substantial portion of these corticosteroids is conjugated as ester-sulphates (5).

Steroidogenesis by Foetal Adrenal

Perfusion studies indicate that the mid-term foetus is capable of forming 4-en-3-one steroids from precursors like acetate and cholesterol (13) and the conversion predominantly occurs in the foetal zone of the adrenal cortex (14). Further reports suggest that the foetal zone of the human foetal adrenal is capable of forming steroids *de novo* or from endogenous precursors (15) and the production is significantly increased by the addition of ACTH (16, 17) or the organ culture media of foetal pituitaries (18). It has also been claimed that the foetal adrenal provides 17α-hydroxypregnenolone sulphate and 17α-hydroxypregnenolone which pass to the placenta and are metabolized to 17α-hydroxyprogesterone (19) to be used by the foetal adrenal for the synthesis of cortisol (20).

Incubation studies with minced tissue of fresh human foetal adrenal (21) showed the conversion of 17α-hydroxyprogesterone to cortisol and 11-deoxycortisol. It has also been claimed that by the eighth week of gestation, all the hydroxylases required to convert progesterone to corticosteroids are present in the foetal adrenal (7, 22). The hydroxylases are almost exclusively found in the foetal compartment and are totally absent from placenta, reaffirming an active corticosteroid biosynthesis by the foetus using maternal progesterone as precursor (23). With pregnenolone as substrate, the recovery of 4-en-3-one steroids was very low indicating a lower activity of 3β-hydroxysteroid dehydrogenase in the foetal adrenal (24). Histochemical evidence suggests that throughout pregnancy, 3β-hydroxysteroid dehydrogenase activity is absent from the foetal zone of the adrenal cortex (25).

Aldosterone was also detected when adrenal homogenate from a 16-week-old foetus was incubated with radioactive progesterone (26). A higher concentration of aldosterone in the foetus near the end of the pregnancy than in the maternal circulation (27) and a late-gestation rise in amniotic fluid concentration of aldosterone (28) support this finding.

Biosynthesis of corticosteroids is significantly diminished in anencephaly in which the foetal zone of the adrenal cortex is markedly hypoplastic (29, 30, 31).

Biosynthesis of Corticosteroid Sulphates - *In Vitro* Studies.

In a series of incubation experiments using adrenal homogenates from 17 to 24 week old foetuses, large amounts of corticosteroid sulphates were isolated when radioactive progesterone was used as a precursor (32). The results (Table 1) showed that the foetal adrenal was capable of synthesizing corticosteroids and has the necessary sulphokinase activity to produce the ester sulphates.

Table 1

Conversion of radioactive progesterone to corticosteroid sulphates by foetal adrenal (as % of total radioactivity added)

Foetal adrenal	Age (weeks)	Sex	Corticosterone sulphates	Cortisol sulphates	Progesterone
1	17	M	26.62	8.32	33.51
2	18	M	31.43	6.91	21.20
3	24	M	33.54	7.81	*
4	22	F	29.23	10.56	26.13
Mean			30.20	8.40	26.95

* Not estimated

Chromatographic analysis showed that 30.2% and 8.4% of total radioactivity were found in corticosterone and cortisol sulphates respectively. Detectable amount of 11-deoxycorticosterone sulphate was also identified. Similarly in the unconjugated fraction, the major metabolite was corticosterone and the most polar one was cortisol. Trace amounts of 17α-hydroxyprogesterone and 11-deoxycorticosterone were also identified. The presence of sulphokinase and 17α-hydroxylase in the foetal zone of the adrenal cortex and a higher conversion to the steroid sulphates in the foetal compared with the adult zone has also been demonstrated (33).

Conversion of corticosteroids to their corresponding sulphate esters was noted when adrenal slices were incubated with cortisol, 11-deoxycortisol, corticosterone and 11-deoxycorticosterone (34). On the basis of substrate concentrations, the conversion to corticosterone and corticosterone sulphate was maximum followed by cortisol, 11-deoxycortisol and 11-deoxycorticosterone sulphates.

Studies with Intact Foetus and Foeto-Placental Unit

Diczfalusy and coworkers (35) using techniques involving whole foetus perfusion and injection into the umbilical vein of [4-^{14}C] progesterone, were able to isolate radioactive corticosterone and 11-deoxycorticosterone sulphates from the adrenals of previable human foetuses of 17 to 21 weeks gestation. In a detailed communication, Solomon (36) reported the isolation and identification of sulphoconjugated metabolites of corticosterone, 11-deoxycorticosterone, 11-dehydrocorticosterone and cortisol after the injection of [4-^{14}C] progesterone into the umbilical vein. These metabolites were found in the adrenal, whereas they could not be detected in the liver or in the residual tissues of the foetus. One of the most abundant unconjugated metabolites in the adrenal was 17α-hydroxyprogesterone. To examine the role of this steroid, radioactive 17α-hydroxyprogesterone was injected into the umbilical vein of two foetuses of 14 and 22 weeks gestation (20). In the adrenal, about 4.9% of the total radioactivity was present as free cortisol and 1.8% as cortisol sulphate.

The sulpho-conjugating mechanism of the foetal adrenal was also observed when a mixture of [^{3}H] deoxycorticosterone and [^{14}C] corticosterone was injected into the intact foeto-placental circulation 15 minutes prior to termination of gestation (37). The majority of radioactive material was found in the adrenal. Both [^{3}H] deoxycorticosterone sulphate and [^{14}C] corticosterone sulphate were identified. Analysis of the placental radioactive steroids showed the presence of a trace amount of [^{14}C] dehydrocorticosterone sulphate, an indication of the conversion of corticosterone sulphate to its 11-dehydro metabolite without losing its sulphate radical. Further studies have confirmed that the foetal adrenal is a much richer source of sulphokinase enzyme than any other organ (38) and the activities are mainly located in the foetal zone of the adrenal cortex (24). The enzyme activities slowly disappear during extra-uterine development (39), suggesting a special role of sulphurylation during uterine and neonatal life.

It is thus assumed that the placenta synthesizes progesterone from endogenous cholesterol, which in the foetal compartment is hydroxylated at various positions with the formation of corticosteroids which are then sulphated.

Corticosteroid Sulphates in Biological Fluids

An extremely high excretion of sulpho-conjugated corticosteroids of the pregn-4-en-3-one series in pregnant women compared to non-pregnant females has been reported (40). The major fraction of the corticosteroid sulphates in urine was the 17-deoxy metabolites (corticosterone, 11-dehydrocorticosterone and 11-deoxycorticosterone) and the finding of these compounds in higher concentration in mixed umbilical plasma than in the maternal plasma (41) indicated a direct relation of these steroid sulphates with the foetus rather than the mother. Furthermore, there was a steady rise in the urinary excretion of corticosteroid sulphates (Table 2) as pregnancy advanced(42), possibly reflecting foetal maturity.

Table 2

The 24-hour excretion (μg) of total corticosteroid sulphates throughout human pregnancy.

Week of pregnancy	10	14	18	22	26	30	34	38
Mean	85	142	215	238	286	340	405	436
SEM	16	15	26	29	24	28	25	37

A steady rise in the maternal urinary excretion of 11-deoxy-corticosterone sulphate near the term has also been reported (43).

Table 3

The mean difference in steroid concentrations in umbilical cord plasma (ng/ml) from 8 full-term deliveries.

Free Corticosteroids			Corticosteroid Sulphates			Progesterone		
Artery	vein	A-V	Artery	vein	A-V	Artery	vein	A-V
158.20	114.75	+43.45	149.12	83.75	+65.37	163.62	387.12	-223.50

The values in Table 3 conclusively suggest that maternal progesterone is retained by the foetus while there is a steady contribution of unconjugated and sulpho-conjugated cortico-steroids by the foetus towards the maternal compartment (32). Studies including isolation and identification of corticosteroid metabolites from either pools or individual samples of mixed cord plasma suggested that corticosterone sulphate concentrations were 4 to 9 times greater than those of corticosterone, but the concentration of 11-dehydrocorticosterone sulphate was 25% to

50% lower than corticosterone sulphate (44). From accumulated evidence, it would appear therefore that the sulphates once formed are almost quantitatively transferred to the maternal side, as the placenta has little or no sulphatase activity for C-21-sulphates (45). The extensive capacity of the foetus to sulphurylate corticosteroids is retained in neonates until a few days after birth. Large amounts of radioactive cortisol-21-sulphate were isolated from urine of two 2-days old neonates after intravenous administration of [^{3}H] cortisol (46).

Conclusion

It has now been well documented that the placenta and the foetus by virtue of a combination of enzyme activities may produce corticosteroids. The significant endogenous pool of cholesterol in the placenta is used as a precursor for the biosynthesis of progesterone, which eventually crosses the foetus and is hydroxylated at various positions to form corticosteroids. These corticosteroids are further esterified to their corresponding sulphates by the sulphokinase activity present in the foetal adrenal. The steroid sulphates are devoid of biologic activity and it can be assumed that the level of biologic activity of the C-21 corticosteroids in the foetal circulation may, in part, be regulated by steroid sulphation.

References

1. Diczfalusy, E.: Steroid metabolism in the human foeto-placental unit. Acta endocr. 61, 649-664 (1969).
2. Drayer, N.M., Giroud, C.J.P.: Corticosteroid sulphates in the urine of the human neonate. Steroids 5, 289-317 (1965).
3. Ducharme, J.R., Leboeuf, C., Sandor, T.: C-21 steroid metabolism and conjugation in the human premature neonate. Urinary excretion and the response to ACTH. J. clin. Endocr. Metab. 31, 96-101 (1970).

4. Hall, C. St. G., Branchaud, C., Klein, G.P., Loras, B., Rothman, S., Stern, L., Giroud, C.J.P.: Secretion rate and metabolism of the sulphate of cortisol and corticosterone in newborn infants. J. clin. Endocr. Metab. 33, 98-104 (1971).

5. Solomon, S., Bird, C.E., Ling, W., Iwamiya, M., Young, P.C.M.: Formation and metabolism of steroids in the foetus and placenta. Recent Prog. Horm. Res. 23, 297-335 (1967).

6. Pasqualini, J.R., Lowy, J., Wiqvist, N., Diczfalusy, E.: Biosynthesis of cortisol from 3, 17, 21-trihydroxypregn-5-en-20-one by the intact human foetus at mid-pregnancy. Biochim. biophys. Acta 152, 648-650 (1968).

7. Villee, D.B.: The development of steroidogenesis. Am. J. Med. 53, 533-544 (1972).

8. Short, R.V., Wagner, G., Fuchs, A.R., Fuchs, F.: Progesterone concentration in the uterine venous blood after intra-amniotic injection of hypertonic saline in mid-pregnancy. Am. J. Obstet. Gynec. 91, 132-141 (1965).

9. Jaffe, R.B., Ledger, W.J.: In vitro steroid biogenesis and metabolism in the human term placenta. In situ placental perfusion with isotopic pregnenolone. Steroids 8, 61-79 (1966).

10. Zander, J.: Gestagens in human pregnancy. In: "Recent progress in the endocrinology of reproduction", ed. Lloyd, C.W., Academic Press, New York, p. 255 (1959).

11. Eberlein, W.R.: Steroids and sterols in umbilical cord blood. J. clin. Endocr. Metab. 25, 1101-1118 (1965).

12. Bengtsson, G., Ullberg, S., Wiqvist, N., Diczfalusy, E.: Autoradiographic studies on previable human foetuses perfused with radioactive steroids. Acta endocr. 46, 544-551 (1964).

13. Telegdy, G., Weeks, J.W., Archer, D.F., Wiqvist, N., Diczfalusy, E.: Acetate and cholesterol metabolism in the human foeto-placental unit at mid-gestation. Acta endocr. 63, 119-133 (1970).

14. Isherwood, D.M., Oakey, R.E.: Cholesterol biosynthesis in vitro in the human foetal adrenal. J. Endocr. 52, xxxi-xxii (1972).

15. Seron-Ferre, M., Lawrence, C.C., Siiteri, P.K., Jaffe, R.B.: Steroid production of definitive and foetal zones of the human foetal adrenal gland. J. clin. Endocr. Metab. 47, 603-609 (1978).

16. Molino, G., Cavanna, A., Marino, M.: Effect of adrenocorticotrophin on 21- and 11-hydroxylase activity in the biosynthesis of cortisol. J. Endocr. 56, 333-334 (1973).

17. Carr, B.R., Parker, C.R., Milewich, L., Porter, J.C., MacDonald, P.C., Simpson, E.R.: Steroid secretion by ACTH-stimulated human foetal adrenal tissue during the first week in organ culture. Steroids 36, 563-574 (1980).

18. Goodyer, C.C., Hall, C. St. G., Guyda, H., Robert, F., Giroud, C.J.P.: Human foetal pituitary in culture. Hormone secretion and response to somatostatin, luteinizing hormone releasing factor, thyrotropin releasing factor and dibutyryl cyclic AMP. J. clin. Endocr. Metab. 45, 73-85 (1977).

19. Belisle, S., Montserrat, M.F., Osathanondh, R., Tulchinsky, D.: Sources of 17α-hydroxypregnenolone and its sulphate in human pregnancy. J. clin. Endocr. Metab. 46, 721-728 (1978).

20. Ling, W., Coutts, J.R.T., MacNaughton, M.C., Solomon, S.: Formation of conjugated metabolites after injection of 4-^{14}C-17α-hydroxyprogesterone into the umbilical vein of the human foetus at mid-pregnancy. J. Endocr. 58, 477-484 (1973).

21. Yoshida, N., Sekiba, K., Shibusawa, H., Sano, Y., Yanaihara, T., Okinaga, S., Arai, K.: Biosynthetic pathways for corticoids and androgen formation in human foetal adrenal tissue in vitro. Endocr. jap. 25, 191-195 (1978).

22. Murphy, B.E.P.: Steroid arteriovenous differences in umbilical cord plasma. Evidence of cortisol production by the human foetus in early gestation. J. clin. Endocr. Metab. 36, 1037-1038 (1973).

23. Lisboa, B.P.: Metabolism of Δ^4-3-OXO steroids in the human foetus at mid-term. Excerpta Medica Int. Cong. Series No.210 Ed. James, V.H.T., Excerpta Medica Foundation, Amsterdam, Abstr. No. 68 (1970).

24. Shirley, I.M., Cooke, B.A.: Sulphokinase and 3β-hydroxysteroid dehydrogenase activities in the separated zones of the human foetal and newborn adrenal cortex. Biochem. J. 112, 29-30 (1969).

25. Cavellero, C., Magrini, U.: Histochemical studies on 3β-hydroxysteroid dehydrogenase and other enzymes in the steroid secreting structure of the human foetus. Proceedings, 2nd International Congress on Hormonal Steroids, Series No. 132, Eds. Martini, L., Fraschini, F., Mota, M., Excerpta Medica Foundation, Amsterdam, pp. 667-674 (1967).

26. Dufau, M.L., Villee, D.B.: Aldosterone biosynthesis by human foetal adrenal in vitro. Biochim. biophys. Acta 176, 637-640 (1969).

27. Bayard, F., Ances, I.G., Tapper, A.J., Weldon, V.V., Kowarski, A., Migeon, C.J.: Transplacental passage and foetal secretion of aldosterone. J. clin. Invest. 49, 1389-1393 (1970).

28. Blankstein, J., Fujida, K., Reyes, F.I., Falman, C., Winter, J.S.D.: Aldosterone and corticosterone in amniotic fluid during various stages of pregnancy. Steroids 36, 161-165 (1980).

29. Fencl, M.M., Osathanondhr, R., Tulchinsky, D.: Plasma cortisol and cortisone in pregnancies with normal and anencephalic foetuses. J. clin. Endocr. Metab. 43, 80-85 (1976).

30. Cawood, M.L., Heys, R.F., Oakey, R.E.: Corticosteroid production by the human foetus. Evidence from analysis of urine from women pregnant with a normal or an anencephalic foetus. J. Endocr. 70, 117-126 (1976).

31. Miyakawa, I., Ikeda, I., Nakayama, M., Maeyama, M.: Plasma concentration of cortisol, progesterone and unconjugated oestradiol and oestriol in women with live anencephalic foetuses before, during and after labour. J. Endocr. 69, 291-292 (1976).

32. Ghosh, P.C.: Unpublished data.

33. Cooke, B.A., Taylor, P.D.: Site of dehydroepiandrosterone sulphate biosynthesis in the adrenal gland of the previable foetus. J. Endocr. 51, 547-556 (1971).

34. Giroud, C.J.P.: Aspects of corticosteroid biogenesis and metabolism during the perinatal period. Clin. Obstet. Gynaecol. 14, 745-763 (1971).

35. Bird, C.E., Solomon, S., Wiqvist, N., Diczfalusy, E.: Formation of C-21 steroid sulphates and glucosiduronates by previable human foetuses perfused with 4-^{14}C-progesterone. Biochim. biophys. Acta 104, 623-626 (1965).

36. Solomon, S.: The formation and metabolism of neutral steroids in the human foetus and placenta. Proceedings 2nd International Congress on Hormonal Steroids, Series No. 132, Eds. Martini, L., Franschini, F., Motta, M., Excerpta Medica Foundation, Amsterdam, pp. 653-662 (1967).

37. Pasqualini, J.R., Marfil, J., Garnier, F., Wiqvist, N., Diczfalusy, E.: Studies on the metabolism of corticosteroids in the human foeto-placental unit. Metabolism of deoxycorticosterone and corticosterone administered simultaneously into the intact umbilical circulation. Acta endocr. 64, 385-397 (1970).

38. Wengle, B.: Distribution of some steroid sulphokinases in foetal human tissues. Acta endocr. 52, 607-618 (1966).

39. Mitchell, F.L.: Steroid metabolism in the foeto-placental unit and in early childhood. Vitam. and Horm. 25, 191-269 (1967).

40. Ghosh, P.C., Lockwood, E., Pennington, G.W.: The solvolysable corticosteroids in human pregnancy urine as determined by competitive protein binding radioassay. Steroids Lipids Res. 3, 75-81 (1972).

41. Schweitzer, M., Branchaud, C., Giroud, C.J.P.: Maternal and umbilical cord plasma concentration of steroids of the pregn-4-en C-21-yl sulphate series at term. Steroids 14, 519-523 (1969).

42. Gowers, H.M.: Corticosteroid patterns in human pregnancy. M. Med. Sc. Thesis, University of Sheffield (1974).

43. Klein, G.P., Kertesz, J.P., Chan, S.K., Giroud, C.J.P.: Urinary excretion of corticosteroid C-21 sulphates during human pregnancy. J. clin. Endocr. Metab. 32, 333-340 (1971).

44. Branchaud, C., Schweitzer, M., Giroud, C.J.P.: Characterization of pregn-4-en-21-yl sulphates in human umbilical cord plasma. Excerpta Medica Int. Cong. Series No. 157, Ed. Gual, C., Excerpta Medica Foundation, Amsterdam, Abstr. No. 428 (1968).

45. Pasqualini, J.R., Cedard, L., Nguyen, B.L., Alsatt, E.: Differences in the activity of human term placenta sulphatases for steroid ester sulphates. Biochim. biophys. Acta 139, 177-179 (1967).

46. Derks, H.J.G.M., Drayer, N.M.: Improved methods for isolating cortisol metabolites from neonatal urine. Clin. Chem. 24, 1158-1162 (1978).

ACTH AND RELATED PEPTIDES IN NORMAL AND ABNORMAL HUMAN TISSUES

Y. Hirata, S. Matsukura, T. Fujita
Third Division, Department of Medicine, Kobe University School of Medicine, Kobe 650, Japan

Introduction

An association of hyperadrenocorticism and certain non-endocrine tumors has long been recognized. It was not well established until 1962 that such association was not coincidental but due to the presence of adrenocorticotropic hormone (ACTH)-like substance(s) in the tumor tissues (1). Since "ectopic ACTH syndrome" was originally coined by Liddle et al. (2), the ectopic ACTH-producing tumors characterized by the elaboration of ACTH-like substances by non-pituitary neoplasms have been well documented (3-5).

Recent technical advances in biochemistry and endocrinology have provided evidence that these tumors elaborate not only ACTH but a variety of related peptides, such as fragments and large molecular weight forms of ACTH ("big" ACTH). It has recently been suggested that such ectopic hormone production is not invariably a peculiar phenomenon of specific tumors but rather a universal concomitant of neoplasms (6).

This paper describes the clinical aspects of the ectopic ACTH syndrome as well as the characterization of ACTH and related peptides ectopically produced by the tumors derived from non-pituitary tissues.

Hormones in Normal and Abnormal Human Tissues, Vol. III

Definition

The ectopic ACTH syndrome has previously been considered to be an uncommon disorder characterized by Cushing's syndrome associated with non-pituitary neoplasms (1-3). However, it has recently been shown that asymptomatic ACTH production by the tumor is not as uncommon as previously thought and ectopic production of ACTH by tumors is not always associated with clinical or biochemical abnormalities (7-10). Thus, the term "ectopic ACTH syndrome" should be only used in cases with excessive hormonal syndromes resulting from ectopic ACTH secretion from the tumor, while ectopic hormone production by tumors without sequelae of hyperadrenocorticism should be defined as asymptomatic "ectopic ACTH-producing tumor". The criteria for the diagnosis of ectopic ACTH syndrome are listed in Table 1. Demonstration of the presence of ACTH in tumor tissues in concentrations significantly higher than either in control tissues or in blood (4) should reasonably satisfy the diagnosis of ectopic ACTH-producing tumor.

Clinical Manifestations

Classical features of Cushing's syndrome, such as moon facies, central obesity, acne, hirsutism and purple striae were observed in only 23% of 30 cases with ectopic ACTH-producing tumors studied at our laboratory (10). Furthermore, none of these cases with primary pulmonary carcinoma had presented Cushingoid features, whereas those with non-pulmonary slowly growing tumors, such as bronchial carcinoid, thymoma, islet cell carcinoma of the pancreas and medullary carcinoma of the thyroid did. The less frequent occurrence of Cushing's syndrome in patients with lung carcinoma may be partly accounted for by rapid tumor growth leading to fatal outcome before the onset of clinically overt hyperadrenocorticism. However, the presence of chemical hyperadrenocorticism, as assessed by high urinary excretion of

Table 1. Criteria for Diagnosis of Ectopic ACTH Syndrome

1. Clinical and biochemical abnormalities due to hyperadrenocorticism in association with the presence of a tumor.
2. Disappearance of these symptoms and signs and/or fall in plasma cortisol levels after removal of the tumor and reappearance after recurrence of the tumor.
3. Demonstration of an arterio-venous gradient of ACTH levels across the tumor or significantly elevated levels of ACTH in drainage veins from the tumor by selective venous catheterization.
4. Demonstration of significant amounts of ACTH in the tumor tissues as determined by radioimmunoassay, bioassay, or radioreceptor assay.
5. Demonstration of ACTH-granules in the tumor cells by immunocytochemical technique and/or intracytoplasmic neurosecretory granules by electron microscopical examination.
6. Demonstration that the tumor can synthesize and secrete ACTH and related peptides either in vitro (labeled amino acid incorporation and tissue culture) or in vivo (transplantation to athymic mice).
7. Demonstration of tumor mRNA-directed ACTH products in cell-free translation system.

17-hydroxycorticosteroids (17-OHCS) and increased plasma levels of cortisol, was found in about 80% of our series of 30 cases. Other symptoms include skin pigmentation (23%), edema (30%), muscle weakness (17%), hypertension (38%), glycosuria (32%) and hypokalemic alkalosis (70%).

Diagnosis

Clinical symptoms associated with the ectopic ACTH syndrome are not specific. Generally, middle-aged male patients with a recognizable or occult tumor in the lung with profound hypokalemic alkalosis (serum potassium less than 2.5 mEq/ℓ and carbon dioxide greater than 30 mEq/ℓ)and/or skin pigmentation should arouse suspicion of the ectopic ACTH syndrome and deserve detailed study. Physicians who suspect this syndrome must always keep in mind the dictum of Dr. Liddle "If one sees hypercortisolism he should look for a tumor; if one sees a tumor he should look for hypercortisolism" (3).

Hypokalemia provides an important clue to this disorder. Aldosterone may not be the major contributory factor because plasma levels are not consistently increased. Elevated levels of plasma cortisol and/or other mineralocorticoids (e.g. 11-deoxycorticosterone and corticosterone) (11) would rather be involved in the development of profound hypokalemia, hypertension and oedema.

The cause of skin pigmentation has been ascribed to β-melanocyte-stimulating hormone (MSH) concomitantly produced by the same tumor (12), thereby the term "ectopic ACTH/MSH syndrome" came in use later (3). It has recently been shown, however, that human β-MSH^{1-22} does not exist in man but is merely artifactually produced from β-lipotropic $hormone^{1-91}$ (LPH) during extraction (13-15). Since both β-LPH and γ-LPH^{1-58} do not possess melanotropic activity, the major factors responsible for pigmentation in the ectopic ACTH syndrome might be either ACTH itself, its N-terminal fragment (? α-MSH^{1-13}) or β-MSH^{1-18} specifically cleaved from ACTH and β-LPH by proteolytic enzymes in some tumors.

To ascertain the presence of hyperadrenocorticism, the endocrinological tests should be performed in patients with suspected ectopic ACTH syndrome. High urinary excretion of 17-OHCS, elevated plasma levels of cortisol without an apparent diurnal rhythm, dexamethasone non-suppressibility and metyrapone unresponsiveness can generally differentiate ectopic ACTH syndrome and adrenocortical tumors from pituitary-dependent Cushing's disease (Figure 1). In patients with pituitary microadenoma, which account for 80-90% of cases of Cushing's disease (16), ACTH secretion is usually suppressed with high-dose dexamethasone and responds to metyrapone. Exceptions to this may occur; dexamethasone suppressed urinary steroids (19%) and metyrapone enhanced them (44%) in some patients with ectopic ACTH-producing tumor (10). These paradoxical phenomena could be explained by several mechanisms (Figure 1). First, periodic hormonogenesis may confuse the evaluation of endocrine tests since some patients with ectopic ACTH-producing tumor show cyclic excretion of urinary steroids (17-19). Second, corticotropin-releasing factor (CRF)-like substances elaborated by the tumor may stimulate ACTH secretion from the pituitary gland; the presence of CRF-like substances was demonstrated first by Upton and Amatruda (20) and subsequently by others (21-24). Third, concomitant production of CRF-like substances may regulate ACTH secretion from the tumor itself as is the case in hypothalamic-pituitary system. We have demonstrated significant release of ACTH from the tumor with simultaneous elevation of intracellular cyclic AMP levels *in vitro* in response to rat median eminence extract in some ectopic ACTH-producing tumors (25, 26) (Figure 2), while others have observed stimulatory effect of lysin-vasopressin on tumor ACTH *in vivo* and *in vitro* (27). Finally, some tumor cells, like the pituitary corticotrophs, may possess cytoplasmic receptors for glucocorticoids. The exact nature of the paradoxical response observed in some patients with ectopic ACTH-producing tumors awaits further investigation.

Determination of plasma ACTH is valuable in distinguishing the ectopic ACTH syndrome from autonomous steroid-secreting adrenocortical tumors (Figure 1); moderately elevated levels of plasma ACTH in the ectopic ACTH syndrome are in contrast to low levels in the adrenal neoplasms. When ectopic ACTH syndrome associated with an occult neoplasm is suspected, selective venous catheterization with simultaneous determination of plasma ACTH may help to localize the site of the tumors (27-30). Measurement of plasma ACTH levels may also serve as a "tumor marker" for the tumor recurrence and the effectiveness of anti-tumor chemotherapy (27, 31) because growth of the tumor mass

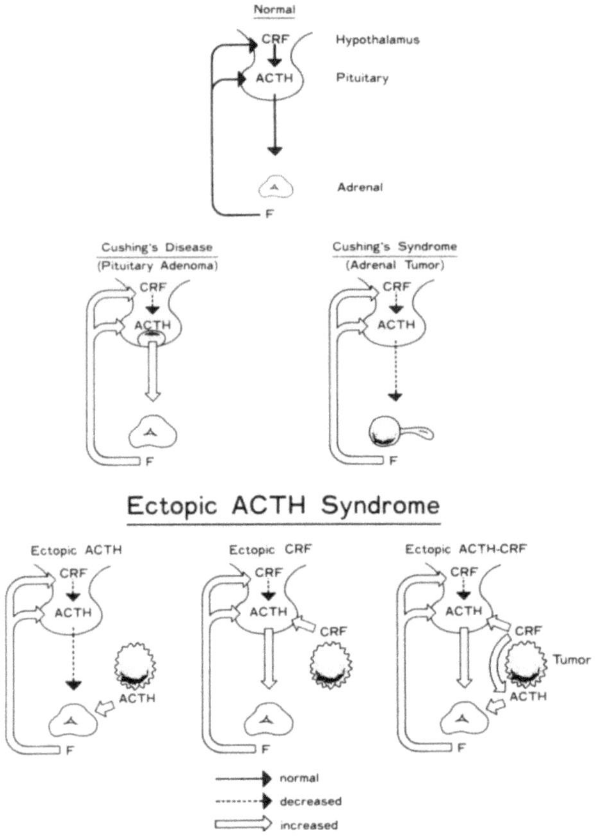

Figure 1. Diagram of the hypothalamic-pituitary-adrenal interrelationships in normal (top), Cushing's syndrome (middle), and the ectopic ACTH syndrome (bottom).

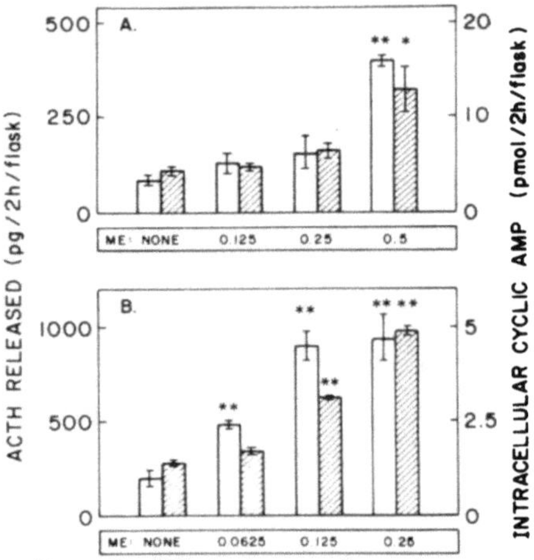

Figure 2. Effect of rat median eminence (ME) extract on ACTH release (open column) from and intracellular cAMP production (shaded column) in dispersed tumor cells from an ectopic ACTH-producing medullary thyroid carcinoma (upper panel) and epithelial thymoma (lower panel).[28]

generally reflects the activity of hormone production by the tumor. Application of radioimmunodetection technique using ^{131}I-labeled anti-ACTH immunoglobulins, as practically used for detection of carcinoembryonic antigen (32), α-fetoprotein (33), and human chorionic gonadotropin (hCG) (34)-producing tumors, may prove useful in tumor detection in the future.

Treatment

The prognosis of patients with ectopic ACTH syndrome appears to be very poor due to rapid growth of the tumor; patients with oat cell carcinoma of the lung, for example, usually do not survive more than a month after initial diagnosis. However, slowly growing tumors, such as carcinoid tumors, medullary carcinoma of the thyroid, thymoma, and islet cell carcinoma of the pancreas may be surgically resectable. We have experienced a patient with an ectopic ACTH-producing gastric carcinoid who presented long-standing Cushing's syndrome which completely abated after successful removal of the tumor (19); she continues to do well without recurrent endocrinologic disturbances eight years postoperatively.

In patients with inoperable neoplasms and severe metabolic disturbances secondary to hypercortisolism, surgical bilateral adrenalectomy or medical treatment to inhibit excessive cortisol production in combination with chemotherapy and/or radiation therapy is preferable. Drugs such as metyrapone, op'-DDD and aminoglutethimide have been used with relatively favorable results (35).

Characterization of ACTH and Related Peptides in Tumor Tissues

ACTH and LPH

Extensive studies by Liddle's group (1-3) have provided substantial evidence that "ectopic" ACTH produced by tumors appears to be biologically, immunologically and physiochemically indistinguishable from pituitary $ACTH^{1-39}$, suggesting the identity of both molecules. However, the presence of more immunoreactivity by antisera against either N-terminal or C-terminal portion of ACTH molecule than bioactivity has been observed in some tumors (8). The apparent discrepancy was later elucidated by the elegant studies by Orth et al.(36) using chromatographic procedures and region-specific ACTH radioimmunoassays; these tumors not only produce authentic $ACTH^{1-39}$, but also N- and C-terminal fragments of the ACTH molecule, while normal pituitary gland only synthesizes $ACTH^{1-39}$. N-terminal and C-terminal fragments, both devoid of steroidogenic activity, may represent α-MSH (N-acetyl $ACTH^{1-13}$) (37) and corticotropin-like intermediate lobe peptide (CLIP: $ACTH^{18-39}$) (38, 39), respectively. Both peptides are confined to the intermediate lobe of the pituitary (38) which man lacks except during the fetal period (40). Thus, specific proteolytic enzymes unique to the tumor and other species with distinct intermediate lobes may participate in the cleavage of ACTH to yield these peptides. Microheterogeneity of tumor ACTH with different isoelectric points on isoelectric focusing has recently been shown, which appears, however, to be identical to that of pituitary ACTH (41). The amino acid composition of ACTH from an ectopic ACTH-producing carcinoid of the thymus has also been demonstrated (42); the tumor ACTH apparently comprised the 2-38 sequence of pituitary $ACTH^{1-39}$. Thus, tumor $ACTH^{2-38}$ may be specifically cleaved from the authentic $ACTH^{1-39}$ or its precursor by the protease present in the tumor but not in the pituitary.

Concomitant production of 'βh-MSH' immunoreactivity (12) by ectopic ACTH-producing tumors has recently been shown to be artifactually derived from larger molecular weight forms, β-LPH^{1-91} and γ-LPH^{1-58}, both containing the sequence of 'βh-MSH^{1-22}, within the molecules (13, 43, 44). We have demonstrated the presence of β-LPH-like peptide in addition to small molecular weight 'β-MSH' in plasma obtained from a patient with the ectopic ACTH syndrome as well as in all eight tumors studied (43) (Figure 3). Our results are consistent with those reported by other investigators (13, 44). Thus, the inclusive term, "ectopic ACTH/LPH-producing tumor", appears to be more appropriate than the "ectopic ACTH-producing tumor". Higher ratio of circulating β-LPH/γ-LPH in the ectopic ACTH syndrome than pituitary-dependent Cushing's disease may suggest the relatively predominant release of β-LPH from the tumor (45). Although βh-MSH^{1-22} does not exist in normal pituitary and plasma of humans, certain tumors may produce β-MSH$^{1-18}$ almost identical to porcine β-MSH, possibly through proteolytic cleavage from γ-LPH (46).

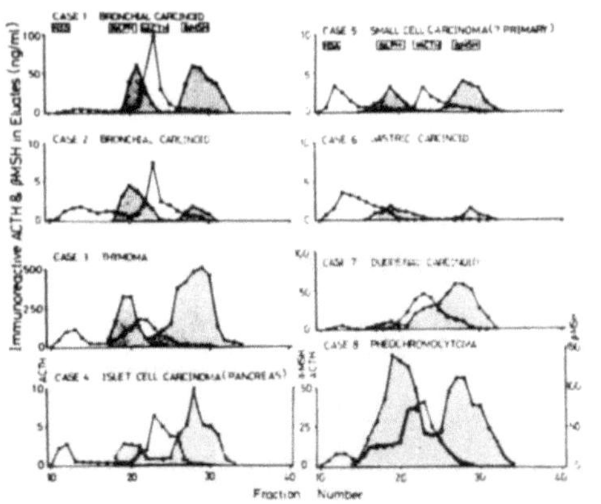

Figure 3. Sephadex G-50 gel chromatography of extracts from the ectopic ACTH-producing tumors[43] : RIA-ACTH (○—○), RIA-'β-MSH' (●—●) with shaded areas.

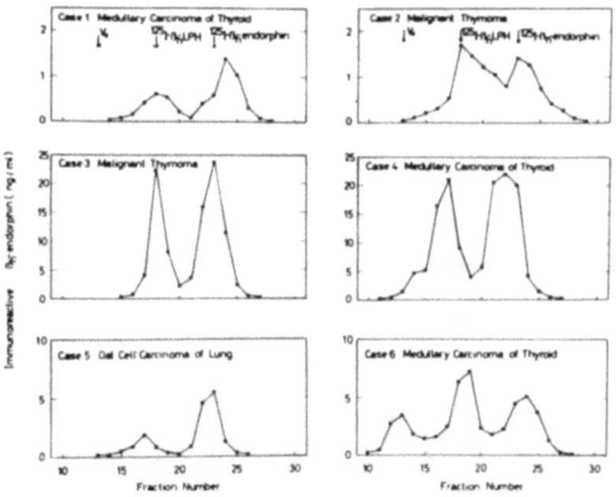

Figure 4. Sephadex G-50 gel chromatography of extracts from the ectopic ACTH-producing tumors[51] : RIA-βh endorphin (●—●).

β-Endorphin, an endogenous opioid peptide, has recently been identified from brain and pituitary gland of many species (47, 48) and found to comprise the C-terminal portion (61-91) of β-LPH molecule. Furthermore, ectopic ACTH-producing tumors concomitantly elaborate β-endorphin in addition to β- and γ-LPH (24, 49-51). We have demonstrated the presence of immunoreactive β-endorphin in all six tumors studied (51) (Figure 4). Thus, these tumors appear to have a similar biosynthetic pathway of β-LPH/β-endorphin to that of the pituitary gland. The mechanism by which ACTH and β-LPH/β-endorphin are always concomitantly elaborated by the pituitary as well as the tumors is discussed in the next section. Pharmacological actions of β-endorphin on the central nervous system, such as analgesic (52) and behavioral effects (53), have been reported.

Thus, elevated levels of β-endorphin secreted from tumors may be partly related to neuropsychiatric manifestations occasionally observed in this disorder. The physiological and pathological functions of β-endorphin, however, await further investigation.

Large Molecular Weight ("Big") ACTH

A large molecular weight form of ACTH ("big" ACTH) was first identified in plasma and tissues of an ectopic ACTH-producing thymoma by Yalow and Berson (54). Big ACTH has less bioactivity (only 3-5% steroidogenic activity of $ACTH^{1-39}$) and is convertible by trypsin to small molecular weight ACTH ("little" ACTH) with full biological activity (55). We have demonstrated that two ectopic ACTH-producing tumors predominantly incorporated labeled phenylalanine into big ACTH which was split into little ACTH after trypsin treatment (25) (Figure 5). Thus, it has been suggested that big ACTH may play a precursor role in the biosynthesis of ACTH. A more prominent production of big ACTH in tumors than in pituitary has also been observed (Figure 3); one case with gastric carcinoid elaborated solely big ACTH (19). Gewirtz and Yalow (9) also demonstrated the asymptomatic production of big ACTH in almost all (93%) lung carcinomas studied. These findings may suggest decreased or absent activity of proteolytic enzymes responsible for conversion of big to little ACTH in tumor tissue.

Further characterization of big ACTH in tumor and pituitary tissues was performed (56). After Sephadex G-100 gel chromatography, an "intermediate" ACTH eluted between big ACTH and little ACTH in both tissues. Both big and intermediate ACTH bound to concanavalin A affinity column and were eluted with α-methylmannopyraminoside, a lectin-specific sugar, suggesting that they have carbohydrate side-chains. Similar observations of the glycoprotein nature of tumor big ACTH have been reported by others (57). SDS-polyacrylamide gel electrophoresis revealed

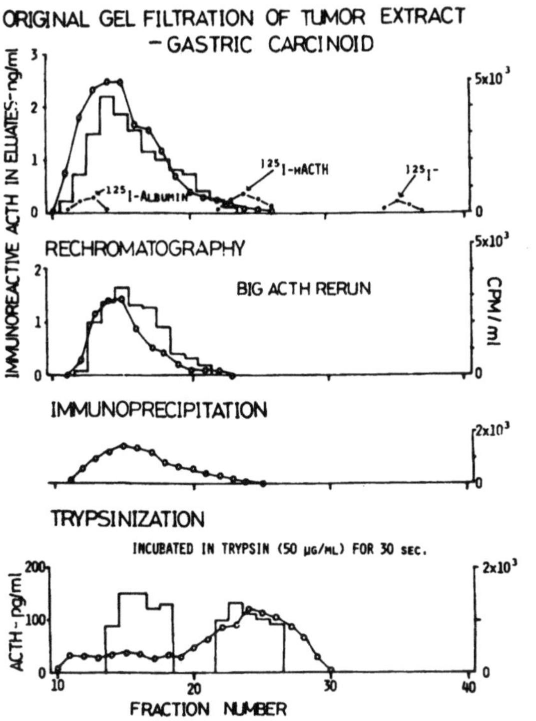

Figure 5. Sephadex G-50 gel chromatography of extract from an ectopic ACTH-producing gastric carcinoid incubated with ^{14}C-phenylalanine[25] : RIA-ACTH (open column), radioactivity of ^{14}C-phenylalanine (o—o), radioactive markers (●—●).

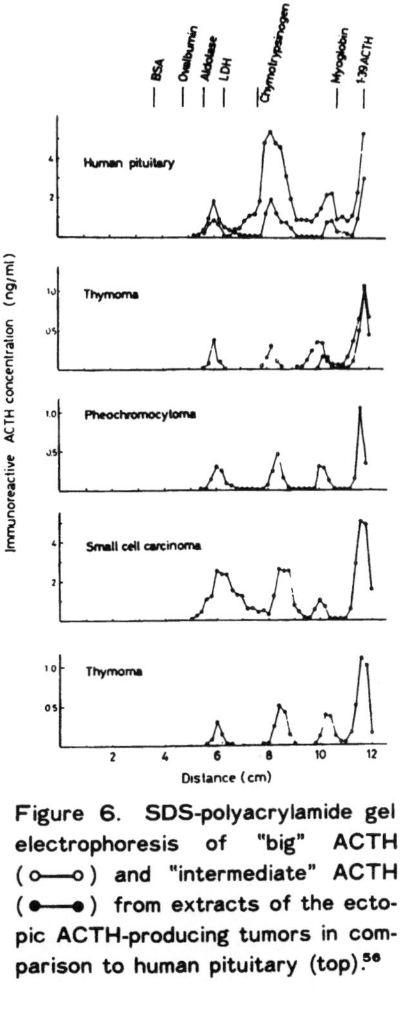

Figure 6. SDS-polyacrylamide gel electrophoresis of "big" ACTH (o—o) and "intermediate" ACTH (●—●) from extracts of the ectopic ACTH-producing tumors in comparison to human pituitary (top).[56]

that the large molecular weight forms of ACTH comprise three distinct peaks with apparent molecular weights of 37,000, 24,000, and 18,000 (56) (Figure 6). Our results are similar to those of mouse pituitary tumor cell line AtT-20 (58-60). Eipper and Main demonstrated that mouse pituitary tumor cells produced three glycosylated large molecular weight forms of

ACTH with apparent molecular weights of 31,000, 23,000, and 13,000, respectively. Thus, these findings suggest that non-pituitary tumors have a biosynthetic pathway for ACTH quite similar to that of the pituitary gland.

A possible common precursor role of big ACTH for both ACTH and β-LPH was suggested by the observation that tumor big ACTH shares both ACTH and β-LPH immunoreactivities within the same molecule (61). Recent elegant studies by Eipper and Mains (62, 63) and Roberts et al. (64, 65) using mouse pituitary tumor cells as well as by Nakanishi's group (66) using bovine pituitary gland, have demonstrated that large molecular weight ACTH represents a common precursor of ACTH and β-LPH/β-endorphin (Figure 7); a 31,000-dalton glycosylated proACTH/β-LPH is post-translationally processed to 23,000-dalton biosynthetic intermediate ACTH and β-LPH^{1-91}. The glycosylated intermediate ACTH is further cleaved to $ACTH^{1-39}$, nonglycosylated or glycosylated, and 16,000-dalton N-terminal fragment, while β-LPH is split into γ-LPH^{1-58} and β-$endorphin^{61-91}$. In intermediate lobe of pituitary and some ectopic ACTH-producing tumors, as stated earlier, ACTH is further converted to α-MSH^{1-13} and $CLIP^{18-39}$, and β-LPH to β-MSH^{1-18}, respectively.

More recently, Nakanishi et al. (67) have successfully sequenced the cDNA coding for the entire ACTH/β-LPH precursor from the bovine pituitary intermediate lobe, thereby elucidating the complete amino acid sequence of proACTH/β-LPH (Figure 7). Unexpectedly, a novel peptide containing a hexapeptide (Met-Gly(Glu)-His-Phe-Arg-Trp) common to both α- and β-MSH, flanked by the paired basic amino acids, has been identified in the N-terminal portion (16K fragment) of the proACTH/β-LPH molecule. They have designated it as "γ-MSH" and its presence has been demonstrated in pituitary (68, 69) as well as in tumors (70). However, the physiological function of γ-MSH is now open to question. Their work has further led to the recent identification of mRNA coding for the common precursor from an ectopic ACTH-producing thymoma with an apparent molecular weight of 38,000 (71) which appears to be consistent with our studies

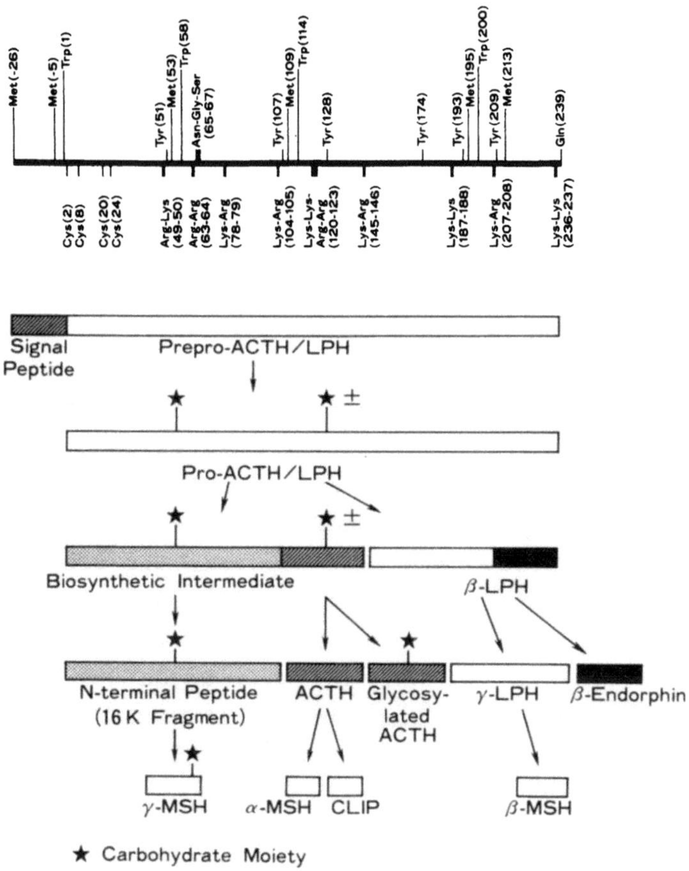

Figure 7. Diagram of biosynthetic pathway of ACTH and related peptides.[67]

(Figure 6). Based on the numerous pieces of evidence recently accumulated, the mechanism of biosynthesis of ACTH/β-LPH in non-pituitary tumors appears to be essentially identical to that in the pituitary, but the post-translational processing, such as enzyme cleavage and glycosylation, may differ in both tissues.

ACTH in Control Tumors and Nontumorous Tissues

Earlier studies revealed a low incidence (7%) of ACTH in unselected tumors (3). However, asymptomatic production of big ACTH has been demonstrated in almost all of the primary pulmonary carcinomas irrespective of tumor types (9). Further, Ratcliffe et al. (8) have demonstrated the presence of ACTH in unselected tumors of various origin, as measured by both radioimmunoassay and cytochemical bioassay. These observations have recently been confirmed by Odell's group (72, 73); extracts from unselected tumors from lung, digestive tract and breast contain significantly greater quantities of both big ACTH and β-LPH than normal tissues. Therefore, ectopic ACTH synthesis may be a universal concomitant of neoplasia as is the case in β-hCG production (6). However, the demonstration of significant amounts of ACTH in the surrounding nontumorous lung tissues comparable to those in lung tumor tissues has been reported (74). This seems unlikely to be due to sequestered blood or incorporation of tumor cells. It might be possible that ACTH production by the endocrine-like cells distributed throughout normal lung tissue may be triggered by the surrounding neoplastic or pre-neoplastic change since pre-cancerous lung tissues of dogs caused by smoking contain ACTH, while normal lung tissues do not (9). Alternatively, such cells might normally synthesize ACTH and related peptides in too low concentrations to be detected by the conventional radioimmunoassays or too widely distributed to be identified by routine immunohistochemical techniques. Their detection, therefore, may be dependent on the sensitivity and specificity of the methods employed at individual laboratories.

Multiple Hormone Production

Ectopic ACTH-producing tumors frequently elaborate a variety of other hormones not derived from the proACTH/β-LPH molecule, such as vasopressin, calcitonin, CRF, biogenic amines etc. (75-78). These polypeptide hormones and amines are normally synthesized by APUD (79) (amine precursor, uptake, and decarboxylation) cells which include corticotrophs of pituitary gland, pineal cells, parafollicular cells of the thyroid, argylophil cells of thymus, Kultschitsky cells of the bronchus, islet cells of the pancreas, adrenal chromaffine cells, entero-chromaffine cells of the gastrointestinal tract, neuroendocrine cells of the brain, melanocytes and so forth. Therefore, tumors derived from APUD series (so-called APUDoma) frequently produce multiple hormones and amines.

Tumor Types of Ectopic ACTH-Producing Tumors

Tumor types associated with the ectopic ACTH syndrome have been classified by Azzopardi and Williams (80) into four categories: oat cell carcinoma of the lung, endocrine tumors of foregut origin, pheochromocytoma and related tumors and certain ovarian tumors. Except for oat cell cancer, the other three categories of tumor belong to the endocrine gland. Thus, it would be reasonable to assume that oat cell cancer of the lung may be derived from the same endocrine-like cells (? Kultschitsky cells) as carcinoid tumor (81, 82). Both tumors share common histochemical and ultrastructural properties; positive argen-taffine or argylophil staining and cytoplasmic neurosecretory granules. Their classification of tumor types appears to be consistent with our studies of 51 cases of ectopic ACTH-producing tumors (5); about half of these cases were broncho-genic carcinoma predominantly consisting of oat cell (or small cell) carcinoma, the others were carcinoid tumors arising from foregut origin (16%), epithelial thymoma (10%), islet cell carcinoma of the pancreas (6%), medullary carcinoma of the thyroid (6%) and miscellaneous tumors (Table 2). Of the tumors 84% were derived from APUD cells (APUDoma), whereas the rest were of non-APUD cell origin, such as squamous cell carcinoma

Table 2. Tumor Types of Ectopic ACTH-Producing Tumors[5]

Tumor histology	No. of cases
Bronchogenic carcinoma	25
Oat cell ca. or small cell ca.	(19)
Large cell ca.	(2)
Adenocarcinoma	(3)
Squamous cell ca.	(1)
Carcinoid	8
Bronchus	(4)
Thymus	(1)
Oesophagus	(1)
Stomach	(1)
Duodenum	(1)
Epithelial thymoma	5
Islet cell ca. of pancreas	3
Medullary ca. of thyroid	3
Oat cell ca. of Oesophagus	3
Squamous cell ca. of larynx	1
Pheochromocytoma of adrenal	1
Plasmacytoma of bone	1
Small cell ca. of unknown origin	1
Total	51

and adenocarcinoma. Therefore, most, if not all, ectopic ACTH-producing tumors comprise APUDoma, possibly originating from neuroectoderm or neural crest (82, 83).

Mechanism of Ectopic ACTH Synthesis

The most probable mechanism for production of ectopic ACTH and related peptides by the tumors would be "derepression" of gene hypothesis (84); the differentiated normal cells retain the 'repressed' genetic information for the production of all proteins (e.g. enzymes and hormones) of which alteration by neoplasms ("derepression") may lead to inappropriate production of specific proteins. However, such derepression of structural genes by the neoplastic change would not occur at random because it could not account for the tumor type specificity and structural similarity of tumor ACTH and related peptides to their normal counterparts of the pituitary. A more satisfactory explanation would be offered by the "APUD" cell hypothesis (79); cells arising from the APUD series with latent capability of producing a variety of hormones and amines could acquire 'switch-on' gene function by neoplastic change resulting in excessive production of hormones of APUD characteristics. The wide distribution of APUD cells and endocrine-like cells (paracrine cells) throughout many normal tissues could easily explain the ectopic ACTH production in most cases derived from APUD tumors and occasional cases arising from a variety of tissues such as prostate, uterine cervix, oesophagus and breast. However, it is difficult to account for ACTH production by tumors derived from nonAPUD cells by this theory. It would be reasonable to assume that normal cells have inherent genes responsible for hormone production which are variably repressed during cellular differentiation (85); APUD cells have easily derepressible genes while undergoing neoplastic transformation or even benign proliferative change, whereas nonAPUD cells have inaccessibly, but not totally repressed genes. An alternative hypothesis would be cell fusion of APUD cells with tumors derived from nonAPUD cells and *vice versa* ("cell hybridization") (86). Elucidation of the exact gene mechanism responsible for the ectopic hormone production by the tumors needs further investigation.

Summary

Ectopic production of ACTH by tumors was previously considered an uncommon phenomenon. However, availability of more sensitive and specific radioimmunoassays to detect hormones as well as an increasing interest of physicians in this particular disorder have led to a better current recognition of ectopic ACTH-producing tumors. Asymptomatic production of ACTH by tumors is not uncommon although clinical and biochemical abnormalities due to hyperadrenocorticism (ectopic ACTH syndrome) occur less frequently. This may be in part accounted for by the predominant production of less bioactive big ACTH, now recognized as a common precursor of ACTH and β-LPH (proACTH β-LPH) and/or ACTH fragments. Recent progress in biochemistry has revealed that ACTH and related peptides synthesized by the tumors appear to be identical to those of the normal pituitary gland although post-translational processing may differ in each tissue. Tumors arising from APUD cells (APUDomas) are likely to elaborate ACTH and related peptides as well as a variety of polypeptide hormones and amines. Therefore, derepression of structural genes coding for proACTH/β-LPH and other hormones in APUD cells by neoplastic transformation might represent a possible mechanism for ectopic hormone production by the tumors.

Acknowledgements

Many of these studies were in part supported by research grants of the Ministry of Health and Welfare, and the Ministry of Education, Science and Culture, Japan. We wish to thank Professor H. Imura, Kyoto University School of Medicine, for helpful advice and encouragement. We are also indebted to Drs. H. Yoshimi and S. Sueoka for their cooperation in these studies.

References

1. Meador, C.K., Liddle, G.W., Island, D.P., Nicholson, W.E., Lucas, C.P., Nuckton, J.G., Leutscher, J.A.: Cause of Cushing's syndrome in patients with tumors arising from 'nonendocrine' tissue. J. clin. Endocrinol. Metab. 22, 693-703 (1962).

2. Liddle, G.W., Givens, J.R., Nicholson, W.E., Island, D.P.: The ectopic ACTH syndrome. Cancer Res. 25, 1057-1061 (1965).

3. Liddle, G.W., Nicholson, W.E., Island, D.P., Orth, D.N., Abe, K., Lowder, S.C.: Clinical and laboratory studies of ectopic hormonal syndromes. Recent Progr. Horm. Res. 25, 283-314 (1969).

4. Rees, L.H.: The biosynthesis of hormones by non-endocrine tumours - a review. J. Endocr. 67, 143-175 (1975).

5. Imura, H.: Ectopic hormone syndrome. Clin. Endocr. 9, 235-260 (1980).

6. Odell, W., Wolfsen, A., Yoshimoto, Y., Weitzman, R., Fisher, D., Hirose, F.: Ectopic peptide synthesis: A universal concomitant of neoplasms. Trans. Ass. Amer. Physns. 90, 204-227 (1977).

7. Hauger-Klevene, J.H.: Asymptomatic production of ACTH. Cancer 22, 1262-1267 (1968).

8. Ratcliffe, J.G., Knight, R.A., Besser, G.M., Landon, J., Stansfeld, A.G.: Tumours and plasma ACTH concentrations in patients with and without ectopic ACTH syndrome. Clin. Endocr. 1, 27-44 (1972).

9. Gewirtz, G., Yalow, R.S.: Ectopic ACTH production in carcinoma of the lung. J. clin. Invest. 53, 1022-1032 (1974).

10. Imura, H., Matsukura, S., Yamamoto, H., Hirata, Y., Nakai, Y., Endo, J., Tanaka, A., Nakamura, M.: Studies on ectopic ACTH-producing tumors II. Clinical and biochemical features of 30 cases. Cancer 96, 1430-1437 (1975).

11. Schanbelan, M., Slaton, P.E., Biglieri, E.G.: Mineralocorticoid production in hyperadrenocorticism: Role in pathogenesis of hypokalemic alkalosis. Am. J. Med. 51, 299-303 (1971).

12. Abe, K., Nicholson, W.E., Liddle, G.W., Island, D.P., Orth, D.N.: Radioimmunoassay for β-MSH in human plasma and tissues. J. clin. Invest. 46, 1609-1616 (1967).

13. Bloomfield, G.A., Scott, A.P., Rees, L.H., Lowry, P.J., Ratcliffe, J.G.: A reappraisal of human β-MSH. Nature 252, 492-493 (1974).

14. Scott, A.P., Lowry, P.J.: Adrenocorticotrophic and melanocyte-stimulating peptides in the human pituitary. Biochem. J. 139, 593-602 (1974).

15. Gilkes, J.J.H., Bloomfield, G.A., Scott, A.P., Lowry, P.J., Ratcliffe, J.G., Landon, J., Rees, L.H.: Development and validation of a radioimmunoassay for peptides related to β-melanocyte-stimulating hormone in human plasma. J. clin. Endocrinol. Metab. 40, 450-457 (1975).

16. Tyrrel, J.B., Brooks, R.M., Fitzgerald, P.A., Coford, P.B., Forsham, P.H., Wilson, C.B.: Cushing's disease: Selective trans-sphenoidal resection of pituitary microadenomas. New Engl. J. Med. 298, 753-758 (1978).

17. Bailey, R.E.: Periodic hormonogenesis - a new phenomenon: Periodicity in function of a hormone-producing tumor in man. J. clin. Endocrinol. Metab. 32, 317-327 (1971).

18. Chajek, T., Ramanoff, H.: Cushing's syndrome with cyclical edema and periodic secretion of corticosteroids. Arch. intern. Med. 136, 441-443 (1976).

19. Hirata, Y., Sakamoto, N., Yamamoto, H., Matsukura, S., Imura, H., Okada, S.: Gastric carcinoid with ectopic production of ACTH and β-MSH. Cancer 37, 377-385 (1976).

20. Upton, G.V., Amatruda, T.T.: Evidence for the presence of tumor peptides with corticotropin-releasing factor-like activity in the ectopic ACTH syndrome. New Engl. J. Med. 285, 419-424 (1971).

21. Yamamoto, H., Hirata, Y., Matsukura, S., Imura, H., Nakamura, M., Tanaka, A.: Studies on ectopic ACTH-producing tumours. IV. CRF-like activity in tumour tissues. Acta Endocrinol. 82, 183-192 (1976).

22. Birkenhäger, J.G., Upton, G.V., Seldenrath, H.J., Krieger, D.T., Tashjian, A.H.: Medullary thyroid carcinoma: Ectopic production of peptides with ACTH-like, corticotropin-releasing factor-like, and prolactin-stimulating activities. Acta Endocrinol. 83, 280-292 (1976).

23. Suda, T., Demura, H., Demura, R., Wakabayashi, I., Nomura, K., Odagiri, E., Shizume, K.: Corticotropin-releasing factor-like, activity in ectopic ACTH-producing tumors. J. clin. Endocrinol. Metab. 44, 440-446 (1977).

24. Hashimoto, K., Takahara, J., Ogawa, N., Yunoki, S., Ofuji, T., Arata, A., Kanda, S., Terada, K.: Adrenocorticotropin, β-lipotropin, β-endorphin, and corticotropin-releasing factor-like activity in an adrenocorticotropin-producing nephroblastoma. J. clin. Endocrinol. Metab. 50, 461-465 (1980).

25. Hirata, Y., Yamamoto, H., Matsukura, S., Imura, H.: In vitro release and biosynthesis of tumor ACTH in ectopic ACTH-producing tumors. J. clin. Endocrinol. Metab. 41, 106-114 (1975).

26. Hirata, Y., Yoshimi, H., Matsukura, S., Imura, H.: Effect of hypothalamic extract and other factors on release of adrenocorticotropin from and cyclic AMP in dispersed non-pituitary tumor cells. J. clin. Endocrinol. Metab. 49, 317-321 (1979).

27. Rees, L.H., Bloomfield, G.A., Gilkes, J.J.H., Jeffcoate, W.J., Besser, G.M.: ACTH as a tumor marker. Ann. N.Y. Acad. Sci. 297, 603-620 (1977).

28. Schteingart, D.E., Conn, J.W., Orth, D.N., Harrison, T.S., Fox, F.E., Bookstein, J.J.: Secretion of ACTH and β-MSH by an adrenal medullary paraganglioma. J. clin. Endocrinol. Metab. 34, 676-683 (1972).

29. Spark, R.F., Connolly, P.B., Gluckin, D.S., White, R., Sacks, B., Landsberg, L.: ACTH secretion from a functioning pheochromocytoma. New Engl. J. Med. 301, 416-418 (1979).

30. Findling, J.W., Aron, D.C., Tyrrell, J.B., Shinsako, J.H., Fitzgerald, P.A., Norman, D., Wilson, C.B., Forsham, P.H.: Selective venous sampling for ACTH in Cushing's syndrome: Differentiation between Cushing's disease and the ectopic ACTH syndrome. Ann. intern. Med. 94, 647-652 (1981).

31. Gropp, C., Havemann, K., Schever, A.: Ectopic hormones in lung cancer patients at diagnosis and during therapy. Cancer 46, 347-354 (1980).

32. Goldenberg, D.M., DeLand, F., Kim, E.E., Bennet, S., Primus, F.J., Van Nagell, J.R., Estes, N., DeSimone, P., Rayburn, P.: Use of radiolabeled antibodies to carcinoembryonic antigen for the detection of diverse cancers by external photoscanning. New Engl. J. Med. 298, 1384-1388 (1978).

33. Goldenberg, D.M., Kim, E.E., DeLand, F., Spremulli, E., Nelson, M.O., Gockerman, J.P., Primus, F.J., Corgan, R.C., Alpert, E.: Clinical studies on the radioimmunodetection of tumors containing alpha-fetoprotein. Cancer 45, 2500-2505 (1980).

34. Goldenberg, D.M., Kim, E.E., DeLand, F., Van Nagell, J.R., Javadpour, N.: Clinical radioimmunodetection of cancer with radioactive antibodies to human chorionic gonadotropin. Science 208, 1284-1286 (1980).

35. Carey, R.M., Orth, D.N., Hartmann, W.H.: Malignant melanoma with ectopic production of adrenocorticotropic hormone: Palliative treatment with inhibitors of adrenal steroid biosynthesis. J. clin. Endocrinol. Metab. 36, 482-487 (1973).

36. Orth, D.N., Nicholson, W.E., Mitchell, W.M., Island, D.P., Liddle, G.W.: Biologic and immunologic characterization and physical separation of ACTH and ACTH fragments in the ectopic ACTH syndrome. J. clin. Invest. 52, 1756-1769 (1973).

37. Abe, K., Island, D.P., Liddle, G.W., Fleischer, N., Nicholson, W.E.: Radioimmunologic evidence for α-MSH in human pituitary and tumor tissues. J. clin. Endocrinol. Metab. 27, 46-52 (1967).

38. Scott, A.P., Ratcliffe, J.G., Rees, L.H., Landon, J., Benett, P.J., Lowry, P.J., McMartin, C.: Pituitary peptide. Nature 44, 65-67 (1973).

39. Ratcliffe, J.G., Scott, A.P., Benett, P.J., Coary, P.J., McMartin, C., Strong, J.A., Walbaum, P.R.: Production of a corticotrophin-like intermediate lobe peptide and of corticotrophin by a bronchial carcinoid. Clin. Endocr. 2, 51 55 (1973).

40. Silman, R.E., Chard, T., Lowry, P.J., Smith, I., Young, I.M.: Human foetal pituitary peptides and parturition. Nature 260, 716-718 (1976).

41. Tanaka, N., Abe, K., Miyakawa, S., Ohnami, S., Tanaka, M., Takeuchi, T.: Analysis of human pituitary and tumor adrenocorticotropin using isoelectric focusing. J. clin. Endocrinol. Metab. 48, 559-565 (1979).

42. Lowry, P.J., Rees, L.H., Tomlin, S., Gilkes, J.J.H., Landon, J.: Chemical characterization of ACTH purified from a malignant carcinoid tumor. J. clin. Endocrinol. Metab. 43, 831-835 (1976).

43. Hirata, Y., Matsukura, S., Imura, H., Nakamura, M., Tanaka, A.: Size heterogeneity of β-MSH in ectopic ACTH-producing tumors: Presence of β-LPH-like peptide. J. clin. Endocrinol. Metab. 42, 33-40 (1976).

44. Tanaka, K., Nicholson, W.E., Orth, D.N.: The nature of the immunoreactive lipotropins in human plasma and tissue extracts. J. clin. Invest. 62, 94-104 (1978).

45. Gilkes, J.J.H., Rees, L.H., Besser, G.M.: Relationship between plasma immunoreactive ACTH and LPH in Cushing's syndrome and Addison's disease. Brit. med. J. 1, 996-998 (1977).

46. Ueda, J., Takeuchi, T., Abe, K., Miyakawa, S., Ohnami, S., Yanaihara, N.: β-Melanocyte-stimulating hormone immunoreactivity in human pituitaries and ectopic adrenocorticotropin-producing tumors. J. clin. Endocrinol. Metab. 50, 550-556 (1980).

47. Hughes, J., Smith, T.W., Kosterlitz, H.W., Fothergill, L.A., Morgan, B.A., Morris, H.R.: Identification of two related pentapeptides from the brain with potent opiate agonist activity. Nature 258, 577-579 (1975).

48. Goldstein, A.: Opioid peptides in pituitary and brain. Science 193, 1081-1086 (1976).

49. Orth, D.N., Guillemin, R., Ling, N., Nicholson, W.E.: Immunoreactive endorphins, lipotropins and corticotropins in a human nonpituitary tumor. J. clin. Endocrinol. Metab. 46, 849-852 (1978).

50. Bertagna, X., Nicholson, W.E., Sorenson, G.D., Pottengill, O.S., Mount, C.D., Orth, D.N.: Corticotropin, lipotropin, and β-endorphin production by a human nonpituitary tumor in culture. Proc. natn. Acad. Sci. U.S.A. 75, 5160-5164 (1978).

51. Yoshimi, H., Matsukura, S., Sueoka, S., Yokota, M., Hirata, Y., Fujita, T.: Concomitant production of β-endorphin in ectopic ACTH/β-LPH-producing tumors. Endocrinol.jap. 27, 129-135 (1980).

52. Loh, H.H., Tseng, L.F., Wei, E., Li, C.H.: β-Endorphin is a potent analgesic agent. Proc. natn. Acad. Sci. U.S.A. 73, 2895-2898 (1976).

53. Bloom, F., Segal, D., Ling, N., Guillemin, R.: Endorphin: Profound behavioral effects in rats suggest new etiological factors in mental illness. Science 194, 630-632 (1976).

54. Yalow, R.S., Berson, R.A.: Size heterogeneity of immunoreactive human ACTH in plasma and in extracts of pituitary gland and ACTH-producing thymoma. Biochem. biophys. Res. Commun. 44, 439-445 (1971).

55. Gewirtz, G., Schneider, B., Krieger, D.T., Yalow, R.S.: Big ACTH: Conversion to biologically active ACTH by trypsin. J. clin. Endocrinol. Metab. 38, 227-230 (1974).

56. Sueoka, S., Matsukura, S., Yoshimi, H., Yokota, M., Hirata, Y., Fujita, T.: High molecular weight forms of immunoreactive ACTH in a human pituitary and ectopic ACTH-producing tumors. Endocrinol. jap. 27, 405-410 (1980).

57. Orth, D.N., Nicholson, W.E.: High molecular weight forms of human ACTH are glycoproteins. J. clin. Endocrinol. Metab. 44, 214-217 (1977).

58. Mains, R.E., Eipper, B.A.: Biosynthesis of adrenocorticotropic hormone in mouse pituitary tumor cells. J. biol. Chem. 251, 4115-4120 (1976).

59. Eipper, B.A., Mains, R.E., Guenigi, D.: High molecular weight forms of adrenocorticotropic hormone are glycoproteins. J. biol. Chem. 251, 4121-4126 (1976).

60. Eipper, B.A., Mains, R.E.: Peptide analysis of a glycoprotein form of adrenocorticotropic hormone. J. biol. Chem. 252, 8821-8832 (1977).

61. Himsworth, R.L., Bloomfield, G.A., Coombes, R.C., Ellison, M., Gilkes, J.J.H., Lowry, P.J., Stechell, K.D.R., Slavin, G., Rees, L.H.: 'Big' ACTH and calcitonin in an ectopic hormone secreting tumour of the liver. Clin. Endocr. 7, 45-62 (1977).

62. Mains, R.E., Eipper, B.A., Ling, N.: Common precursor to corticotropins and endorphins. Proc. natn. Acad. Sci. U.S.A. 54, 3014-3018 (1977).

63. Mains, R.E., Eipper, B.A.: Coordinate synthesis of corticotropins and endorphins by mouse pituitary tumor cells. J. biol. Chem. 253, 651-655 (1978).

64. Roberts, J.L., Herbert, E.: Characterization of a common precursor to corticotropin and β-lipotropin: Cell-free synthesis of the precursor and identification of corticotropin peptides in the molecule. Proc. natn. Acad. Sci. U.S.A. 74, 4826-4830 (1977).

65. Roberts, J.L., Herbert, E.: Characterization of a common precursor to corticotropin and β-lipotropin: Identification of β-lipotropin and their arrangement relative to corticotropin in the precursor synthesized in a cell-free system. Proc. natn. Acad. Sci. U.S.A. 74, 5300-5304 (1977).

66. Nakanishi, S., Inoue, A., Taii, S., Numa, S.: Cell-free translation product containing corticotropin and β-endorphin encoded by messenger RNA from anterior lobe and intermediate lobe of bovine pituitary. FEBS Lett. 84, 105-109 (1977).

67. Nakanishi, S., Inoue, A., Kita, T., Nakamura, M., Chang, A.C.Y., Cohen, S.N., Numa, S.: Nucleotide sequence of cloned cDNA for bovine corticotropin-β-lipotropin precursor. Nature 278, 423-427 (1979).

68. Tanaka, I., Nakai, Y., Jingami, H., Fukata, J., Nakao, K., Oki, S., Nakanishi, S., Numa, S., Imura, H.: Existence of γ-melanotropin-like immunoreactivity in bovine and human pituitary glands. Biochem. biophys. Res. Commun. 94, 211-217 (1980).

69. Shibasaki, T., Ling, N., Guillemin, R.: Pituitary immunoreactive γ-melanotropins are glycosylated oligopeptides. Nature 285, 416-417 (1980).

70. Nakai, Y., Tanaka, I., Fukata, J., Nakao, K., Oki, S., Takai, S., Imura, H.: Evidence for γ-MSH-like immunoreactivity in ectopic ACTH-producing tumors. J. clin. Endocrinol. Metab. 50, 1147-1148 (1980).

71. Tsukuda, T., Nakai, Y., Jingami, H., Imura, H., Taii, S., Nakanishi, S., Numa, S.: Identification of the mRNA coding for the ACTH-β-lipotropin precursor in a human ectopic ACTH-producing tumor. Biochem. biophys. Res. Commun. 98, 535-540 (1981).

72. Wolfsen, A.R., Odell, W.D.: ProACTH: Use for early detection of lung cancer. Am. J. Med. 66, 765-772 (1979).

73. Odell, W.D., Wolfsen, A.R., Bachelot, I., Hirose, F.M.: Ectopic production of lipotropin by cancer. Am. J. Med. 66, 631-638 (1979).

74. Bloomfield, G.A., Holdaway, I.M., Corrin, B., Ratcliffe, J.G., Rees, G.M., Ellison, M., Rees, L.H.: Lung tumours and ACTH production. Clin. Endocr. 6, 95-104 (1977).

75. Rees, L.H., Bloomfield, G.A., Rees, G.M., Corrin, B., Franks, L.M., Ratcliffe, J.G.: Multiple hormones in a bronchial tumor. J. clin. Endocrinol. Metab. 38, 1090-1097 (1974).

76. Hirata, Y., Matsukura, S., Imura, H., Yakura, T., Ihjima, S., Nagase, C., Itoh, M.: Two cases of multiple hormone-producing small cell carcinoma of the lung: Coexistence of tumor ADH, ACTH, and β-MSH. Cancer 38, 2575-2582 (1976).

77. Coscia, N., Brown, R.D., Miller, M., Tanaka, K., Nicholson, W.E., Parks, K.R., Orth, D.N.: Ectopic production of antidiuretic hormone (ADH), adrenocorticotrophic hormone (ACTH) and beta-melanocyte stimulating hormone (β-MSH) by an oat cell carcinoma of the lung. Am. J. Med. 62, 303-307 (1977).

78. Abe, K., Adachi, I., Miyakawa, S., Tanaka, M., Yamaguchi, K., Tanaka, N., Kameya, T., Simosato, Y.: Production of calcitonin, ACTH and β-MSH in tumors derived from amine precursor uptake and decarboxylation cells. Cancer Res. 37, 4190-4194 (1977).

79. Pearse, A.G.E.: Common cytochemical and ultrastructural characteristics of cell producing polypeptide hormones (the APUD series) and their relevance to thyroid and ultimobranchial C cells and calcitonin. Proc. roy. Soc. B 170, 71-80 (1969).

80. Azzopardi, J.G., Williams, E.D.: Pathology of 'nonendocrine' tumors associated with Cushing's syndrome. Cancer 22, 274-286 (1968).

81. Besch, K.G., Corrin, B., Pariente, R., Spencer, H.: Oat-cell carcinoma of the lung: Its origin and relationship to bronchial carcinoid. Cancer 22, 1163-1172 (1968).

82. Skrabanek, P., Powell, D.: Unifying concept of non-pituitary ACTH-secreting tumors - evidence of common origin of neural-crest tumors, carcinoids and oat-cell carcinoma. Cancer 42, 1263-1269 (1978).

83. Weichert, R.F. III.: The neural ectodermal origin of the peptide-secreting endocrine glands: A unifying concept for the etiology of multiple endocrine adenomatosis and the inappropriate secretion of peptide hormones by nonendocrine tumors. Am. J. Med. 49, 232-241 (1970).

84. Britten, R.J., Davidson, E.H.: Gene regulation for higher cells - a theory. Science 165, 349-357 (1969).

85. Williams, E.D.: Tumours, hormones, and cellular differentiation. Lancet 2, 1108 (1969).

86. Warner, T.F.C.S.: Cell hybridisation in the genesis of ectopic hormone-secreting tumours. Lancet 1, 1259-1260 (1974).

PARATHYROID HORMONE IN HUMAN TISSUES

H. W. Minne and R. Ziegler
Abteilung Innere Medizin VI - Endokrinologie - Universitäts-kliniken Heidelberg, Luisenstrasse 5, D 6900 Heidelberg, Federal Republic of Germany

Introduction

Parathyroid Hormone (PTH) is produced by both normal and hyperplastic parathyroid glands, and also by parathyroid tumours. These tissues secrete the hormone directly into the blood stream, which transports it to target tissues via the circulation. Specific receptors then bind the hormone, and this results in a cascade of specific cell functions. At the same time, the hormone molecule is cleaved into fragments; this fragmentation accompanies either activation or inactivation of the hormone - the exact details, however, remain largely unsolved.

Certain malignant tumours also synthesize and secrete PTH or PTH-like peptides, thus causing paraneoplastic hypercalcemia. This aggravates the clinical course of the malignant tumour. Tumour PTH seems to differ from parathyroid tissue PTH as far as immunoreactivity is concerned; its biological properties, however, resemble those of the endogenous hormone.

This review deals with both endogenous and tumour PTH, and describes:

- parathyroid hormone synthesis and secretion by parathyroid tissues, and the interaction of the hormone with target tissues;

- paraneoplastic PTH secretion by malignant tumours of non-endocrine origin.

Hormones in Normal and Abnormal Human Tissues, Vol. III

1. Synthesis, Secretion, and Peripheral Metabolism of Parathyroid Tissue PTH

Transfer of information from the parathyroid cell genome to the secretory granule leads to the synthesis of "pre-pro-parathyroid hormone" (1, 2, 3). It is transformed to the 90 aminoacid "pro-parathyroid hormone", following the cleaving off of 25 amino-acids from the aminoterminus of the molecule. A further six aminoacids are cleaved from the prohormone during its transport to the Golgi apparatus (4) and subsequently into secretory granules (5). This process takes 20 to 30 minutes (6).

The newly synthesised hormone, consisting of 84 aminoacids, is then secreted into the blood stream in a calcium dependent manner (7, 8). This has been demonstrated many times in vivo (9, 10) as well as in vitro (11, 12); low concentrations of extracellular calcium stimulate, and high concentrations inhibit PTH release from the parathyroid cell. This applies not only to normal parathyroid tissue, but also to tumorous parathyroid tissue - where the secretion of the hormone is inhibited to the same extent, but by higher than normal calcium concentrations (13, 14).

Besides calcium, a variety of other factors have been demonstrated to modulate PTH release from the parathyroid cell, both in vivo and in vitro (15, 16, 17, 18, 19); β-adrenergic agents, vitamin D and its metabolites, gastrointestinal hormones and other compounds are examples of such agents.

Hanson (20) and Collip (21) were the first to extract PTH from bovine parathyroid tissue in 1925; 34 years later, the bovine hormone was isolated in a highly purified state (22, 23), which was a prerequisite for analysis of the hormone's aminoacid sequence (24, 25). Whereas the bovine PTH was isolated from parathyroid glands, human hormone preparations are derived from parathyroid adenomas and hyperplastic parathyroid glands. Human PTH has been analysed step by step, firstly the aminoterminal fragment 1-34 (26, 27), and then the whole molecule. Full information about the composition and aminoacid sequence of human, bovine and porcine PTH is now at our disposal (28, 29, 30).

The three parathyroid hormones (human, bovine and porcine) are identical in length, but different in aminoacid composition and sequence. These differences are responsible for divergent immunoreactivity, thus creating incomplete cross-reactivity of one PTH with antibodies raised against the other. Human PTH has less bioactivity than the other two. A PTH peptide chain, consisting of the first 27 aminoterminal aminoacids is required to develop any biological activity at all. A PTH peptide consisting of the first 34 aminoterminal aminoacids has a biological activity equivalent to the complete PTH molecule, which consists of 84 aminoacids (31). The biological function of the carboxyterminal region of the PTH molecule is at present unknown.

Radioimmunological serum PTH analyses, at first gave confusing results. Berson and Yalow (32) demonstrated in 1968 that different radioimmunoassay techniques detected not only different levels of hormone, but also differences in disappearance rates; the latter also changed after removal of the parathyroid gland or tumour, if different radioimmunoassay procedures were applied. This heterogeneity of circulating immunologically detectable PTH (iPTH) as well as the demonstration that the biological activity of the hormone is represented by a mere 34 of the 84 amino acid peptide chain, gave rise to extensive research.

The injection of intact hormone to animals and the follow-up of the biochemical pathways did not contribute much to the solution, because the results described exogenous hormone degradation, which does not necessarily equate with endogenous hormone physiology. Nevertheless, it allowed the conclusion that the organism is able to produce PTH fragments from intact radioiodinated exogenous PTH (33). This cleavage at the sequence positions 33-34 and 36-37 produces both the aminoterminal and the carboxyterminal PTH fragments. The carboxyterminal fragment was identified as being around 4000 to 6000 Daltons. These carboxyterminal fragments were dominant in the peripheral circulation. The occurrence of peripheral hormone cleavage was obvious as the parathyroid gland itself is known to secrete, more or less exclusively, intact 1-84 PTH. However, this was true in a limited sense only, and one has to stress again that experiments involving labelled hormone injections demonstrate exogenous hormone pathways, and not endogenous hormone metabolism. Moreover, radioiodinated hormone is of doubtful biological relevance, if the Hunter and Greenwood Chloramine T procedure (34) has been applied, as has been done in the study referred to.

The analyses of iPTH in rat, chicken, and dog have never demonstrated such an accumulation of fragments under normal conditions; the percentage of fragments did not rise to above 20% of the intact hormone concentration in these animals (35, 36). In hypersecretory states and under hormone secretion stimulating conditions, parathyroid glands and tumours not only release intact PTH 1-84 but also carboxyterminal PTH fragments to a remarkable extent (14, 37, 38, 39).

Therefore, under normal conditions, parathyroid glands release intact PTH; in hyperfunctioning states the tissue releases intact PTH as well as PTH fragments. The latter seems to be independent of the reasons for hyperfunction: one finds it in parathyroid adenomas as well as in normal glands reacting to a decrease in circulating ionized calcium (37, 38, 39, 40). This contributes to heterogeneity of iPTH in serum samples of patients with hyperparathyroidism. Another source derives from peripheral cleavage of the intact PTH 1-84 (see below).

PTH action on target tissues is linked to its binding to specific cell receptors. This initiates a cascade of cellular metabolic processes. Therefore, target tissue receptors are bifunctional: firstly, they <u>recognize</u> a hormone, and then after recognition and binding, they <u>cause</u> hormone mediated cell activity (41).

The study of hormone - receptor interactions requires the use of isotope labelled hormone preparations. The integrity of such tracer bioactivity is of great importance as in the studies designed to follow up biochemical pathways of PTH. Three different approaches have been described in this respect:

- non-oxidative preparation of tritiated PTH derivatives (42, 43, 44),
- hormone iodination using the lactoperoxidase reaction (45) or electrolytic labelling (46, 47, 48),
- the synthesis of bovine PTH 1-34 with norleucine instead of methionine at positions 8 and 18, which is biologically stable even after chloramine T labelling (49) or with iodinated thyrosinamine at position 34 (50).

The labelled peptide needs additional purification to remove biologically inactive products of the reaction or synthesis prior to receptor studies (41). This is performed applying receptor binding to renal cell membranes (51).

Other possible sources of error concern membrane (i.e. receptor) preparation. In addition, one has to prove that the binding of the hormone preparation to the receptor does in fact cause a specific response, namely, activation of adenylate cyclase to produce cyclic AMP, which serves as the second messenger in the target tissue. Studies also permit analysis of mechanisms of hormone - receptor adenylate cyclase coupling; such experiments provided evidence initially that a membrane associated GTP binding protein exists, and modulates the response to hormone binding (41, 52).

Renal PTH receptors have been studied extensively (41, 52). They have two functions: they recognize (i.e. bind) the appropriate hormone (discriminator function), and, after hormone binding, they initiate specific actions (coupling function). The specificity of the reaction has been proven: the binding of a PTH antagonist (53), which is an analogue of PTH 1-34, to a PTH receptor occurs without stimulation of the specific response (i.e. activation of adenylate cyclase).

Whereas _in vivo_ studies (isolated perfused canine bone) have pointed to a difference in principle between skeletal and renal PTH receptors, initial studies with bone cells, isolated from embryonic chick calvaria, have demonstrated that these receptors possess affinity and selectivity properties similar to those of renal PTH receptors (41, 54, 55). A distinctive characteristic of skeletal PTH receptors remains to be established (41).

Synthesis and secretion on the one hand, and receptor binding and adenylate cyclase activation by target tissue on the other hand, show the path followed by PTH from its formation to the biological function transmitted by the hormone. The peripheral metabolism of the hormone itself is again the product of interaction between tissues and PTH. In part, the tissues which bind the hormone as first messenger are the same as the tissues which bind the hormone to metabolize it. Nevertheless, there is no obvious link between hormone cleavage and hormone mediated activation of the second messenger.

Besides the parathyroid glands, which in hyperfunctioning states contribute to the circulating PTH fragments (14, 37, 38, 39), target tissues and cells, located in the liver (which possibly are target cells too), cleave the PTH molecule. Analyses of serum samples applying gel filtration have demonstrated that the size of the fragments, which occur after the injection of exogenous PTH, is the same as that of the fragments which are produced by cleavage of the endogenous hormone. The measurable fragments consist primarily of middle and carboxyterminal parts of the molecule (56, 57, 58, 59, 60, 61).

The liver contributes more than other organs to this PTH cleavage (33, 57, 61, 62, 63). The fact that this cleavage is calcium dependent, means that high calcium levels inhibit the production of fragments, whereas low calcium levels enhance it (57). The first autographs of liver sections following contact with isotope labelled PTH showed a tendency of hormone accumulation near the sinusoids (47). Further studies demonstrated that the Kupffer cells accumulated the hormone (64). Whether Kupffer cells initiate PTH cleavage, or whether this process describes Kupffer cells as PTH target cells, remains open to question. The latter points towards possible PTH mediated activation of macrophages to ingest bone particles (36).

The kidney removes both the PTH fragments and intact hormone from the circulation. First observations concerning arterio-venous gradients through the organ were revealed after injection of bovine PTH extracts into normal dogs (59, 61), and also by means of iPTH analyses in serum samples of patients with primary hyperparathyroidism, who had undergone selective venous catheterisation for parathyroid adenoma localisation (65).

Following the injection of synthetic bovine PTH 1-34 into dogs, the kidneys account for about 45% of the metabolic clearance rate of the hormone fragments (59). The biologically active intact PTH molecule and the aminoterminal PTH fragment are both removed by peritubular uptake, whereas glomerular filtration eliminates the carboxyterminal PTH fragment (66). Studies in patients with renal transplantation confirmed this in man. One has to keep in mind that these processes are possibly independent of specific PTH actions on the kidneys which are receptor mediated. Nevertheless, the importance of renal function for the removal of carboxyterminal PTH fragments is obvious. In renal insufficiency, these fragments accumulate independently of the PTH bioactivity detectable in the organism; this gives high iPTH values in serum samples, if radioimmunoassays for the carboxyterminal PTH fragments are applied. Under such conditions, there is an enormous discrepancy between PTH C - immunoreactivity on the one hand, and PTH bioactivity on the other. This has been substantiated by bioassay determinations in comparison with the analyses of PTH immunoreactivity (67, 68). The establishment of PTH bioassays, which are able to measure PTH bioactivity in serum samples, had been a prerequisite for these investigations.

Isolated perfused bone (canine tibia) takes up a significant amount of aminoterminal PTH fragment; at the same time, cyclic AMP release from bone increases. Intact PTH is ineffective in this respect. Activation of bone adenylate cyclase is receptor mediated (41, 54). Osteoblastic and progenitor cells, which form a layer at the external surface of incubated mouse calvaria, bind aminoterminal PTH fragments specifically, and then the activation of the adenylate cyclase occurs (54, 55). Bone has not been described as being of importance for PTH cleavage or degradation and elimination from the circulation.

In brief, parathyroid tissue synthesizes and secretes PTH, which is bound by target tissue receptors; the specific effect is thus mediated. Extraction of the hormone is worth while only from parathyroid glands or parathyroid tumours. The hormone is cleaved by cells located in the liver; the hormone and its fragments are eliminated from the circulation by the kidney.

2. Paraneoplastic PTH Secretion by Malignant Tumours of Non-Endocrine Origin

In the communication by F. Albright in 1941, the opening sentence referred to the factor which is responsible for paraneoplastic hypercalcemia in malignant tumour diseases; it stated "I suspected that the tumour (a renal cancer, which had caused hypercalcemia and hypophosphatemia in the patient) might be producing parathyroid hormone. I therefore had it assayed by Dr. J.B. Collip, but no hormone was found" (69). Fifteen years after the first removal of a parathyroid tumour which had caused von Recklinghausen's "Ostitis fibrosa generalisata"(i.e. primary hyperparathyroidism) by Mandl (70), Albright speculated on the ability of malignant tumours of non-endocrine origin to synthesize and secrete PTH. Collip, however, was unable to demonstrate PTH-like bioactivity in the tumour extracts, but which he had been able to do in parathyroid gland extracts (21, 71).

The significance of such paraneoplastic hyperparathyroidism as the origin of paraneoplastic hypercalcemia was in doubt for many years. After a lengthy period of inactivity, prostaglandins and the Osteoclast Activating Factor, which had previously dominated the scene as supposed originator of this paraneoplastic hypercalcemia, PTH or PTH-like bioactivity again placed itself in the foreground.

In the beginning, the unfolding of knowledge seemed to happen in a plausible way: in 1923, Klemperer observed a patient with mammary cancer who suffered from a bone disease (72), which was similar to that described by Strada (1909) (73), Bauer (1911) (74) and Tomaszewski (1914) (75), who had studied Recklinghausens Ostitis fibrosa generalisata. In 1926, Mandl removed the first parathyroid adenoma (70); in 1930, Barr and Bulger drew attention to the concept of hyperparathyroidism (76) and in 1931, Mason and Warren applied this concept to malignant tumour dependent bone disease, believing that a tumour might stimulate endogenous PTH release. Finally, Albright postulated that a tumour might produce PTH by itself and independently from the parathyroids. Collip's lack of success in demonstrating the hormone by bioassay did not impede this.

Albright's idea was again confirmed 15 years later (77), and, subsequently, a large variety of malignant tumours were blamed for paraneoplastic PTH secretion; among those quoted were cancers of the pharynx (78), oesophagus (79), colon (80), liver (81), bladder (82), ovaries (83), vagina (84), vulva (85), and uterus (86), sarcoma of the uterus (87), pheochromocytoma (88), Hodgkin's disease (89), leukaemia (90) and others.

It cannot be excluded that, in some of the patients described, there could have been coincidence of a malignant tumour and primary hyperparathyroidism. The list just quoted does, however, give some impression regarding the variety of such tumours. A synopsis of 50 (91), and another of an additional 23 (92) patients with paraneoplastic hyperparathyroidism describe a prevalence of bronchus and renal cancers (60% of the 73 tumours).

Some findings in such patients make conclusive statements difficult:

- one finds relatively low or even suppressed iPTH values in serum samples, irrespective of the actual radioimmunoassay applied (93, 94, 95, 96),

- extraction of PTH from such tumours yields only very small quantities of the hormone (97). This is in agreement with findings in patients who suffer from ACTH secreting bronchial cancer (98).

Therefore, the secretion of abnormal PTH by malignant tumours has been discussed. The search for humoral hypercalcemic tumour products other than PTH has been successful. The competing candidates are:

- prostaglandins, which have been demonstrated to cause hypercalcemia in patients (95, 96) and a respective animal model (99, 100),
- Vitamin D-like steroids (101),
- the Osteoclast Activating Factor (OAF), which has been demonstrated in patients with myeloma (102, 103) and was accepted as being a lymphokine of physiological importance (104).

Recently, Stewart and coworkers have published data obtained in patients and they returned to Albright's hypothesis - which was that a tumour might produce a peptide which acted like PTH with respect to calcium phosphate and renal cAMP excretion. The only problem is missing PTH immunoreactivity (105). Similar data were found in a respective animal model (106). This points to the possibility that tumours secrete a type of PTH which lacks or possesses decreased immunoreactivity (93, 94); this has been demonstrated in patients, and also in rats with the transplantable hypercalcemic Walker carcinosarcoma 256 (107) (which serves as a useful model for the disease) (108). This also reminds one that radioimmunoassays sometimes create more problems than they solve.

The animal models for paraneoplastic hypercalcemia (99, 109, 110), which have now been established, will allow additional work to be carried out in order to further analyse the disease, but it seems as if there will be a long way to go before all the viewpoints of v. Virchows (1855) on paraneoplastic bone disease (111) are elucidated.

References

1. Dorner, A.J., Kemper, B.: Formation in vitro of membrane-bound polysomes containing parathyroid hormone messenger ribonucleic acid. Biochemistry 24, 5496-5501 (1979).

2. Kemper, B., Habener, J.F., Mulligan, R.C., Potts, J.T., Rich, A.: Preparathyroid hormone: A direct translation product of parathyroid messenger RNA. Proc. natn. Acad. Sci. U.S.A. 71, 3731-3735 (1974).

3. Potts, J.T., Kronenberg, H.M., Habener, J.F., Rich, A.: Biosynthesis of parathyroid hormone. Ann. N.Y. Acad. Sci. 343, 38-55 (1980).

4. Cohn, D.V., MacGregor, R.R., Chu, L.L.H., Kimmel, J.R., Hamilton, J.W.: Calcemic fraction A: biosynthetic peptide precursor of parathyroid hormone. Proc. natn. Acad. Sci. U.S.A. 69, 1521-1525 (1972).

5. Chu, L.L.H., MacGregor, R.R., Hamilton, J.W., Cohn, D.V.: Conversion of proparathyroid hormone to parathyroid hormone: The use of amines as specific inhibitors. Endocrinology 95, 1431-1438 (1974).

6. Cohn, D.V., Morrissey, J.J., Hamilton, J.W., Chu, L.L.H., MacGregor, R.R.: Secretion of parathyroid hormone from two independently controlled intracellular pools. In: "Hormonal Control of Calcium Metabolism", Eds. Cohn, D.V., Talmage, R.V., Les Matthews, J.L., International Congress Series 511, Excerpta Medica, Amsterdam-Oxford-Princeton, pp. 28-34 (1981).

7. Sherwood, L.M., Mayer, G.P., Ramberg, C.F., Kronfeld, D.S., Aurbach, G.D., Potts, J.T.: Regulation of parathyroid hormone secretion: proportional control by calcium, lack of effect of phosphate. Endocrinology 83, 1043-1051 (1968).

8. Sherwood, L.M., Potts, J.T., Care, A.D., Mayer, G.P., Aurbach, G.D.: Evaluation by radioimmunoassay of factors controlling the secretion of parathyroid hormone. Nature (London), 209, 52-55 (1966).

9. Arnaud, C.D., Littledike, T., Tsao, H.S.: Calcium homeostasis and the simultaneous measurement of calcitonin and parathyroid hormone in the pig. In: "Calcitonin", Eds. Taylor, S.F., Foster, G., Proceedings of the Second International Symposium, London 21-24 July, 1969, William Heinemann Medical Books Ltd., London, pp. 95-101 (1970).

10. Arnaud, C.D., Tsao, H.S., Littledike, T.: Radioimmunoassay of human parathyroid in serum. J. clin. Invest. 50, 21-34 (1971).

11. Au, W.Y., Poland, A.P., Stern, P.H., Raisz, L.G.: Hormone synthesis and secretion by rat parathyroid glands in tissue culture. J. clin. Invest. 49, 1639-1646 (1970).

12. Hamilton, J.W., Cohn, D.V.: Studies on the Biosynthesis in vitro of parathyroid hormone. J. biol. Chem. 244, 5421-5429 (1969).

13. Brown, E.M., Brennan, M.F., Hurwitz, S., Windeck, R., Marx, S.J., Spiegel, A.M., Koehler, J.O., Gardner, D.G., Aurbach, G.D.: Dispersed cells prepared from human parathyroid glands: District calcium sensitivity of adenomas vs. primary hyperplasia. J. clin. Endocrinol. Metab. 46, 267-275 (1978).

14. Habener, J.F.: Responsiveness of neoplastic and hyperplastic parathyroid tissues to calcium in vitro. J. clin. Invest. 62, 436-450 (1978).

15. Brown, E.M., Hurwitz, S., Aurbach, G.D.: Beta-Adrenergic stimulation of cyclic AMP content and parathyroid hormone release from isolated bovine parathyroid cells. Endocrinology 100, 1696-1702 (1977).

16. Brown, E.M., Hurwitz, S., Woodward, C.J., Aurbach, D.: Direct identification of beta-adrenergic receptors on isolated bovine parathyroid cells. Endocrinology 100, 1703-1709 (1977).

17. Canterbury, J.M., Lerman, S.: Inhibition of parathyroid hormone secretion by 25-Hydroxycholecalciferol in the dog. J. clin. Invest. 61, 1375-1383 (1978).

18. Fischer, J.A., Blum, J.W.: Acute parathyroid hormone response to epinephrine in vivo. J. clin. Invest. 52, 2434-2440 (1973).

19. Peck, W.A., Klahr, S.: Cyclic nucleotides in bone and mineral metabolism. In: "Advances in Cyclic Nucleotide Research", vol. 11, Eds. Greengard, P., Robinson, G.A., Raven Press, New York, pp. 89-124 (1979).

20. Hanson, A.M.: The hormone of the parathyroid glands. Proc. Soc. exp. Biol. Med. 22, 560 (1925).

21. Collip, J.B.: The extraction of a parathyroid hormone which will prevent or control parathyroid tetanie. J. biol. Chem. 113, 395 (1925).

22. Aurbach, G.D.: Isolation of parathyroid hormone after extraction with phenol. J. biol. Chem. 234, 3179-3181 (1959).

23. Rasmussen, H., Craig, L.C.: Purification of parathyroid hormone by use of counter-current distribution. J. Amer. chem. Soc. 81, 5003 (1959).

24. Brewer, H.B., Ronan, R.: Bovine parathyroid hormone: Aminoacid sequence. Proc. natn. Acad. Sci. U.S.A. 67, 1862-1869 (1970).

25. Niall, H.D., Keutmann, H.T., Sauer, R.T., Hogan, M.L., Dawson, B.F., Aurbach, C.T., Potts, J.T.: The aminoacid sequence of bovine parathyroid hormone. Hoppe-Seyler's Z. physiol. Chem. 94, 367 (1970).

26. Brewer, H.B., Fairwell, T., Ronan, R., Sizemore, G.W., Arnaud, C.D.: Human parathyroid hormone: amino acid sequence of the amino-terminal residues 1-34. Proc. natn. Acad. Sci. U.S.A. 69, 3585-3588 (1972).

27. Niall, H.D., Sauer, R.T., Jacobs, J.W., Keutzmann, H.T., Segre, G.V., O'Riordan, J.L.H., Aurbach, G.D., Potts, J.T.: The amino-acid sequence of the amino-terminal 37 residues of human parathyroid hormone. Proc. natn. Acad. Sci. U.S.A. 71, 384 (1974).

28. Arnaud, C.D., Drusa, T., Sizemore, G.W., Ritte, W., Fairwell, T., Ronan, R., Brewer, H.B.: Aminoterminal human parathyroid hormone. Biological properties and specific radioimmunoassay. J. clin. Invest. 52, 5 (1973).

29. Arnaud, C.D., Sizemore, G.W., Oldham, S.B., Fischer, J.A., Tsao, H.S., Littledike, E.T.: Human Parathyroid Hormone: Glandular and secreted molecular species. Am. J. Med. 50, 630-638 (1971).

30. Keutmann, H.T.: Chemistry of parathyroid hormone. In: "Endocrinology"2,Eds. DeGroot, L.J., Cahill, C.F., Martini, L., Nelson, D.H., Odell, W.D., Potts, J.T., Steinberger, E., Winegrad, A.I., Grune & Stratton, New York, pp. 593-597(1980).

31. Tregear, G.W., van Rietschoten, J., Greene, E., Keutmann, H.T., Niall, H.D., Reit, B., Parsons, J.A., Potts, J.T.: Stimulation of the adenyl cyclase - cycle AMP system in the thyroid of the rat. Endocrinology 93, 1349-1353 (1973).

32. Berson, S.A., Yalow, R.S.: Immunochemical heterogeneity of parathyroid hormone in plasma. J. clin. Endocrinol. Metab. 28, 1037-1047 (1968).

33. Neuman, W.F., Neuman, M.W., Lane, K., Miller, L.L., Sammon, P.J.: The metabolism of labeled parathyroid hormone. V. Collected biological studies. Calc. Tiss. Res. 18, 271-287 (1975).

34. Hunter, W.M., Greenwood, F.C.: Preparation of iodine - 131 labelled human growth hormone of high specific activity. Nature (London) 194, 495-496 (1962).

35. Neuman, M.W., Neuman, W.F., Lane, K.: Formation of serum disappearance of fragments of parathyroid hormone in the infused dog. Calc. Tiss. Res. 28, 79-81 (1979).

36. Teitelbaum, A.P., Schneider, N., Neuman, W.F.: Relation between peripheral cleavage of parathyroid hormone and its biological activity in kidney. Metab. Bone Dis. Rel. Res. 2, 25-31 (1979).

37. Flueck, J.A., DiBella, F.P., Edis, A.J., Kehrwald, J.M., Arnaud, C.D.: Immunoheterogeneity of parathyroid hormone in venous effluent serum from hyperfunctioning parathyroid glands. J. clin. Invest. 60, 1367-1375 (1977).

38. Hanley, D.A., Takatsuki, K., Sultan, J.M., Schneider, J.M., Sherwood, L.M.: Direct release of parathyroid hormone fragments from functioning bovine parathyroid glands in vitro. J. clin. Invest. 62, 1247-1254 (1978).

39. Mayer, G.P., Keaton, J.A., Hurst, J.G., Habener, J.F.: Effects of plasma calcium concentration on the relative proportion of hormone and carboxyl fragments in parathyroid venous blood. Endocrinology 104, 1778-1884 (1979).

40. Silvermann, R., Yalow, R.S.: Heterogeneity of parathyroid hormone. J. clin. Invest. 52, 1958-1971 (1973).

41. Nissensen, R.A., Teitelbaum, A.P., Abbott, S.R., Pliam, N., Silve, C., Zitzner, L., Nyiredy, K., Arnaud, C.D.: Parathyroid hormone receptors in kidney and bone: relation to adenylate cyclase activation. In: "Hormonal Control of Calcium Metabolism", Eds. Cohn, D.V., Talmage, V.R., Les Matthews, J., International Congress Series 511, Excerpta Medica, Amsterdam-Oxford-Princeton, pp. 44-54 (1981).

42. Chansel, D., Sraer, J., Morgat, J.L., Hesch, R.D., Ardaillou, R.: Preparation of biologically active tritium-labelled 1-34 human parathyroid hormone. FEBS Lett. 78, 237-243 (1977).

43. Zull, J.E., Malbon, C.C., Chuang, J.: Binding of tritiated bovine parathyroid hormone to plasma membranes from bovine kidney cortex. J. biol. Chem. 252, 1071-1078 (1972).

44. Zull, J.E., Repke, D.W.: Studies with tritiated polypeptide hormones. J. biol. Chem. 247, 2183-2188 (1972).

45. Sutcliffe, H.S., Martin, T.J., Eisman, J.A., Pilczyk, R.: Binding of parathyroid hormone to bovine kidney cortex plasma membranes. Biochem. J. 134, 913-921 (1973).

46. diBella, F.P., Drusa, T.P., Miller, S.S., Arnaud, C.D.: Parathyroid hormone receptors of renal cortex. Proc. natn. Acad. Sci. U.S.A. 71, 723-726 (1974).

47. Neuman, W.F., Neuman, M.W., Sammon, P.J., Cararett, G.W.: The metabolism of labeled parathyroid hormone. IV. Autoradiographic studies. Calc. Tiss. Res. 18, 263-270 (1975).

48. Sammon, P.J., Brand, J.S., Neuman, W.F., Raisz, L.G.: Metabolism of labeled parathyroid hormone. I. Preparation of biologically active ^{125}I labeled parathyroid hormone. Endocrinology 92, 1596-1603 (1973).

49. Rosenblatt, M., Goltzman, D., Keutman, H.T., Tregear, G.W., Potts, J.T.: Chemical and biological properties of synthetic, sulfur-free analogues of parathyroid hormone. J. biol. Chem. 251, 159-164 (1976).

50. Segre, G.V., Rosenblatt, M., Reiner, B.L., Mahaffey, J.E., Potts, J.T.: Characterization of parathyroid hormone receptors in canine renal cortical plasma membranes using a radioiodinated sulfur-free hormone analogue. J. biol. Chem. 254, 6980-6986 (1979).

51. Nissensen, R.A., Arnaud, C.D.: Properties of the parathyroid hormone receptor-adenylate cyclase system in chicken renal plasma membranes. J. biol. Chem. 254, 1469-1475 (1979).

52. Rodbell, M.: The role of nucleotide regulatory components in the coupling of hormone receptors and adenylate cyclase. In: "Molecular Biology and Pharmacology of Cyclic Nucleotides" Eds. Folco, G., Paoletti, R., Elsevier, North Holland, Amsterdam, pp. 1-12 (1978).

53. Rosenblatt, M., Callahan, E.N., Mahaffey, J.E., Pont, A., Potts, J.T.: Parathyroid hormone inhibitors: Design, synthesis and biologic evaluation of hormone analogues. J. biol. Chem. 252, 5847-5851 (1977).

54. Pliam, N.B., Nyiredy, K.O., Silve, C.M., Arnaud, C.D.: The parathyroid hormone receptor in bone cells: Properties and regulation. Proc. 3rd Ann. Meet. Am. Soc. Bone Min. Res. p. 38A, Cincinnati (1981).

55. Silve, C.M., Hradik, G., Jones, A., Arnaud, C.D.: Parathyroid hormone receptors in intact bone: Identification and cellular localization. Proc. 3rd Ann. Meet. Am. Soc. Bone Min. Res. P. 39A, Cincinnati (1981).

56. Arnaud, C.D., Goldsmith, R.S., Bordier, P.J., Sizemore, G.W., Larson, J.A., Oldham, S.B.: Influence of immunoheterogeneity of circulating parathyroid hormone on results of radioimmunoassays of serum in man. Am. J. Med. 56, 785-793 (1974).

57. Canterbury, J.M., Bricker, L.A., Levey, G.S., Kozlovskis, R.L., Ruis, E., Zull, J.E., Reiss, E.: Metabolism of bovine parathyroid hormone. J. clin. Invest. 55, 1245-1253 (1975).

58. Fischer, J.A., Binswanger, U., Dietrich, F.M.: Human parathyroid hormone: Immunological characterization of antibodies against a glandular extract and the synthetic amino terminal fragments 1-12 and 1-34 and their use in the determination of immunoreactive hormone in human sera. J. clin. Invest. 54, 1382-1394 (1974).

59. Hruska, K.A., Kopelman, R., Rutherford, W.E., Klahr, S., Slatopolsky, E.: Metabolism of immunoreactive parathyroid hormone in the dog. The role of the kidney and the effects of chronic renal disease. J. clin. Invest. 56, 39-48 (1975).

60. Segre, G.V., d'Amour, P., Potts, J.T.: Metabolism of radioiodinated bovine parathyroid hormone in rat. Endocrinology 99, 1645-1652 (1976).

61. Singer, F.R., Segre, G.V., Habener, J.F., Potts, J.T.: Peripheral metabolism of bovine parathyroid hormone in the dog. Metabolism 24, 139-144 (1975).

62. Fang, V.S., Tashjian, A.H.: Studies of the role of the liver in the metabolism of parathyroid hormone. Endocrinology 90, 1177-1184 (1972).

63. Martin, K.J., Hruska, K., Greenwald, A., Klahr, S., Slatopolsky, E.: Selective uptake of intact parathyroid hormone by the liver differences between hepatic and renal uptake. J. clin. Invest. 58, 781-788 (1976).

64. D'Amour, P., Segre, G.V., Roth, S.I., Potts, J.T.: Analysis of parathyroid hormone and fragments in rat tissues. J. clin. Invest. 63, 89-98 (1979).

65. Minne, H., Raue, F., Ziegler, R.: Cleavage of parathyroid hormones in kidney. Proc. 5th International Congr. Endocrinol. Hamburg, Abstract No. 555 (1976).

66. Martin, K.J., Hruska, K.A., Lewis, J., Anderson, C., Slatopolsky, E.: The renal handling of parathyroid hormone role of peritubular uptake and glomerular filtration. J. clin. Invest. 60, 808-814 (1977).

67. Goltzman, D., Henderson, B., Loveridge, N.: Cytochemical bioassay of parathyroid hormone. J. clin. Invest. 65, 1309-1317 (1980).

68. Nissensen, R.A., Abbott, S.R., Teitelbaum, A.P., Clark, O.H., Arnaud, C.D.: Endogenous biologically active human parathyroid hormone: Measurement by a guanyl nucleotide-amplified renal adenylate cyclase assay. J. clin. Endocrinol. Metab. 52, 840 (1981).

69. Albright, F., Aub, J.C., Hampton, A.O., Mallory, T.B., Cope, O.: Case record of the Massachusetts General Hospital - Case 27461. New Engl. J. Med. 225, 789-791 (1941).

70. Mandl, F.: Therapeutischer Versuch bei einem Fall von Ostitis fibrosa generalisata mittels Exstirpation. Tentralblatt Chirurgie 53, 264 (1926).

71. Collip, J.B.: The parathyroid glands. 1st Harvey Lectures, Balliere, Tindall and Cox, London, 21, 113-172 (1926).

72. Klemperer, P.: Parathyroid hyperplasia and bone destruction in generalized carcinomatosis. Surg. Gynec. Obstet. 36, 11 (1923).

73. Strada, F.: Le paratirioidi nell' osteomalacia et nell' osteoporosi senile. Pathologica 17, 423 (1909).

74. Bauer, Th.: Über das Verhalten der Epithelkörperchen bei der Osteomalacie. Frankfurt Z. Pathol. 7, 321 (1911).

75. Tomaszewski, Z.: Untersuchungen über das Verhalten der Glandulae parathyreoidea des Menschen beim Vorhandensein von Kalkablagerungen im Organismus. Frankfurt Z. Pathol. 21, 38 (1914).

76. Barr, D.P., Bulger, H.A.: The clinical syndrome of hyperparathyroidism. Am. J. med. Sci. 179, 449 (1930).

77. Connor, T.B., Thomas, W.C., Howard, J.E.: The etiology of hypercalcaemia associated with lung carcinoma. J. clin. Invest. 35, 697-698 (1956).

78. Terz, J.J., Estep, H., Bright, R., Lawrence, W., Curutchet, H.P., Kay, S.: Primary oropharyngeal cancer and hypercalcemia. Cancer 33, 334-339 (1974).

79. Snedecor, P.A., Baker, H.W.: Pseudohyperparathyroidism due to malignant tumors. Cancer 17, 1492-1496 (1964).

80. Case record of the Massachusetts General Hospital. New Engl. J. Med. 269, 801-813 (1963).

81. Samuelson, S.M., Werner, I.: Hepatic carcinoma simulating hyperparathyroidism. Acta med. scand. 173, 539-547 (1963).

82. Lipsett, M.B., Odell, W.D., Rosenberg, L.D., Waldman, T.A.: Humoral syndromes associated with nonendocrine tumors. Ann. intern. Med. 61, 733 (1964).

83. Ross, L., Shelley, E.: Mesonephric carcinoma of the ovary producing hypercalcemia. Am. J. Obstet. Gynec. 100, 418-421 (1968).

84. O'Neill, R.T., Mikuta, J.J.: Reversible hypercalcemia in squamous cell carcinoma of the vagina. Report of a case. Obstet. and Gynec. 36, 458 (1970).

85. Schatten, W.E., Ship, A.G., Pieper, W.J., Bartter, F.C.: Syndrome resembling hyperparathyroidism associated with squamous cell carcinoma. Ann. Surg. 148, 890-894 (1958).

86. Plimpton, C.H. Gellhorn, A.L.: Hypercalcemia in malignant disease without evidence of bone destruction. Am. J. Med. 21, 750 (1956).

87. Seftel, L.A., Gusberg, S.B.: Hyperparathyroid states in gynecological malignancy. Review of literature and report of a case. Obstet. and Gynec. 25, 693-698 (1965).

88. Kukreja, S.C., Hargesm, G.K., Rosenthal, I.M., Williams, G.A.: Pheochromocytoma causing excessive parathyroid hormone production and hypercalcemia. Ann. intern. Med. 79, 838 (1973).

89. Scholz, D.A., Riggs, B.L., Purnell, D.C., Goldsmith, R.S., Arnaud, C.D.: Ectopic hyperparathyroidism with renal calculi and subperiostal bone resorption. Mayo Cl. Proc. 48, 124 (1973).

90. Neimann, R.S., Li, H.C.: Hypercalcemia in undifferentiated leukemia. Cancer 30, 942-944 (1972).

91. Lafferty, F.W.: Pseudoparathyroidism. Medicine 45, 247 (1966).

92. Omenn, G.S., Roth, S.J., Baker, W.J.: Hyperparathyroidism associated with malignant tumors of non parathyroid origin. Cancer 24, 1004 (1969).

93. Benson, R.C., Riggs, B.L., Pickard, B.M., Arnaud, C.D.: Immunoreactive forms of circulating parathyroid hormone in primary and ectopic hyperparathyroidism. J. clin. Invest. 54, 175-181 (1974).

94. Riggs, B.L., Arnaud, C.D., Reynolds, J.C., Smith, L.H.: Immunologic differentiation of primary hyperparathyroidism from hyperparathyroidism due to nonparathyroid cancer. J. clin. Invest. 50, 2079-2083 (1971).

95. Seyberth, H.W., Segre, G.V., Hamet, P., Sweetman, B.J., Potts, J.T., Gates, J.A.: Characterization of the group of patients with hypercalcemia of cancer who respond to treatment with prostaglandin synthesis inhibitors. Trans. Ass. Amer. Phycns. 89, 92-104 (1976).

96. Seyberth, H.W., Segre, G.V., Morgan, J.L., Sweetman, B.J., Potts, J.T.: Prostaglandins as mediators of hypercalcemia associated with certain types of cancer. New Engl. J. Med. 293, 1278-1283 (1975).

97. Roof, B.S., Carpenter, B., Tink, D.J., Gordan, G.S.: Some thoughts on the nature of ectopic parathyroid hormones. Am. J. Med. 50, 686-691 (1971).

98. Holdaway, I.M., Bloomfield, G.A., Ratcliffe, J.G., Hinson, K.W.F., Rees, G.M., Rees, L.H.: Adrenocortical corticotrophin levels in normal and neoplastic lung tissue. In: Proc. 4th Int. Symp. Endocrinol., William Heinemann Medical Books Ltd., London, pp. 309-315 (1974).

99. Goldhaber, P.: Enhancement of bone resorption in tissue culture by mouse fibrosarcoma. Proc. Amer. Ass. Cancer Res. 3, 113 (1960).

100. Tashjian, A.H., Voelkel, E.F., Levin, L., Goldhaber, P.: Evidence that the bone resorption-stimulating factor produced by mouse fibrosarcoma cells is prostaglandin E_2. J. exp. Med. 136, 1329-1443 (1972).

101. Gordon, G.S., Fitzpatrick, M.E., Lubich, W.P.: Identification of osteolytic sterols in human breast cancer. Trans. Ass. Amer. Phycns. 80, 183-189 (1967).

102. Mundy, G.R., Luben, R.A., Raisz, L.G., Oppenheim, J.J., Buell, D.N.: Bone-resorbing activity in supernatants from lymphoid cell lines. New Engl. J. Med. 290, 867-871 (1974).

103. Mundy, G.R., Raisz, L.G., Cooper, R.A., Schechter, G.P., Salmon, S.E.: Evidence for the secretion of an osteoclast stimulating factor in myeloma. New Engl. J. Med. 291, 1041-1046 (1974).

104. Raisz, L.G., Luben, R.A., Mundy, G.R., Dietrich, J.W., Horton, J.E., Trummel, C.L.: Effect of osteoclast activating factor from human leukocytes on bone metabolism. J. clin. Invest. 56, 408-413 (1975).

105. Stewart, A.F., Horst, R., Deftos, L.J., Broadus, A.E.: Biochemical and clinical classification of patients with malignancy-associated hypercalcemia. In: "Hormonal Control of Calcium Metabolism", Eds. Cohn, D.V., Talmage, R.V., Les Matthews, J.L., International Congress Series 511, Excerpta Medica, Amsterdam-Oxford-Princeton, pp. 79-86 (1981).

106. Saxe, A., Brennan, M., Deftos, L., Spiegel, A.: Humoral hypercalcemia caused by a rat Leydig cell tumor is associated with increased urinary cAMP and suppressed PTH. Proc. 3rd Ann. Meet. Am. Soc. Bone Min. Res. Cincinnati p. 39A (1981).

107. Minne, H., Ziegler, R., Arnaud, C.D.: Paraneoplastic parathyroid hormone production by the hypercalcemic Walker carcinosarcoma 256 of the rat. In: "Endocrinology of Calcium Metabolism", Proc. 6th Parathyroid Conference Vancouver, 1977, Eds. Copp, D.H., Talmage, R.V., Excerpta Medica, Amsterdam, p. 385 (1978).

108. Minne, H., Raue, R., Bellwinkel, S., Ziegler, R.: The hypercalcaemic syndrome in rats bearing the Walker carcinosarcoma. Acta endocr. 78, 613-624 (1975).

109. Hilgard, P., Schmitt, W., Minne, H., Ziegler, R.: Acute hypercalcemia due to Walker carcinoma 256 in the rat. Hormone Metab. Res. 2, 255 (1970).

110. Young, D.M., Fioravanti, J.L., Prieur, D.J., Ward, J.M.: Hypercalcemic VX-2 carcinoma in rabbits. Laboratory Invest. 35, 30-46 (1977).

111. von Virchow, R.: Kalkmetastasen. Virchows Arch. Path. Anat. 8, 103 (1855).

EFFECTS OF GOSSYPOL ON MALE REPRODUCTION

G. W. Sang
Department of Pharmacology, Zhejiang Academy of Experimental Hygiene, Hangchow, China

I. Introduction

In a World Health Symposium report a brief introductory survey (1) stressed "the need for men to assume greater responsibility for fertility control" obviously linked "at least with the limited variety of methods available... since only periodic abstinence, condoms and vasectomy are open to them". Since that time, much work has been carried out in the human male in a search for an effective male contraceptive. Some potential compounds such as α-chlorohydrin, cyproterone acetate, Win-18446, ORF-1616 and some oestrogens, progestins or androgens have been considered. However, their use as contraceptive agents for men was precluded by their side-effects. Thus, so far we still lack a reliable male antifertility agent that shows real promise of widespread practical application.

Recently, there has been much interest in the Chinese finding that cooking with crude cotton-seed oil induced sterility in males and the active principal that induced sterility was identified as gossypol. Studies on gossypol have provided a new lead in research of drugs for male fertility control (2).

Feeding of crude cotton-seed oil for contraception had been suggested early in 1957 (3). In the late 1960's, investigators were puzzled by the extremely low birth rates in a particular geographic area and eventually related the phenomenon to the resident's exclusive use of crude cotton-seed oil for cooking . Subsequently, experiments on animals with highly purified gossypol showed that the antifertility constituent in crude

Hormones in Normal and Abnormal Human Tissues, Vol. III

cotton-seed oil was gossypol. Furthermore, the Chinese workers demonstrated the remarkable antifertility effect of gossypol in male rat, hamster, guinea-pig, pig and monkey (2, 4, 5). On this basis, gossypol was tested for its antifertility action in more than 8000 men in the People's Republic of China. At present gossypol, gossypol acetic acid and gossypol formic acid are being used for clinical and animal studies.

The clinical information shows that gossypol given orally at a dose of 20 mg/kg for 2 months followed by a maintenance dose of 150-220 mg/month induces a reversible infertility in 99.8% of men as assessed by the incidence of necrospermia or sperm count below 4 million per ml (2, 6). However, further research is needed to solve several disadvantages, such as the slow onset of the antifertility effect and the danger of sterility after longterm administration. It is necessary to indicate that gossypol is far from being an ideal contraceptive because it possesses some important side-effects, especially hypokalaemia and the damage on liver function. Since this agent is new, the issues of toxicity, effectiveness, reversibility and mode of action remain serious topics of research.

Broader aspects of its effect on fertility, its metabolism and toxicity have been extensively reviewed (7, 8, 9). The present paper emphasizes the pharmacological effects of gossypol and its site and mechanism of action and contains some information on its clinical trials and endocrine activities.

II. Chemistry of Gossypol

1. Chemical structure

Gossypol is a polyphenolic compound occurring in the pigment glands of the seed, leaf, stem, laproot bark and roots of the cotton plant. Gossypol has a molecular weight 518.54 and a molecular formula of $C_{30}H_{30}O_8$. Gossypol, (2,2'-binaphthalene)-8,8'-dicarboxaldehyde-1,1',6,6',7,7',-hexahydroxy-5,5'-diisopropyl-3,3'dimethyl, occurs in three tautomeric forms: the aldehyde I, the hemiacetal II, and its phenolic quinoid tautomer III (Fig. 1).

Gossypol constitutes 20-40% of the weight of the pigment glands in cotton-seed, which usually contains 0.4-1.7% gossypol. The total world production of cotton-seed is about 25 million tons per year, containing approximately 78000 tons of gossypol.

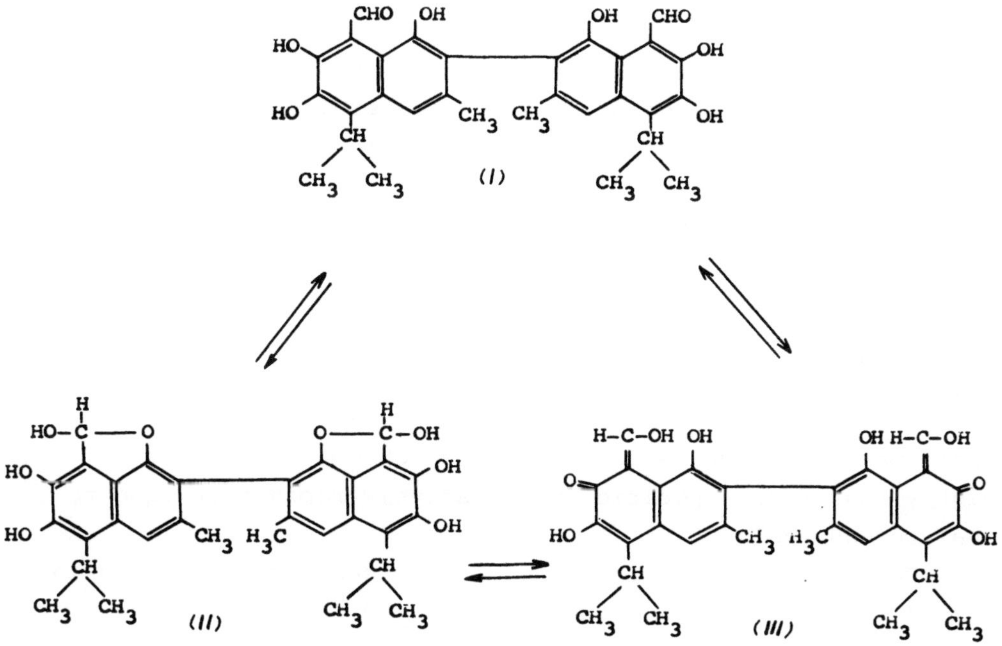

Fig. 1. Tautomer forms of gossypol
(from M.B. Abou-Donia, 1976)

2. Isolation, analysis and the optical activity of gossypol

The principal method for manufacture of gossypol is extraction of tho ground cotton seed kernels with low boiling petroleum ether to remove the oil, followed by extraction with diethyl ether to remove the gossypol. The pigment can be separated as a gossypol acetic acid complex after addition of acetic acid to the concentrated ether solution (9). Gossypol is insoluble in water but forms salts in alkaline solutions. Gossypol is soluble in most organic solvents.

Since other gossypol-related compounds, such as gossypurpurin, gossyfulvin, gossycaerulin and gossyverdurin, are present in pigment glands, it is essential to develop an analytical procedure that ensures the purity of the product used. Various analytical methods have been used to determine gossypol: gravimetric, titrimetric and spectrophotometric. These methods are not specific since gossypol and other related pigments may react similarly to the same analytical reagents. Chromatographic methods, including paper, thin-layer and gas-liquid , have been developed to analyse gossypol. The paper and the thin-layer chromatographic procedures lack sensitivity, however, and the gas-liquid chromatographic method requires prior conversion to the trimethylsilyl ether derivative of gossypol. Compared to these methods, high-performace liquid chromatography is a highly sensitive, specific and relatively rapid technique to analyze gossypol (10).

Gossypol isolated from the cotton-seed pigment is the inactive racemate but the product extracted from a tropical tree Thespesia Populnea Corr. is strongly dextrorotatory (+) (11). The optical activity of the Thespesia gossypol must arise through restricted rotation around the bond which joins the naphthalene nuclei. Oral administration of (+) gossypol at dose levels varying from 6 mg/kg/day to 12 mg/kg/day for 5 weeks did not affect the epididymal sperm motility, suggesting that (+) gossypol had no antifertility effect (4). Therefore, the antifertility action of gossypol isolated from the cotton-seed might be related to its levo-rotatory form.

However, recently, (+) gossypol showed promising post-coital anti-implantation activity in fertile female albino rats at a dose level of 10 mg/kg body weight intraperitoneally and at a dose of 30 mg/kg orally. Thus (+) gossypol may possess slight oestrogenic activity (12).

Synthesis of gossypol derivatives for screening for anti-fertility activity was also conducted in China. However, the antifertility effect was lost when the -CHO and -OH groups in the structure of gossypol were replaced by other groups. Derivatives of gossypol, including imino compounds, esters and metallic complexes, have been prepared but none has shown anti-fertility activity better than gossypol acetic acid (4). Change of the aldehyde group of gossypol to a Schiff's base, oxime, hydrazone or transforming the hydroxyl group to methoxyl, acetate and ethyl acetate ether or modifying the naphthol ring to naphthaquinone, showed no biological activity in rats even at doses higher than gossypol itself.

It was reported that ferrous sulphate may reduce the toxicity of gossypol in pigs. However, the ferrous salt was inactive (13) and the aluminium and magnesium salts possessed some activity but were not as effective as gossypol.

It is therefore clear that the whole molecule of gossypol is important for its antifertility effect.

III. Pharmacological and Toxicological Studies on Gossypol

1. Species and strain differences in the antifertility action of gossypol

There are obvious species differences between rats, hamsters, monkeys, dogs, rabbits, mice, guinea-pigs and pigs in terms of the antifertility effect of gossypol. Rats and hamsters appear to be the most sensitive species. After oral administration of gossypol in a daily dose of 15-30 mg/kg, adult Wistar male rats became infertile in approximately 3-5 weeks (5, 14, 16, 17). The antifertility effects were determined by the presence of dead sperm in the cauda epididymis and abnormal sperm in the testis. The results of mating experiments agreed with the results of semen examination.

The oral minimal effective antifertility dose of gossypol for male rats was reported to be 7.5 mg/kg/day for 12 weeks (14). Wang et al.(4) found that the minimal effective dose of gossypol was 10-12 mg/kg/day for 5 weeks when administered to rats orally. Chang et al.(15) reported that pregnancy was still possible, although the implantation sites were significantly decreased when females were mated with male rats fed daily with gossypol at 10 mg/kg for 12 weeks. Lin et al.(18) demonstrated that 5 weeks of treatment with gossypol acetic acid given orally at 30 mg/kg/day was sufficient to render male rats incapable of impregnating proestrus females, although intromission had taken place as verified by vaginal smears.

At different time intervals after gossypol acetic acid administration to male rats at 30 mg/kg/day for two weeks, the sperm count of cauda epididymis was found to fluctuate within the normal range, even though fertility may be lost. However, after treatment the motility of the sperm began to decrease gradually in the caput epididymis and then in the cauda epididymis. Recovery of motility of the sperm followed the same sequence: first in the caput and then in the cauda (14).

It is true that loss and restitution of activity of sperm in the vas deferens and epididymis seem to follow a definite sequence after treatment with gossypol. However, Shi et al. in my laboratory found that loss of activity took the following order: sperms in vas deferens and cauda epididymis-corpus-caput whereas restitution took the reverse order: caput epididymis-corpus-cauda and vas deferens (16).

Chang et al.(15) found that male hamsters were more sensitive than male rats to the antifertility effect of gossypol because none of the female hamsters became pregnant after mating with male hamsters fed gossypol at a dose as low as 5 mg/kg for

12 weeks. Reversible male antifertility activity was obtained with orally administered gossypol acetic acid in hamsters at 10 mg/kg/day for 6 weeks (17).

Hahn et al.(17) also demonstrated that gossypol acetic acid was an effective and reversible male antifertility agent in rats and hamsters but not in mice. In male rats, a daily dose of 10 mg/kg for 14 weeks did not alter fertility, but at 20 mg/kg, infertility occurred after 6 weeks of treatment and lasted for the eight-week treatment period. Infertility was observed after 6 and 4 weeks of treatment at 10 and 20 mg/kg, respectively in male hamsters. On the other hand, oral administration of gossypol at 40 mg/kg/day for 8 weeks did not alter the fertility of male mice even though this dose induced obvious toxicity (17).

Shi and Chang found that gossypol given orally at 20 mg/kg/day for 8 weeks had no antifertility effect in mice. When gossypol suspension was injected subcutaneously in immature mice at 8.3 mg/kg for 4 weeks, no obvious effects were observed on the motility of sperm in the seminiferous tubules and epididymis. However, there was a significant reduction in the weight of the accessory reproductive organs and levator ani muscle (19).

Gossypol fed at a dose of 10-80 mg/kg/day for up to 35 weeks failed to induce sterility in the Dutch-belted rabbit. Gossypol at these dose levels is fatal (20). Chang et al. also indicated that oral administration of gossypol acetic acid at dose levels varying from 1.25 to 10 mg/kg given for 5 to 14 weeks did not affect the average number of sperm per ejaculate in male rabbits, although the motility of sperm was poor during treatment in some bucks. The pregnancy rates and the proportion of implantation sites were also not affected by insemination of female rabbits with sperm from males during treatment with this dose of gossypol (15).

Dogs are very sensitive both to the antifertility effect and the toxicological actions induced by gossypol. Spermatogenesis was inhibited for between 63 and 81 days in dogs treated with 2 or 4 mg/kg/day (2). Of 6 dogs given gossypol orally at a daily dose of 2-5 mg/kg, 4 died of cardiac toxicity on day 42, 63, 77 and 86 respectively. Histopathological examination revealed that the seminiferous tubules were depopulated to a marked degree and became atrophic, with only a single layer of Sertoli cells and spermatogonia left in the tubules. Nuclear vacuolation, karyorrhexis and cytolysis were observed. Spermatocytes disappeared almost completely. However, there was no detecable damage to the interstitial cells. The surviving animals were autopsied 40 and 396 days after cessation of treatment. Histological examination showed that spermatogenesis had been restored. The morphology of the testes and the epididymis exhibited no conspicuous changes as seen under a light microscope (21).

In male monkeys, spermatogenesis was significantly suppressed after oral administration of gossypol at a dose of 4 mg/kg/day for 2 years. Histological examination revealed severe damage to most of the seminiferous tubules; spermatids and spermatocytes disappeared almost completely and only spermatogonia and sertoli cells remained. A few normal spermatids and spermatozoa were still present in some tubules in one monkey (21).

Table 1. Relative potency of the antifertility effect of gossypol in different species.

Species	Dose (mg/kg/day)	Duration of treatment (weeks)	Fertility
Hamster	5	12	0
	20	4	0
Rat	10	12	decreased
	20	6	0
Mouse	20	8	normal
Rabbit	10	35	normal
Dog	2-4	9-12	decreased
Monkey	4	2 (years)	decreased
	80	5-7	normal

Recently, Shandilya and Clarkson observed the anti-reproductive and hypolipidaemic effects of gossypol in male cynomolgus monkeys (Macaca facicularis) (22). The monkeys were treated with 5 or 10 mg/kg/day of gossypol for 6 months. Suppression of sperm production and motility was observed without any significant decrease in plasma levels of testosterone. A sudden increase in sperm count was observed after attaining azoospermia although the sperm motility remained very sluggish. Spermatozoa observed by light microscopy showed more sperm with coiled or broken tail pieces and an occasional detached head and tail and ultrastructurally, disruption of axial complexes was often observed. At 10 mg/kg/day, the entire axial complex was frequently destroyed, suggesting an impairment of sperm motility. In addition, gossypol had a hypolipidaemic effect, a previously unreported property. Changes were observed in low density lipoproteins, with only insignificant differences in high density lipoprotein-cholesterol concentrations. In general, no serious pathological findings were observed in any of the monkeys except diarrhoea and loss of appetite among the high dose group. The mean body weight of the animals did not change. Results of measurements of liver enzyme concentrations (SGOT, SGPT, γ-GT)were within normal range in all animals. Kidney function tests as evaluated by blood urea nitrogen and serum creatinine showed no impairment. The haematological data revealed normal haematopoiesis. There were no changes in serum protein levels and plasma levels of sodium and potassium nor in blood pressure. The risk of "break through" in sperm concentrations, particularly when the sperm motility is very poor, requires further study, as does the exact mechanism and site of action of gossypol in achieving its antifertility and hypolipidaemic effects (22).

Chang(23) reported that the effect of gossypol differed in different strains of rats. Four strains, Sprague-Dawley, Wistar, Long-Evans and Fisher, were fed 40 mg/kg of gossypol daily by gavage for 2 weeks. There was no mortality in Sprague-Dawley, but 4/15 Long-Evans and 4/15 Fisher rats died during the first 3 days of treatment. The Fisher strain lost weight in 2 weeks. The antifertility effect was evident in all four strains.

2. Antifertility effects of gossypol and its impurities

Some investigators have speculated that part or all of the toxicity and antifertility effects of gossypol are a result of impurities. Recently, Waller et al.(24) prepared purified gossypol and a fraction containing the total impurities. Only pure gossypol produced a decrease in fertility of the male hamster after six weeks of dosing. A full recovery of fertility in the pure gossypol group was observed four weeks after cessation of treatment. These data supported the claim that gossypol is indeed the active antifertility agent. The impurities, however, may have the ability to block or decrease the efficacy of gossypol.

3. Dose-response and time-response relationship of the antifertility action of gossypol

The speed of onset of antifertility induced by gossypol seems to be dose related. Male rats fed with gossypol acetic acid at 60, 30, 15 or 7.5 mg/kg/day for 1, 2, 4 or 12 weeks lost their fertility. However, 3 mg/kg/day given for 16 weeks was ineffective (14). In our laboratory, it was shown that daily oral administration of gossypol acetic acid at a dose of 6 mg/kg to adult male rats for 5 weeks, produced no effect on fertility. When the dosage was raised to 12 mg/kg/day for 5 weeks, a definite antifertility effect was produced. If the dosage was further raised to 24 mg/kg/day for 3 weeks, 100% antifertility effect was observed. Hence, in rats, the minimum effective dose to achieve antifertility was 12 mg/kg/day (16). But Zhou et al. (25) found that administration of 7.5 mg/kg/day of gossypol for over a year led to infertility without gross degenerative changes in the testis and mating behaviour. Xue et al.(26) suggested that there were variations among animals in response to gossypol.

A series of cytologic changes occur in the seminiferous

epithelium of rat testis after administration of gossypol. The earliest sign of drug effect was seen in the spermatids which displayed nuclear vacuolation and swelling. With the increase in dose and duration of drug administration, the effects became more pronounced and extended to the spermatocytes. Obvious changes such as pyknosis, karyorrhexis or cytolysis were present in an appreciable number of these 2 classes of cells. Exfoliation of the cells of the germinal epithelium with resultant desquamation and formation of multinucleated giant cells of spermatid and spermatocytic derivation were readily discernible. The germinal epithelium underwent a progressive reduction in cell layers and asynchrony of cellular association was noted in most of the tubules. Finally, the seminiferous tubules were depopulated to a marked degree and became atrophic. The degenerating cells disappeared completely and only a layer of Sertoli cells and spermatogonia was left in the tubules (2).

The degree of damage caused by gossypol acetic acid in the seminiferous epithelium of rat testis increased with the dose as well as with the duration of administration. The most pronounced effect was seen about 2 weeks after stopping the drug (16). Lin et al.(18) also found that sperm counts, determined from vaginal washings showed a decrease directly related to treatment time.

The antifertility effect of gossypol persisted for 3 to 5 weeks after withdrawal of treatment and thereafter fertility gradually recovered (2). Wang et al.(4) reported that male rats recovered their fertility 4-5 weeks after cessation of the gossypol treatment (10-12 mg/kg/day for 4-5 weeks). Lin et al.(18) reported re-establishment of normal fertility by 6 weeks post-treatment (gossypol acetic acid, 30 mg/kg/day for 5 weeks). Similar results were observed in our laboratory. After cessation of dosing (gossypol acetic acid, 24 mg/kg for 3 weeks) the antifertility effect was maintained for 5-6 weeks; thereafter fertility was gradually restored (16). Recovery of spermatogenesis and fertility is related to the dose and the duration of treatment. Recovery is possible only in such cases where the spermatogonia are not damaged; prolonged treatment with gossypol and damage to seminiferous epithelium leads to permanent sterility (25, 27). Gossypol acetic acid given orally caused a dose- and time- dependent temporary infertility in the male hamster. Daily treatment with 10 mg/kg/day of gossypol induced total sterility within 10 weeks, whereas with 15 mg/kg/day sterility occurred in 7 to 8 weeks. The reversal process, however, was inversely proportional to the dose administered. A period of 5 to 7 weeks was needed for animals to regain fertility after treatment with 10 or 15 mg/kg/day of gossypol (28).

4. Site and mechanism of the antifertility action of gossypol

Many theories have been put forward to explain gossypol-induced sterility in the male. After ligation of the epididymis of rats fed with gossypol, Dai and Dong (29) reported that the site of action was not in the epididymis but in the testes. Electron microscopic examination of rat testis revealed vacuolated mitochondria in the middle piece of the spermatids and led Dai et al.(30) to conclude that the effect of gossypol was directly on the spermatids during maturation.

After treatment with gossypol acetic acid at 30, 15 and 7.5 mg/kg/day for 2, 10 and 12 weeks respectively, the morphology of the testes and the epididymis exhibited no conspicuous change as seen under a light microscope. After prolonged treatment with gossypol acetic acid at a dose of 30 mg/kg/day for 7 weeks, formation of multinucleated giant cells and asynchrony of cellular association were observed in most of the seminiferous tubules. In some rats the spermatids and the spermatocytes disappeared completely. It appears that the mechanism of the antifertility action of gossypol acetic acid might vary with the dose and duration of treatment (14).

Xue et al.(26) reported that the earliest damage was seen in the spermatids and pachytene spermatocytes 2 to 3 weeks after treatment, showing different pathological changes such as pycnosis, nuclear vacuolation, swelling or displacement of head

Table 2. Induction of sterility by oral administration of gossypol acetic acid and its reversal in the male Syrian hamster
(from: Saksena and Salmonsen, 1982)

Treatment	and dose	Test of fertility	Females pregnant left for mating	%	Number of viable embryos[c]
Vehicle	Control	5 weeks after	5/5	100	16, 14, 12, 10, 14
Gossypol	10 mg/kg/day	treatment	3/6	50	6, 0, 8, 0, 0, 13
	15 mg/kg/day		2/6	33	12, 9, 0, 0, 0, 0
Vehicle	Control	7-8 weeks after	5/5	100	11, 13, 11, 9, 10
Gossypol	10 mg/kg/day	treatment	3/6	50	9, 3, 10, 0, 0, 0
	15 mg/kg/day		0/6	0	0, 0, 0, 0, 0, 0
Vehicle	Control	10 weeks after	5/5	100	12, 15, 13, 11, 14
Gossypol	10 mg/kg/day	treatment	3/6	50	9, 3, 0, 0, 10, 0
	15 mg/kg/day		0/6	0	0, 0, 0, 0, 0, 0
Gossypol	10 mg/kg/day[b]	12 weeks after	0/6	0	0, 0, 0, 0, 0, 0
	15 mg/kg/day[a]	treatment	0/6	0	0, 0, 0, 0, 0, 0
Gossypol	10 mg/kg/day[b]	16 weeks after	0/6	0	0, 0, 0, 0, 0, 0
	15 mg/kg/day[a]	treatment	0/6	0	0, 0, 0, 0, 0, 0
Vehicle	Control	20 weeks after	5/5	100	12, 10, 13, 13, 10
Gossypol	10 mg/kg/day[b]	treatment	6/6	100	13, 13, 9, 15, 9, 10
	15 mg/kg/day[a]		3/5[d]	60	9, 12, 0, 0, 7
Control		22 weeks after	5/5	100	11, 10, 11, 13, 12
Gossypol	15 mg/kg/day[a]	treatment	5/5	100	14, 12, 7, 8, 12

a. Treatment for 8 weeks. b. Treatment terminated in the 10th week. c. Females were caged with males individually for 8 days and then killed 7 days later. d. One male died.

cap and karyorrhexis. Four weeks after treatment, metamorphosing spermatids with their heads and tails separated were evident. Finally, spermatids of 7 to 19 steps and spermatocytes of mid- and late-stages almost disappeared completely and only a single layer of Sertoli cells and spermatogonia were left in the tubules. It was concluded that the spermatids and spermatocytes were the most sensitive and vulnerable to gossypol. They were the first to show detectable damage, the first to degenerate and the most intensive ^{131}I-gossypol labelled cells in the seminiferous epithelium (Fig. 2, from 26).

Waller et al. (24) reported that spermatozoa were present in vaginal smears 6 to 9 weeks after treatment of hamsters with gossypol at a time when the fertility rate was zero. It was suggested that complete inhibition of spermatogenesis was probably not the primary action of gossypol. Cellular damage to the seminiferous epithelium of rats, monkeys and men were encountered during gossypol-induced infertility but no noticeable damage to interstitial cells or epithelium of the epididymis was detected (26, 21).

Electron microscopic studies showed swelling, dissociation and fragmentation of the acrosome and head caps of spermatids and swelling and derangement of the mitochondrial cristae (2, 26, 31). Hadley et al.(32) found that epididymal spermatozoa of gossypol treated rats show degeneration of the mitochondrial sheath. Nadakavukaren et al.(33) reported disorganization of the motor apparatus and damage to the mitochondrial system of the rat spermatozoa after gossypol treatment.

Loss of motility of spermatozoa may be due to disorganization of the mitochondrial sheath, missing cell element from the middle piece, missing members of both outer fibres and inner microtubules of the principal piece and disrupted cell membranes of sperm head. Wang and Lei found that the motility of the sperm in the testes was not markedly different before and after administration of gossypol, although the rats were infertile. The sperm tail was able to wave slowly in Ringers solution, which indicated that the sperm were still alive.

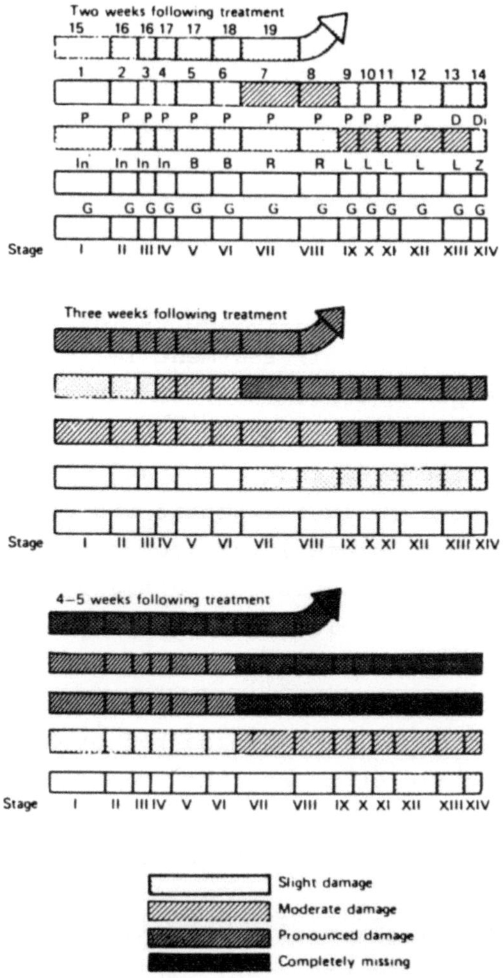

Fig. 2. The kinetics of cell types damaged and the stages within the cycle of the seminiferous epithelium at which damage is observed after 2,3 and 4 weeks of gossypol administration (30 mg/kg per day). B: B-type spermatogonia; D: diakinesis of spermatocytes; Di: reduction division; G: A-type spermatogonia; In: intermediate-type spermatogonia; L: leptotene spermatocyte; P: pachytene spermatocyte; R: resting spermatocyte; Z: zygotene spermatocyte (from 26)

They suggested that the infertility may be due to changes in the epididymal spermatozoa which were non-motile and showed separation of head and tail or in the epididymal milieu interfering with maturation of spermatozoa. Recently, Hadley and Burgos (34) have shown that introduction of gossypol into the epididymal fat pads of rats inhibits epididymal sperm motility and alteration of sperm morphology within 24 hours of administration.

The lower zinc concentration of the atrophied testis and epididymis after gossypol treatment led Yu et al.(35) to suggest that gossypol chelates zinc in the male reproductive system.

Gu et al. reported that light and electron microscopic changes were observed in the testis and epididymis of rats and hamsters which had become infertile after treatment with gossypol (36). Spermatogenesis was partially inhibited in both animals but the germ cells were disordered. The earliest changes after gossypol treatment were noted in the early stage of spermatid with changes in the mitochondrial sheath of the mid-piece. Epididymal spermatozoa had broken membranes, outer fibres or inner microtubules. The epididymal epithelium also showed ultrastructural changes and in some of the principal cells of the epididymal duct there appeared to be degenerated mitochondria.

So far the biochemical mechanism of the antifertility effect of gossypol is not clear. Zhou and Xue (37) reported that the nuclear DNA content of primary spermatocytes of treated rats was markedly reduced and the main peak of DNA in a distribution histogram was shifted to the left compared to that of controls. The synthetic rate of DNA in cell-free systems was inhibited by gossypol at a concentration of 6 μM (37). However, it was also reported that there was no change in the DNA and total protein content of the testis after gossypol treatment (38) and no significant change in the incorporation of ^{3}H-TdR into DNA of the thymus, small intestine and liver in gossypol-treated rats and mice (38, 39). Gossypol did not inhibit the incorporation of ^{3}H-lysine and ^{3}H-uridine into spermatogenic cells either *in vivo* or *in vitro* but the activity as well as frequency of labelling of ^{3}H-arginine in spermatids of 11-19 stages were decreased (40). Spermatids of late stages which incorporated ^{3}H-arginine selectively for the synthesis of arginine-rich histone were the most sensitive to gossypol.

Gossypol has been reported to act by uncoupling oxidative phosphorylation (41). Gossypol inhibited ATPase activity in human spermatozoa and testis (38, 42). Damage to the mitochondrial system of rat and human spermatozoa has been observed at the submicroscopic level (2, 33). Sugar utilisation was profoundly inhibited when freshly ejaculated human sperm cells were exposed to increasing concentrations of gossypol in the presence of uniformly labelled fructose (43). Gossypol inhibits respiration of isolated testicular mitochondria *in vitro*, indicative of interference with oxidative phosphorylation (44).

Gossypol did not significantly affect ^{3}H-thymidine incorporation into DNA of germ cells (38, 39) suggesting that gossypol does not interact with the genetic material. Negative results obtained in the AMES-salmonella-microsome test with gossypol indicate that it is not mutagenic (45).

Although gossypol appears to inhibit several lactate dehydrogenases to some extent, its greatest inhibitive effect is on lactate dehydrogenase X, which is found only in sperm and testes (46). Lee and Malling (47) showed a similar selective inhibition of gossypol on LDH-X from mouse, human and other rodent species. In rodents, but not in humans, it can cause irreversible inactivation of malate dehydrogenase.

An *in vitro* spermicidal effect of gossypol on human spermatozoa has been reported (43, 48, 49, 50). Spermatozoa were rapidly immobilized by gossypol, possibly due to a direct effect of the drug on the mitochondria and/or pronounced depression of spermatozoal fructose utilization. Gossypol-PVP coprecipitate prevented sperm motility when applied intravaginally in Macaca arctoides (51). Because the concentration of gossypol required for a direct spermicidal effect is low, because it is effective in the presence of cervical mucus, and because its systemic toxicity is low, the use of gossypol as a vaginal spermicidal agent has been suggested (43, 48, 51).

Recently, Tso et al.(52) classified the sensitivity of various spermatozoal enzymes to gossypol inhibition into three groups: (1) Enzymes not affected by gossypol, (2) enzymes affected only at high gossypol concentration (10^{-4} M or higher); many of this class may even show a slight stimulation of the enzyme activity at subthreshold inhibition concentrations, and (3) enzymes very susceptible to gossypol inhibition (Table 3).

Table 3. Gossypol effect on spermatozoal enzymes

Enzyme	Stimulation		Inhibition	
	Concentration*	Response	Concentration*	Response
Hexokinase	-	-	high	steep
LDH (total)	high	slight	high	steep
LDH	-	-	low	gradual
Carnitine acetyltransferase	-	-	-	-
Citrate synthase	-	-	high	steep
NAD-isocitrate dehydrogenase	-	-	low	gradual
α-Ketoglutarate dehydrogenase	low	slight	-	-
Succinyl-CoA synthetase	-	-	low	gradual
Succinate dehydrogenase	high	slight	high	steep
Fumarase	-	-	low	steep
NAD-malate dehydrogenase	-	-	high	steep
Acrosin	-	-	low	gradual

*Concentration of gossypol: high=at or above 10^{-4}M, low=below 10^{-4}M.

5. Endocrinological effects of gossypol

There are still some discrepancies regarding gossypol action on the pituitary-gonadal system. Wang et al.(4) reported that gossypol neither altered the mating behaviour and the function of accessory glands in rats nor affected plasma testosterone levels in rats and rhesus monkeys.

A. Effects of gossypol on morphology of the interstitial cells and testicular steroidogenesis. There were no detectable morphological or histochemical changes in interstitial cells, no change in libido and no significant change in weight of the seminal vesicles, prostate and coagulating gland in rats treated with 30 mg/kg/day of gossypol orally for 4 weeks (26). There was also no detectable difference in the ultrastructure of the interstitial cells between the gossypol treated and the control groups (2). It was also reported that there was no significant change in testicular levels of 3β-hydroxysteroid dehydrogenase, lipids and cholesterol (44).

However, Lin et al. reported that Leydig cells from treated rats produced less testosterone than controls when incubated with LH and suggested that gossypol may have a direct effect on steroid production (18). Saksena et al.(20) also found that testosterone release from testis mince in the presence of hCG was reduced significantly when high amounts of gossypol were present in the incubation medium.

Recently, Lin et al.(53) clearly demonstrated that gossypol had a direct inhibitory effect on steroidogenesis. Testosterone formation in response to LH stimulation was blocked by gossypol (Fig. 3).

B. Effect of gossypol on blood levels of gonadal and pituitary hormones. Plasma testosterone and dehydrotestosterone levels were not significantly altered in men by gossypol (26, 54). Gossypol did not significantly influence plasma LH levels and pituitary response to LHRH in rats (55). However, Lin et al. (18) reported that in rats serum testosterone levels decreased

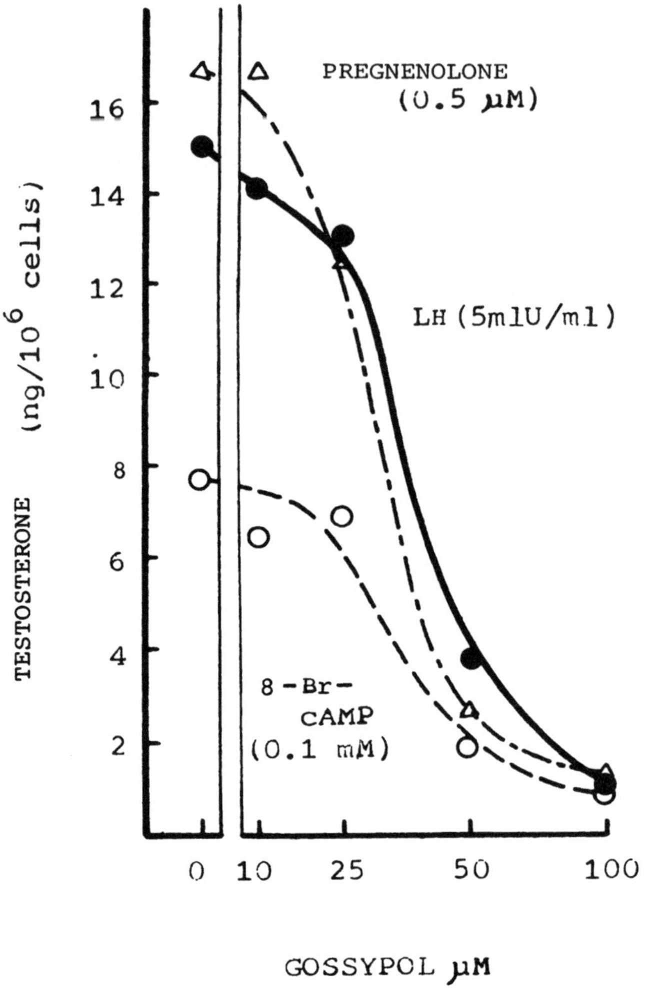

Fig. 3. Effect of gossypol on testosterone formation. Each point represents the mean of three incubations. Interstitial cells from mature Sprague-Dawley rats were incubated for 3 h. in medium 199-bovine serum albumin with 0.1 mM 1-methyl-3-isobutyl xanthine and various concentrations of gossypol, LH (●), 8-bromo-cyclic AMP (8-Br-cAMP) (O) and pregnenolone (Δ) at 34°C, under $95\%O_2/5\%CO_2$.

significantly from a pretreatment value of 5.25 ± 0.46 to 1.18 ± 0.25 ng/ml after 5 weeks of gossypol treatment (30 mg/kg/day); serum LH was decreased from a pretreatment value of 1185 ± 85 to 700 ± 60 pg/ml but serum FSH levels were unchanged. Saksena et al.(20) found substantially reduced levels of testosterone in bucks and in other experiments male hamsters treated with 10 mg/kg/day of gossypol were sterile after 10 weeks of treatment and testosterone concentration and total sperm population along the reproductive tract were significantly reduced (28). In spite of this, the sterile males induced pseudopregnancy in females suggesting that the suppressed testosterone level after gossypol treatment was adequate to maintain sexual behaviour.

Serum concentrations of testosterone (56) decreased significantly in immature and mature rats by treatment with gossypol for different time intervals; however, there was no change in serum LH levels.

These discrepancies could represent a species difference or could reflect the use of different doses of gossypol for varying times and by different routes of administration.

C. Endocrine activities of gossypol and its effect on androgen-dependent organs. Hahn et al.(17) found that gossypol did not have oestrogenic, anti-oestrogenic, androgenic or anti-androgenic activities in several standard endocrine bioassays; however, gossypol did potentiate the androgenicity of methyltestosterone. It is possible that gossypol enhanced the absorption or affected the metabolism of methyltestosterone.

A significant reduction in the weight of the accessory reproductive organs and levator ani muscle after a subcutaneous injection of 8.3 mg/kg/day of gossypol for 4 weeks in immature mice and rats has been reported (16) and this effect could not be antagonised completely in gonadectomized animals by the injection of 20 µg testosterone propionate. However, these androgen-dependent organs were not responsive to gossypol injection in adult mice and rats.

Wu et al.(57) reported that oral administration of 5-20 mg/kg/day of gossypol acetic acid altered pituitary and ovarian hormones during proestrus and estrus in hamsters. Administration of gossypol was mostly associated with a rise in serum FSH. Gossypol administered for 40 days at a dose of 10 mg/kg resulted in a significant decrease in ovarian progesterone concentration during proestrus and estrus. However, these changes were not accompanied by alteration in the serum levels of progesterone nor did gossypol compete for receptor binding sites.

A recent report on the usefulness of gossypol in treatment of certain uterine dysfunctions has suggested that gossypol inhibits ovarian secretion of estrogens in humans (58).

6. Toxicity of gossypol

There are obvious species differences between animals in regard to the toxic effects of gossypol. Animals such as dogs, mice, rabbits, pigs and guinea-pigs appear to be very susceptible. Toxic effects are usually manifest before the occurrence of damage to the germinal epithelium. Rats and monkeys are relatively more tolerant and usually show no marked toxic reactions with an antifertility dose (44). However, tolerance to gossypol in rats is determined by the amount and quality of protein in the diet (9).

(1) Acute toxicity of gossypol. The LD_{50} in mice given a single dose is 2200 mg/kg for gossypol acetic acid and 4623 mg/kg for gossypol formic acid. The LD_{50} at a daily dose for 6 days is 412 mg/kg (i.e. 70 mg/kg per day) for gossypol acetic acid and 1042 mg/kg (i.e. 170 mg/kg per day) for gossypol formic acid. We found that the LD_{50} in rats for a single dose of gossypol in oil is 2590 $\pm$ 310 mg/kg. If gossypol is given in aqueous suspension, the LD_{50} in rats is 2480 $\pm$ 450 mg/kg. According to Abou-Donia, the values of LD_{50} in rat, mice, rabbit, guinea-pig and pig were 2400-3000 mg/kg, 900-950 mg/kg, 350-600 mg/kg, 280-300 mg/kg and 550 mg/kg respectively (9).

(2) Subacute and chronic toxicity of gossypol. Gossypol had no obvious toxic effect at antifertility doses in rats. Gossypol (30 mg/kg/day) was given to male rats and after 60 days of treatment, only a few of the treated animals showed oedema, cloudy swelling, acidocytosis and focal inflammation of liver and cardiac muscle. Gossypol acetic acid fed to male rats at the minimal antifertility dose of 7.5 mg/kg/day for a year had no significant effect on the blood picture, bone marrow, SGPT, blood urea nitrogen and electrocardiogram. Histological examination of the various organs, with the exception of the testis, revealed no pathologic changes (2). For gossypol acetic acid 7.5-15 mg/kg per day is a reliable and safe antifertility dose for rats. Administration of these doses for more than six months resulted in no mortality and no pathological or histochemical changes in liver, kidney and of adrenal (44). When the dose was increased to 20-30 mg/kg, except for individual weak animals that showed slight transitory pathological changes in the liver and cardiac muscle, the majority of animals survived the treatment and became infertile (44).

We found marked differences between the toxicity of gossypol in dogs and monkeys. After four weeks of daily doses of 2-5 mg/kg of gossypol orally to 6 dogs, the ECG showed abnormalities, but the blood picture, hepatic function and renal function tests remained normal (Fig. 4). However, acute effects such as anorexia, vomiting, diarrhoea, weakness, decrease in heart rate were noted. Four dogs died of cardiac toxicity on day 42, 67, 77 and 86 respectively. Autopsy examination revealed severe pathological changes, such as heart dilatation and hypertrophy, endocarditis, congestion of the kidneys and spleen, fatty degeneration and necrosis of the liver, and oedema and haemorrhage of the lungs. No obvious damage was seen in the seminiferous epithelium of the testes. In the dogs which survived, the toxic cardiac signs and histological changes disappeared 1 year after withdrawal of gossypol (Fig. 4).

In monkeys all biochemical parameters and ECG remained normal during oral medication for 2 years at a daily dose of

4 mg/kg. Histochemical studies on liver, kidneys, heart, spleen, stomach, intestine and adrenal gland revealed no obvious difference between 3 treated monkeys and 2 control monkeys. Heart muscle showed slight congestion, with changes in LDH but not in SDH or ATPase. Liver showed slight distension of hepatic sinusoids partial vacuolation in central zones of liver lobules but no changes in LDH isoenzymes, G6PDH, ATPase and RNA. The kidney showed cloudy swelling in the proximal renal tubules, a decrease in ATPase but no change in G6PDH or juxtaglomerular cell granules (21, 44).

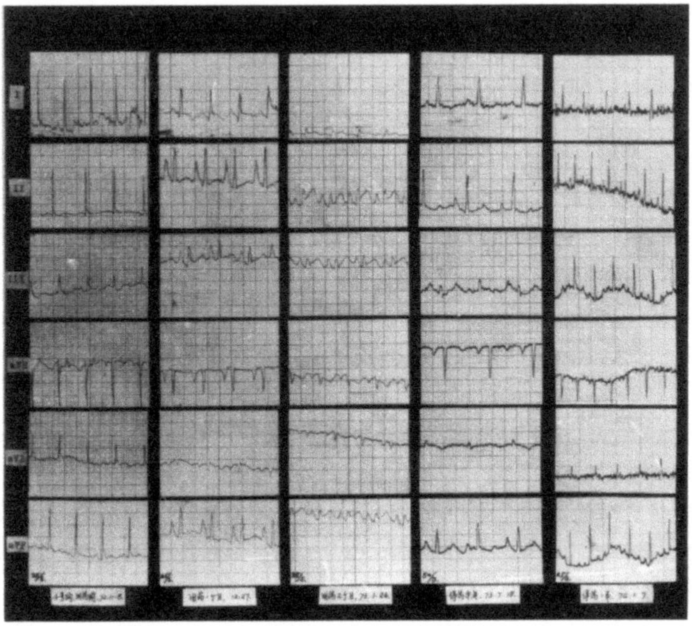

A B C D E

Fig. 4. The electrocardiographic changes produced by treatment of gossypol (2 mg/kg/day) in dogs.

A: before medication;
B: 4 weeks after the beginning of treatment;
C: 8 weeks after the beginning of treatment;
D: 6 months later stopping medication;
E: 1 year later stopping medication.

There were marked differences in absorption and excretion of gossypol between dogs and monkeys. Gossypol was less well absorbed and more was excreted in monkeys than in dogs and this may be one reason for the difference in toxicity (21).

(3) Genetic effects of gossypol (44)

a. Chromosomal aberration. In rats treated with gossypol (20 mg/kg per day for 9 days), there were no significant differences, compared to control animals, in the frequency of metaphase chromosomal aberrations (including the incidence of breakages, gaps, and polyploidy) in the spermatogonia and spermatocytes or in lymphocyte micronuclei. The chromosome mutation frequency in the leucocytes in 16 volunteers also showed no significant deviation from normal (Institute of Genetics, Fu-Dan University, unpublished data).

b. Dominant lethal mutagenic effect. Male rats received a dose of 20 mg/kg of gossypol for one month and were allowed to mate with untreated females at 10-day intervals, commencing one month after withdrawal of gossypol treatment. The dominant lethal effect on the resulting embryos was then determined. The frequency of dead embryos in the first two rounds of mating was significantly higher in treated rats ($P < 0.01-0.05$) than in controls, but was not significantly increased in the third mating period. These data suggest that the genetic damage to the spermatozoa is transitory (Institute of Genetics, Fu-Dan University, unpublished data).

c. Frequency of sister chromatid exchange. *In vivo* experiments were carried out on sister chromatid exchange in the bone marrow cells of mice (strain ICR) after treatment with 10 times the clinical dose of gossypol acetic acid (4 mg/kg per day for 4 days). No significant differences were noted in the average sister chromatid exchange per cell between treated (3.09 ± 0.27) and control (2.96 ± 0.29) animals. No deviations were seen either in *in vitro* experiments with the Chinese hamster cell strain CHO k-1 treated with two doses of gossypol (0.23

and 2.3 µg/ml) in the culture medium for 24 hours (44).

d. Ames in vitro test. Gossypol acetic acid and gossypol formic acid, at concentrations of 0.1-1000 µg/plate (incorporation assay) and 0.5-500 µg/paper sheet (spot test), were employed for mutagenicity studies on Salmonella typhimurium using nitrosoguanidine, aflatoxin B, mepacrine, sodium azide and 9-aminoacridine as positive controls. Both assay methods gave negative results, indicating that gossypol was not mutagenic. Similar data have been reported by De Peyster and Wang (45).

e. Offspring observation. Gossypol-treated male rats were mated with untreated females after recovery from the antifertility effect. The offspring in the F_1 and F_2 generations appeared normal and healthy on gross examination. Of 260 women that became pregnant after their husbands had ceased taking gossypol, 53 carried their pregnancies to term and gave birth to normal children (44).

On the basis of the above tests and examinations no significant genetic damage resulting from gossypol treatment could be detected.

IV. Clinical Trials of Gossypol

Gossypol was first employed clinically as a male antifertility agent in 1972 in the People's Republic of China. To date, 8806 men in 14 provinces of China have been treated, 2100 men with gossypol, 5280 men with gossypol acetic acid, and 1426 men with gossypol formic acid (2, 6, 59). The dose administered was 20 mg daily. It usually took 60 to 70 days to reduce sperm counts below 4 million/ml and subjects were then given a maintenance dose of 150-220 mg per month in divided doses. Efficacy evaluated by semen analysis was 99%.

The first change noticed in the ejaculates was a decrease in the percentage of motile spermatozoa and increase in malformed spermatozoa followed by a gradual drop in sperm count until severe oligospermia and azoospermia were achieved. The ejaculate consisted of exfoliated and degeneration spermatozoa. Ultrastructural changes in spermatozoa included decondensation of the nucleus, loss of axial filaments, swelling of the mitochondria and absence of cristae and degeneration of the acrosome and head cap; succinic dehydrogenase and lactic dehydrogenase in the midpiece were decreased, while acrosomal proteinase was unchanged (2). The exfoliated cells (60) were spermatids (45.3%), a mixture of spermatids and spermatocytes (34.0%), sperms (16.9%, including abnormal sperms) and spermatocytes (3.8%). The sequence of exfoliation of immature cells of the germinal line was: spermatid-spermatocyte-spermatogonium. After maintenance dose of 40 mg/week for 4-24 months (60) the cells in the semen from 42 men (Fig. 5) were spermatocytes (33.3%), spermatids (28.7%) and a mixture of spermatocytes and spermatogonia (38.0%).

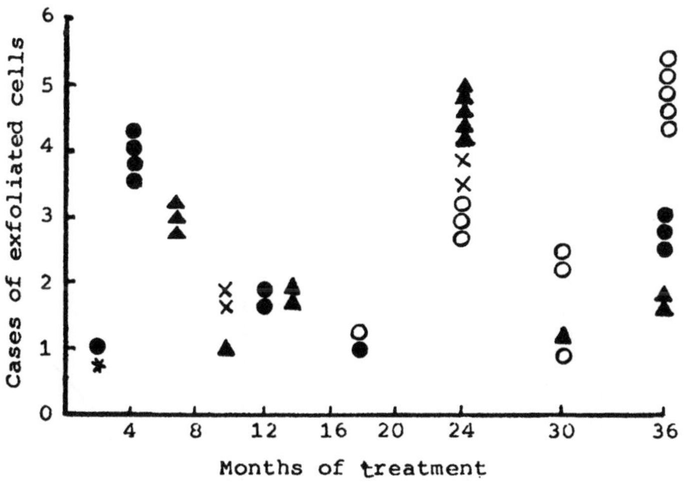

Fig 5. Exfoliated cells in 42 human ejaculates during maintenance with gossypol acetic acid 40 mg/wk
✱ abnormal spermatozoa; ● spermatid; ✕ sperm; ▲ spermatocytes; ○ spermatogonia

Of 13 men treated continuously for 10-24 months, 8 showed spermatocytes, 4 spermatogonia and 1 a mixture of spermatocytes and spermatids. Three months after cessation of gossypol spermatogenesis was gradually restored in 10 men but was not restored to the original number and activity after withdrawal of gossypol for 12 months. In 3 of 4 men spermatogonia remained the same even after cessation of gossypol for 24 months and it was suggested (60) that the restoration in sperm count and activity was related to the damaged spermatogonia (Fig. 6).

Recovery

Semen analysis in 2067 men 6 months to 4.5 years after cessation of gossypol administration indicated that in 73.7% the effect was reversible (sperm count over 4 million/ml), 16.4% had incomplete recovery (appearance of sperm but count below

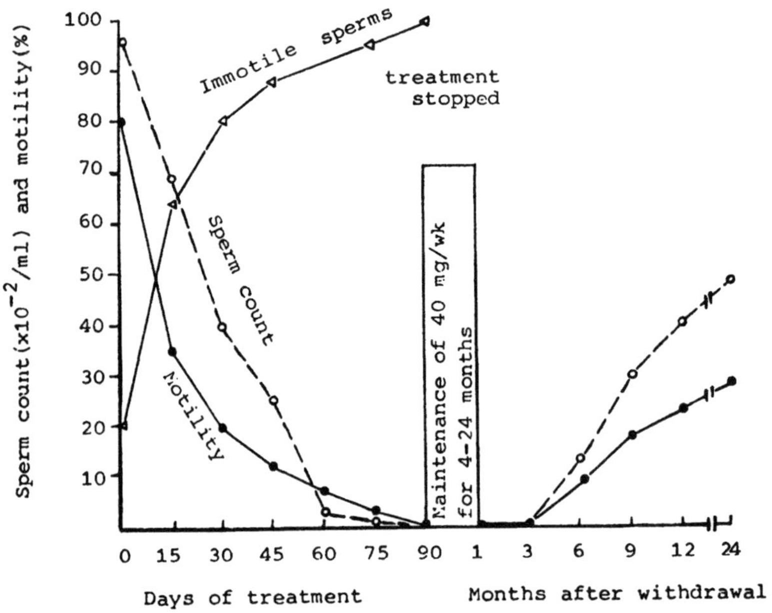

Fig 6. Effect of gossypol acetic acid (20 mg/d) on sperms of 13 men

4 million/ml), while 9.9% remained azospermic at the time of the last semen examination. In subjects taking gossypol for less than 2 years, the recovery rate was much higher than in those taking it for more than 2 years. Therefore, it was suggested that if the aim of gossypol treatment was not to produce sterility, its duration should be restricted to less than 2 years. In addition, it is worth pointing out that the earliest evidence of sperm recovery may occasionally be delayed for as long as 3 years after withdrawal of gossypol. Therefore, the actual recovery rate must be higher than the figures mentioned above, as these figures include subjects in whom the posttreatment withdrawal period was less than 3 years.

Side-effects of gossypol

Common side-effects include fatigue (12.6%), gastrointestinal symptoms (7.3%), decreased libido and potency (5.0%), dizziness (3.8%) and dryness of the mouth (3.0%). Occasionally there may be other manifestations, such as sleepiness, palpitations, oedema of the eyelids, decreased perspiration, increased libido and potency, and skin rash. Most of these side-effects occur initially and are generally transient. A minority of cases may require symptomatic treatment or cessation of the drug. Fatigue may be related to potassium deficiency and can usually be alleviated by potassium administration.

Of all the side-effects, hypokalaemic paralysis is the most important. Among the 8806 volunteers, 66 (0.75%) such cases were found. Most of them recovered promptly after potassium repletion but a few recover only after prolonged potassium therapy. Total body potassium in patients with gossypol-induced hypokalaemia was low (61) due to renal potassium loss; aldosterone activity of such patients is not increased. In rats after intravenous injection of ^{42}K, the urinary ^{42}K excretion was significantly higher in the gossypol-treated than in the control group (62).

Similarly in rats, the increased elimination of urinary potassium and depletion of intracellular potassium may be unrelated to levels of circulating mineralocorticoids since the levels of aldosterone were not increased. The potassium-losing effect of gossypol may be due to an inhibitory action on Na-K-ATPase activity (63). Gossypol inhibits Na-K-ATPase and other magnesium dependent enzyme systems and potassium transport in the isolated rabbit heart and skeletal muscle (64, 65). In animals fed a low potassium or potassium-free diet, tissue potassium levels were decreased but there is, as yet, no animal model in which hypokalemic paralysis similar to that in man can be induced (44, 46). Recently, Qian (66) postulated the involvement of prostaglandins in induction of hypokalemia and the anti-spermatogenic action of gossypol. In view of the fact that the literature on effects of prostaglandins on testicular function and sperm motility are replete with contradictions, a great deal more study will be required before this suggestion can be accepted.

In the first clinical study outside China, carried out by Coutinho et al. (67), eight Brazilian men with normal sperm count and motility were treated with gossypol for periods of 6-12 months. A dose of 20 mg daily for 4 months followed by 20 mg on alternate days resulted in azoospermia at the end of 4 months of treatment with no change in semen volume. The response to LH-RH and hCG was normal during treatment. Testosterone levels remained within the normal range. None of the subjects reported loss of libido or potency. Blood chemistry was normal. There were no significant changes in blood pressure or body weight. Reversibility was faster in men who took the drug for short periods of time. These observations confirm those reported by Chinese scientists.

References

1. Kessler, A., Standley, C.C.: The WHO programme of research in fertility regulation. In: "Regulation of Human Fertility" Ed. Diczfalusy, E., Copenhagen, pp. 11-19 (1977).

2. National Coordinating Group on Male Antifertility Agents. Gossypol. A new antifertility agent for males. Chin. Med. J. (English edition) 4, 417-428 (1978).

3. Liu, B.S.: Suggestions of feeding crude cottonseed oil for contraception. Shanghai Acta Med. 6, 43 (1957).

4. Wang, Y.E., Luo, Y.G., Tang, X.C.: Studies on the antifertility actions of cottonseed meal and gossypol. Acta Pharmaceutica Sinica 14, 663-669 (1979).

5. Dai, R.X., Pang, S.N., Lin, X.K., Ke, Y.B., Liu, Z.L., Dong, R.H.: A study of antifertility of cottonseed. Acta Biol. Exp. Sinica. 11, 1-14 (1978).

6. Liu, Z.Q., Liu, G.Z., Hei, L.S., Zhang, R.A., Yu, C.Z.: Clinical trial of gossypol as a male antifertility agent. In: "Recent Advances in Fertility Regulation", Eds. Chang, C.F., Griffin, D., Woolman, A., Atar S.A., Geneva, pp. 160-163 (1981).

7. Lei, H.P.: Review and prospect of gossypol research. Acta Pharmaceutica Sinica 17(1): 1-4 (1982).

8. Prasad, M.R.N., Diczfalusy, E.: Gossypol. International Journal of Andrology, Suppl. 5, pp. 53-70 (1982).

9. Abou-Donia, M.B.: Physiological effects and metabolism of gossypol. Residue Reviews 61, 124-159 (1976).

10. Abou-Donia, S.A., Lasker, J.M., Abou-Donia, M.B.: High-performance liquid chromatographic analysis of gossypol. J. Chromat. 206, 606-610 (1981).

11. King, T.J., de Silva, L.B.: Optically active gossypol from Thespesia populnea. Tetrahedron Letters 3, 261 (1968).

12. Murthy, R.S.R., Basu, D.K., Murti, V.V.S.: Antifertility activity of (+) gossypol. Current Science 50, 64-66 (1981).

13. Lu, G.S.: Purification of gossypol and preparation of derivatives. In: Workshop on Gossypol, Chicago 11 March, 1980. Abstract 11.

14. Wang, N.G., Lei, H.P.: Antifertility effect of gossypol acetic acid on male rats. Chin. Med. J. 59, 402-405 (1979).

15. Chang, M.C., Gu, Z.P., Saksena, S.K.: Effects of gossypol on the fertility of male rats, hamsters and rabbits. Contraception 21, 461-469 (1980).

16. Shi, Q.X., Zhang, Y.G., Yuan, Y.Y.: Studies on antifertility effect of gossypol. II. The effects of gossypol acetic acid on the spermatogenesis in rats. Acta Zoologica Sinica 27(1) 22-28 (1981).

17. Hahn, D.W., Rusticus, C., Probst, A., Homm, R., Johnson, A.N.: Antifertility and endocrine activity of gossypol in rodents. Contraception 24(1) 97-105 (1981).

18. Lin, Y.C., Hadley, M.A., Klingener, D., Dym, M.: Effects of gossypol on the reproductive system of male rats. Biology of Reproduction 22(1) 95A (Suppl.) (1980).

19. Shi, Q.X., Zhang, Y.G.: Studies on antifertility effect of gossypol. I. Effects of gossypol on androgen-dependent organs in mice and rats. Acta Zoologica Sinica 26(4), 311-316 (1980).

20. Saksena, S.K., Salmonsen, M.A., Lau, I.F., Chang, M.C.: Gossypol: Its toxicological and endocrinological effects in male rabbits. Contraception 24(2) 203-214 (1981).

21. Sang, G.W., Zhang, Y.G., Shi, Q.X., Shen, K.Y., Lu, F.Y., Zhao, X.J., Wang, M.Q., Liu, X.L., Yuan, Y.Y.: Chronic toxicity of gossypol and the relationship to its metabolic fate in dogs and monkeys. Acta Pharmacologica Sinica 1(1), 39-43 (1980).

22. Shandilya, L.N., Clarkson, T.B.: Antireproductive and hypolipidemic effects of gossypol in male cynomolgus monkeys. Contraceptive Delivery Systems 3 (3/4), Abstract 277 (1982).

23. Chang, C.C.: Studies to evaluate effects of gossypol obtained from different sources on different strains of rats. In: Workshop on Gossypol, Chicago, Abstract 6, March 1980.

24. Waller, D.P., Fong, H.H.S., Cordell, G.A., Soejarto, D.D.: Antifertility effects of gossypol and its impurities on male hamsters. Contraception 23(6), 653-659 (1981).

25. Zhou, L.F., Chen, C.C., Wang, N.G., Lei, H.P.: Observations on long-term administration of gossypol acetic acid to rats. Chin. Med. J. 60, 343-344 (1980).

26. Xue, S.P., Zong, S.D., Su, S.Y., Wu, Y.W., Liu, Y., Zhou, Z.G., Ma, X.X.: Antifertility effect of gossypol on the germinal epithelium of the rat testis. A cytological, autoradiographical and ultrastructural observation. Scientia Sinica (English edition) 23(5), 642-657 (1980).

27. Zhou, L.F., Lei, H.P.: Recovery of fertility in rats after gossypol treatment. In: "Recent Advances in Fertility Regulation", Eds. Chang, C.F., Griffin, D., Woolman, A., Atar S.A., Geneva, pp. 147-151 (1981).

28. Saksena, S.K., Salmonsen, R.A.: Antifertility effects of gossypol in male hamsters. Fertility and Sterility 37(5), 686-690 (1982).

29. Dai, R.X,, Dong, R.H.: Studies on antifertility effects of gossypol. I. An experimental analysis by epididymal ligature. Acta Biol. Exp. Sinica 11(1), 15-22 (1978).

30. Dai, R.X., Pang, S.Y.: Studies on the antifertility effects of gossypol. VI. Observations of testicular atrophy of rats administered with gossypol for long-terms. Acta Biol. Exp. Sinica 13(2), 193-199 (1980).

31. Dai, R.X., Pang, S.N., Liu, Z.L.: Studies on the antifertility effect of gossypol. II. A morphological analysis of the antifertility effect of gossypol. Acta Biol. Exp. Sinica 11(1), 27-36 (1978).

32. Hadley, M.A., Lin, C.Y., Dym, M.: Effects of gossypol on the reproductive system of male rats. J. Andrology 2, 190 (1981).

33. Nadakavukaren, M.J., Sorensen, R.H., Tone, N.J.: Effect of Gossypol on the ultrastructure of rat spermatozoa. Cell Tissue Res. 204, 293-296 (1979).

34. Hadley, M.A., Burgos, M.H.: Inhibition of rat epididymal sperm by gossypol. Paper presented at the New York Academy of Sciences Meeting on the Cell Biology of the Testis, April 1981.

35. Yu, T.H., Chang, H.T., Hsieh, P.L.: The in vivo effect of gossypol on zinc, iron and manganese concentrations in rats. Acta Physiologica Sinica 33(1), 17-23 (1981).

36. Gu, Z.P., Tsong, S.D., Chang, C.C.: Effect of gossypol on the testis and epididymis of rat and hamster. In: Contraceptive Delivery Systems 3 (3/4), Abstract 279 (1982).

37. Zhou, W.Y., Xue, S.P.: Effect of gossypol acetate on the DNA content of primary spermatocytes in rats. Reproduction and Contraception 1(3), 26-29 (1981).

38. Kalla, N.R., Vasudev, M.: Studies on the male antifertility agent, gossypol acetic acid. III. Effect of gossypol acetic acid on rat testis. Andrologia 13(3), 242-249 (1981).

39. Ye, Y.X., Liang, D., Gao, H.Y., Ye, G.Y.: The effect of gossypol on the incorporation of ^{3}H-thymidine in the liver, testis and small intestine of experimental animals. Acta Pharmaceutica Sinica 16(5), 390-393 (1981).

40. Ye, W.S., Liu, Y., Shao, T.S., Liu, Z.H., You, M.M., Guo, Y., Xue, S.P.: Observations of the gossypol effects on the protein and nucleic acid synthesis in spermatogenic cells of rat testis in vivo and in vitro. Acta Anatomica Sinica, 13(1), 92-96 (1982).

41. Abou-Donia, M.B., Dickert, J.W.: Gossypol: uncoupling of respiratory chain and oxidative phosphorylation. Life Science 14, 1955-1963 (1974).

42. Kalla, N.R., Vasudev, M.: Studies on male antifertility agent, gossypol acetic acid. II. Effect of gossypol acetic acid on the motility and ATPase activity of human spermatozoa. Andrologia 13(2), 95-98 (1981).

43. Poso, H., Wichmann, K., Janne, J., Luukkainen, T.: Gossypol, a powerful inhibitor of human spermatozoa metabolism. Lancet 19, 885-886 (1980).

44. Xue, S.P.: Studies on the antifertility effect of gossypol, a new contraceptive for males. In: "Recent Advances in Fertility Regulation", Eds. Chang, C.F., Griffin, D., Woolman, A., Atar S.A., Geneva, pp. 122-146 (1981).

45. Peyster, A.D., Wang, Y.Y.: Gossypol - proposed contraceptive for men pass the AMES test. New Engl. J. Med. 301, 275-276 (1979).

46. Maugh, T.H.: Male "Pill" blocks sperm enzyme. Science 212, 314 (1981).

47. Lee, C.Y., Malling, H.Y.: Selective inhibition of sperm-specific lactate dehydrogenase X by an antifertility agent, gossypol. Fed. Proc. 40, 718 (1981).

48. Waller, D.P., Zaneveld, L.J.D., Fong, H.H.S.: In-vitro spermicidal activity of gossypol. Contraception 22, 183-187 (1980).

49. Kalla, N.R., Vasudev, M.: Studies on the male antifertility agent, gossypol acetic acid. I. In-vitro studies on the effect of gossypol acetic acid in human spermatozoa. IRCS Med. Sci. Biochemistry 8, 375-376 (1980).

50. Ridley, A.J., Blasco, L.: Testosterone and gossypol effects on human sperm motility. Fertility and Sterility 36(5), 638-642 (1981).

51. Cameron, S.M., Waller, D.P., Zaneveld, L.J.D.: Vaginal spermicidal activity of gossypol in the Macaca arctoides. Fertility and Sterility 37(2), 273-274 (1982).

52. Tso, W.W., Lee, C.S., Tso, M.Y.W.: Sensitivity of various spermatozoal enzymes to gossypol inhibition. Contraceptive Delivery Systems 3, (3/4), Abstract 280 (1982).

53. Lin, T., Murono, E.P., Osterman, J., Nankin, H.R., Coulson, P.B.: Gossypol inhibits testicular steroidogenesis. Fertility and Sterility 35(5), 563-566 (1981).

54. Wang, Y.E., Luo, Y.D., Shen, L.I., Tan, X.C.: Plasma testosterone levels in Chinese normal males, endocrinopath and gossypol receivers. Reproduction and Contraception 1(1), 41-44 (1981).

55. Wang, H.Y., Xu, Y.S., Jiang, L.G., De, S.L., Shi, Y.Q., Zhou, Z.M.: The effects of sex steroid hormones and gossypol on LH secretion of rat pituitary by radioimmunoassay. Acta Physiologica Sinica, 31(4), 337-343 (1979).

56. Liang, S.X., Pang, S.N., Dong, R.H., Dai, R.X.: Radioimmunoassay of serum concentration of testosterone and LH in male rats administered with gossypol. Acta Biol. Exp. Sinica 14 (2), 191-197 (1981).

57. Wu, Y.M., Chappel, S.C., Flickinger, G.L.: Effects of gossypol on pituitary-ovarian endocrine function, ovulation and fertility in female hamsters. Contraception 24(3), 259-268 (1981).

58. Han, M.L.: Gossypol treatment for menopausal functional bleeding, myoma of uterus and endometrosis. Acta Acad. Med. Sinica 2, 167-170 (1980).

59. Qian, S.Z., Hu, J.H., Ho, L.X., Sun, M.X., Huang, Y.Z., Fang, J.H.: The first clinical trial of gossypol on male antifertility. In: "Clinical Pharmacology and Therapeutics" Proceedings of First World Conference on Clinical Pharmacology and Therapeutics, Ed. Turner, P., Macmillan, London, pp. 489-492 (1981).

60. Shi, Q.X., Qiu, J.X., Zhang, G.Y.: Analysis on exfoliated cells in human semen after oral administration of gossypol acetic acid. Acta Pharmacologica Sinica 2(4), 262-266 (1981).

61. Qian, S.Z., Jing, G., Wu, X.Y., Xu, Y., Li, Y.Q., Zhou, Z.H.: Gossypol related hypokalemia. Clinico-pharmacological studies. Chinese Med. J. 93, 477-482 (1980).

62. Xue, S.P., Liang, D.C., Shao, T.S., Wu, Y.W., Liu, Y., Zhou, Z.H., Wang, N.Y.: Studies on the effect of gossypol on ^{42}K metabolism of rat. Acta Anat. Sinica 10, 78-87 (1979).

63. Qian, S.Z., Xu, H.: The effect of gossypol on potassium and prostaglandin metabolism. Reproduction and Contraception 1(1), 6-9 (1981).

64. Qian, S.Z., Xu, Y., Chen, Z.C., Cao, L.M., Sun, S.C., Tang, X.C., Wang, Y.E., Shen, L.Y., Zhu, M.K.: The influence of gossypol on the potassium metabolism of rats and the effect of some possible contributing factors. Acta Pharmaceutica Sinica 14, 513-520 (1979).

65. Bi, X.F., Aheng, Y.J., Yang, H.F., Zhang, Z.Y.: The effect of gossypol on renal ATPase activity. Sci. Sinica 9, 914-919 (1980).

66. Qian, S.Z.: Effect of gossypol on potassium and prostaglandin metabolism and mechanism of action of gossypol. In: "Recent Advances in Fertility Regulation", Eds. Chang, C.F., Griffin, D., Woolman, A., Atar S.A., Geneva, pp. 152-159 (1981).

67. Coutinho, E.M.: Clinical studies with gossypol. Contraceptive Delivery Systems 3 (3/4), Abstract 271 (1982).

THE RENIN ANGIOTENSIN SYSTEM IN THE EXTRARENAL VASCULAR WALLS: AN APPROACH TO STUDIES IN HUMANS

H. Dahlheim, I. C. M. Jacob, J. Pschorr and J. Rosenthal *
Department of Physiology, University of Munich, Pettenkofer-strasse 12, D-8000 Munich 2, and * Ulm University Medical Center, D-7900 Ulm, Federal Republic of Germany

Introduction

Renal renin

The first component of the renin angiotensin system (RAS) to be described was renin; this compound was detected in the kidney. Its existence and pressor effect was demonstrated in 1898 by Tigerstedt and Bergman (1). They measured the increase of arterial blood pressure following intravenous injection of extracts of rabbit kidney cortex. These observations were reproduced several times by other investigators (2, 3, 4). However, four decades went by before it was recognized that renin was an important link in a complex system, the RAS, and that it was involved in the pathogenesis of (renal) hypertension (5, 6, 7). It is still not clear whether the RAS participates in the development and/or maintenance of essential hypertension, which is the most common form of hypertensive disease.

Extrarenal renin

Jiménez-Díaz and colleagues were the first to detect extrarenal renin-like activity; it was found in arterial walls. They suggested, therefore, that this enzyme may play a role in blood pressure regulation, and could also be involved in the development of essential hypertension (8, 9, 10). They performed cross-circulation experiments in dogs and observed that stimulation

Hormones in Normal and Abnormal Human Tissues, Vol. III

of the central endings of the vagus nerve in one dog generated blood pressure elevation in both animals. In order to further investigate this phenomenon, they developed an operation technique which they called "perro partido" (sectioned dog); in this procedure, the circulation of the upper part of one dog was separated from the lower part, so that the spinal cord was the only remaining functional connection. Following stimulation of the vagus nerve, blood pressure elevation occurred in both parts. However, when the lower circulation was perfused with Ringer's solution instead of blood, blood pressure rose only in the upper section. This led to the assumption that nervous stimulation induced the release from vascular walls of a substance which generated a vasopressor agent, only in the presence of plasma. They postulated that the vascular component was renin-like and reacted with "hypertensinogen" (renin substrate) in plasma. In order to further investigate this hypothesis, they prepared extracts of kidney cortex and arterial wall according to the method described by Braun-Menéndez and colleagues (5), and compared their effects on blood pressure. Neither hypertensinogen, nor the arterial or kidney extracts by themselves caused blood pressure elevation; however, following incubation with the renin substrate preparation, both arterial and renal extracts increased blood pressure in a comparable way. Jiménez-Dîaz assumed that the vasopressor formed in plasma, which he called "arteriohypertensin", was similar to the vasoactive reaction product of renin (10). He believed that renin-like substances could be found not only in the kidney, but also in all other parts of the vascular system (9).

It is beyond doubt that Jiménez-Dîaz was the first to have suggested the existence of renin or a renin-like substance in the extrarenal arterial wall; moreover, he drew attention to its possible role in essential hypertension. Some years later, the author replaced his own hypothesis by the assumption that norepinephrine had caused the observed vasoconstriction (11). However, in the latter case, the role of plasma, whose pressure was necessary to produce the effect on blood pressure just described, was not explained. Today, the RAS is known to interfere with catecholamine release, and there is evidence for an intrinsic vascular RAS. Therefore, both norepinephrine and the vascular RAS may well have played some role in Jiménez-Dîaz's experiments.

Physiological Aspects

These studies were continued by Dengler (12), in order to obtain more information on vasoactive substances in the arterial wall, irrespective of possible participation in the reflex mechanism described by Jiménez-Dîaz. The author performed perfusion experiments on isolated rabbit ears. He observed a marked vasoconstriction lasting up to 30 minutes when arterial extracts from hogs and hog plasma or globulin were perfused together. Agreeing with Jiménez-Dîaz, Dengler concluded that the vascular extract, which was not effective by itself, contained an enzyme catalyzing formation of a vasoconstrictor substance in the presence of whole plasma, or of the globulin fraction only. Analogous to renal renin (1), the vasoactive component was not dialyzable and was thermolabile above 56°C. Biological measurements with isolated guinea-pig intestine or rat uterus further ascertained the constricting properties of the vascular extracts when incubated with plasma or globulin. In addition, experiments on anaesthetized rats showed that the long-lasting blood pressure response is comparable to that of renal renin. The author suspected that the substance from the arterial extracts catalyzed the release of the actual vasoactive compound from a plasma protein contained within the globulin fraction. However, he did not consider this enzyme to be altogether identical with renin; the response of the rabbit ear vasculature to arterial extracts was more pronounced than the reaction to renin, whereas the effect on rat blood pressure was the opposite. On the other hand, Dengler noted similar electrophoretic behaviour of plasma and arterial extracts. He suggested therefore that the plasma protein fraction containing the substrate for the enzyme might also be present in the vascular wall, so that the vasoconstricting substance could be formed in loco. This assumption may be fundamental for the understanding of the physiological role of the vascular RAS. It has not yet, however, been confirmed whether the renin substrate itself is present in sufficient amounts in the vascular wall, and if so, from where it originates. Moreover, based on our present knowledge, it should be considered that the plasma angiotensinogen content is extremely low, as compared with the total globulin fraction. Probably the electrophoretic measurements performed do not allow any conclusions as to the presence of renin substrate in vascular tissue.

Due to the long-lasting blood pressure effect described by the author, the vasoactive compound is likely not to be angiotensin, but rather renin, since intravenous injections of this enzyme produce such a prolonged pressure response.

In the meantime, the RAS was further characterized, and in 1953, Skeggs and coworkers recognized the existence of two "hypertensins" (angiotensins) (13): one form of hypertensin (angiotensin I, A I) is converted into the other (angiotensin II, A II) by an enzyme present in plasma, which they called "hypertensin converting enzyme"(angiotensin I converting enzyme, ACE). Earlier, Kahn and associates (14) had found that high levels of angiotensin occur in the arterial blood of patients with malignant hypertension, as opposed to those with the benign form of disease. Skeggs (15) pointed out that if A II was formed through the local action of renin in the vascular walls, plasma renin activity or plasma A II levels would be no measure of peripheral vascular resistance. Thus, hypertension might be caused by activation of the vascular RAS.

Distribution and site of synthesis of renin

In 1964, Gould, Skeggs and Kahn(16) determined the distribution of specific renin activities of various tissue extracts, in particular those of arterial walls and kidney. The question then arose as to whether the renin measured in vasculature was synthesized locally or whether it originated from the plasma. The authors measured specific renin activities of artery, liver, lung, placenta, spleen, blood, skeletal muscle, heart, and brain, as well as of the pregnant and non-pregnant uterus of the hog. In addition, renin activity was determined for the first time in venous walls. Enzymatic activity was demonstrated in the media and especially in the adventitia (75% of arterial renin activity). Renin activity was easily measurable in the liver also, but in the heart, brain, and non-pregnant uterus, renin activity could not be demonstrated by this method.

Biochemical studies

In order to characterize the arterial wall enzyme, the activation energy and Michaelis constants (Km) of A I formation, and the effect of pH on enzymatic activity were investigated. In addition, inhibition experiments with antirenin were performed in vitro.

The authors were probably the first to demonstrate the existence of extrarenal vascular renin or renin-like activity by means of systematically applied biochemical methods, although they were not able to differentiate the arterial enzyme from renal renin.

Basso and Taquini (17) studied the behaviour of renin activity in the vascular walls of bilaterally nephrectomized and normal dogs; they also determined the Km values, velocity constants, and activation energies for this enzyme and for purified hog kidney renin. Their enzyme-kinetic studies did not allow them to discriminate between arterial wall and kidney renin. However, arterial wall renin could not be affected by bilateral nephrectomy.

The authors calculated an activation energy of 12,900 cal/mol for the arterial wall extract and 13,700 cal/mol for the kidney enzyme. In comparison, Gould and coworkers determined 15,300 cal/mol for both preparations. Although they also measured reaction velocities and Km values, the results of Basso and Taquini were difficult to compare with those of other authors (16, 18, 19), because the species studied, the methods used for renin extraction and incubation, and the units in which the results were expressed were different (17).

Gould et al. (16) assumed that, even though the concentration of arterial wall renin is very small, it may be far more effective on blood pressure than the plasma enzyme. The experiments did not allow the authors to draw any conclusions as to the origin of extrarenal renin.

Action of renin

Based on their experiments with aminopeptidases, Daum, Uehleke and Klaus (20) found that the decrease in pressure effect of renin following intravenous injection of aminopeptidases is far less pronounced than that of angiotensin. They suggested that renin was bound to the arteriolar walls, which may result in angiotensin formation next to their receptors. Schaechtelin, Regoli and Gross (21) also assumed that plasma renin may accumulate in the arteriolar muscle cells. They performed cross-circulation experiments and studied the effect of intravenously injected renin on the blood pressure of nephrectomized rats. The blood pressure response was far more prolonged than could be explained by the disappearance rate of renin from the circulation.

Factors influencing renin

Rosenthal and coworkers (18) postulated that accumulation of renin at the site of the vascular angiotensin receptors could account for the low plasma renin activities occurring in some hypertensive states. They assumed that more precise knowledge of the relationship between aortic and plasma renin would provide a better basis for the interpretation of plasma renin activity measurements in hypertensive patients. Therefore, they simultaneously determined aortic and plasma renin activity, and renin substrate concentration in the rat under different pathophysiological conditions. Following bilateral nephrectomy, plasma as well as arterial renin activity decreased rapidly;

after 24 h, plasma renin was undetectable, whereas aortic renin activity was very low. Renin substrate concentration rose and reached a plateau after about 12 h. Water deprivation for 3 days increased plasma and aortic renin activities, whereas renin substrate concentration was significantly lower than that of control animals. The behaviour of the enzymatic activities after water deprivation for 3 days followed by bilateral nephrectomy was similar to that of nephrectomized animals with normal access to water. Bilateral adrenalectomy elevated plasma renin activity significantly, aortic renin increasing six-fold compared with the controls and three-fold compared with water-deprived animals; plasma renin substrate was undetectable. From these findings the authors concluded that arterial bound renin responds to the same stimuli as those which are known to influence plasma renin activity. They emphasized that aortic renin activity is still detectable after bilateral nephrectomy, whereas plasma renin is not; they thought this might be caused by the postulated accumulation of renin in arterial tissue.

In a subsequent investigation (19), Genest and associates studied the distribution of norepinephrine and renin in arterial tissues from different vascular beds in the dog. The study was based on the assumption that the mesenteric vasculature plays a role in the regulation of systemic blood pressure, as can be seen in the splanchnic vasoconstriction response to the upright posture, or in the high incidence of arteriosclerotic lesions in the splanchnic region of hypertensive patients. The norepinephrine and renin measurements were noted to be roughly parallel in that the highest activities were measured in tissue of the mesenteric artery branches, in contrast to those of other arteries of similar diameter. The content of both substances in corresponding mesenteric veins was comparable to that in the arteries. In dogs with experimental congestive heart failure, Hayduk et al. found an increase of renin activity in the mesenteric artery (22, 23); norepinephrine content, however, remained the same, although it increased markedly in the mesenteric vein (23). This fact was considered by them to be of great importance, since it might represent the biochemical substrate of the active venous vasoconstriction in congestive heart failure. Recently, this assumption was supported by investigations with ACE blocker captopril, which showed that this drug has a beneficial therapeutic effect in congestive heart failure. The sodium content of all investigated arteries except for the carotid was increased in animals with congestive heart failure. It remains unclear whether the sodium content of the vasculature is correlated with its renin activity.

Pathophysiological conditions affecting renin levels

The same investigators also studied other (patho-) physiological conditions in the dog: severe haemorrhage (24), Clipping of one renal artery (22, 25) or of the superior mesenteric artery (25, 26), sodium restriction (22, 27), and nephrectomy (22, 25, 26). Renin was measured in several samples of vascular tissues of dogs, and additionally in plasma, kidney, heart, lung, liver, spleen, skeletal muscle, and the adrenal glands. Ganten and colleagues (24) performed haemorrhage experiments on bilaterally nephrectomized dogs and determined renin activity in mesenteric arteries and blood from the aorta and portal vein. The renin content of mesenteric artery branches was elevated three-fold, whereas plasma renin activity increased gradually in aortic and even more markedly in the portal venous blood. The authors therefore suggested that the plasma renin as measured following nephrectomy originates from the splanchnic vasculature.

Experimental renovascular hypertension did not affect the renin content of vascular tissue, regardless of whether the contralateral kidney was removed or not. However, mesenteric and aortic renin activities increased significantly in normotensive dogs with clipped renal arteries (22, 26). The authors were unable to explain this phenomenon at that time.

The effect of moderate constriction of the superior mesenteric artery of dogs on vascular renin activity was also studied by Ganten et al. (25, 26). In addition, the animals were bilaterally nephrectomized 24 h prior to plasma and tissue sampling. Renin increased in the mesenteric branches, but decreased in the aorta, and was undetectable in plasma. The authors excluded the possibility that the elevation of renin levels in mesenteric tissue could be due to an uptake of renin from plasma, since renin had disappeared from the circulation following nephrectomy. They suggested that ischemia stimulated renin formation in the peripheral branches of the mesenteric artery. This assumption was supported by the finding that aortic renin remained unchanged after bilateral nephrectomy (26).

Nutritional factors affecting renin

Severe sodium chloride restriction caused elevation of renin activity in saphenous and mesenteric vasculature, but not in the aorta (22). Moreover, renin activity was increased in plasma, renal cortex, heart, lung, liver, spleen, and skeletal muscle, but not in the adrenals. The authors concluded that in most tissues of the dog, renin is the limiting factor for angiotensin formation. In a subsequent study (27), the control dogs were kept on a diet containing less sodium; it was found that the increases of vascular renin activity in the sodium restricted animals were not significant. Norepinephrine values in vascular tissue decreased, but not significantly, and blood pressure remained constant. However, the vascular response to exogenous renin and angiotensin was attenuated. The authors also observed a decrease in sodium content of the vascular tissues, except for that of the renal artery, which remained the same. They concluded that the response and receptor sensitivity of the renal artery to various stimuli remained normal following sodium restriction.

Strewler and associates (28) studied the effect of dietary sodium deprivation in rabbits on vascular smooth muscle preparations (in vivo and in vitro experiments), and found a reduced response to angiotensin. They postulated that changes in sodium intake affected the smooth muscle cell membranes, and thereby the affinity of their angiotensin receptors. Brunner et al.

came to similar conclusions by means of their experiments on rats with different sodium diets (29, 30). They pointed out that the pressor effect of exogenous angiotensin in animals, whose RAS had been stimulated by sodium deprivation, was suppressed by much smaller amounts of antiserum than in controls. In contrast, following a high sodium chloride diet, large amounts of antiserum were necessary to inhibit the angiotensin effect. Swales and Thurston confirmed these experimental results (31, 32). However, they interpreted them differently; they assumed that the experimental data could not exclusively be explained by a sodium-dependent alteration of A II receptor sensitivity, but rather by local A II synthesis in the vascular walls. These workers measured, in different groups of anaesthetized rats, the amount of A II antiserum needed to compensate a blood pressure rise caused by a given dose of intravenously infused A II. Smaller amounts of antiserum were required under the following conditions: sodium deprivation, sodium loading with additional intravenous administration of exogenous rat renin, one-clip-two-kidney hypertension, peritoneal dialysis (predominantly stimulatory measures), versus sodium loading or bilateral nephrectomy. They assumed that the antibody molecules could not reach the site of local A II formation due to their high molecular weight. In addition, bilaterally nephrectomized rats were submitted to peritoneal dialysis, and compared with sodium restricted, anephric animals; both groups required similar amounts of antibodies as untreated bilaterally nephrectomized animals. Thus, the authors concluded that the kidney was necessary for sodium-dependent changes in response to A II.

Experimental Studies

Arterial renin and nephrectomy

The above results, together with several observations of other researchers (21, 33, 34, 35) induced Thurston and Swales to continue their investigations. Schaechtelin et al. (21) had assumed that accumulation of plasma renin occurred in the vascular wall of the rat, since blood pressure was not affected by bilateral nephrectomy. Several authors supported this by the observation that, in bilaterally nephrectomized dogs, arterial renin also remained constant. Both Rosenthal et al. (18) and Thurston and coworkers (36) measured a distinctive decrease in arterial renin content in the rat following bilateral nephrectomy, even though the enzymatic activity was still measurable. This discrepancy may be due to the different species used for the experiments. Weiser, Johnson and Hoobler (33) found that the effect of exogenous rat renin can be abolished by the application of antirenin, but only partially by anti-A II, as observed by Bing and Poulson (34). Bumpus and coworkers (35) indicated that, in some experimental hypertension models, A II antagonists were more effective than antisera. The hypothesis that vascular renin generates A II in the vascular wall was again supported by Thurston and Swales, with their experiments on bilaterally nephrectomized rats (37, 38, 39). The blood pressure rise observed following intravenous injection of purified hog renin and A II could be partly neutralized by anti-A II, and completely so by A II antagonists. The authors concluded that the antagonists had better access to the site of the A II receptors due to their smaller molecular weight.

In addition, some experiments were performed, in which A II antiserum was injected prior to the renin infusion. In this case, the blood pressure rise was less pronounced. Under an additional infusion of an A II antagonist, blood pressure returned to normal, and even if this was followed by further renin or A II administration, no additional blood pressure response occurred.

In an attempt to clarify the pathophysiological role of arterial wall renin, Thurston and colleagues (40) studied its behaviour in several forms of hypertension. In rats with Goldblatt hypertension, aortic renin activity increased in the initial stage, and fell with prolonged duration of the disease; at all times, however, the enzymatic levels remained significantly above normal. The authors did not detect elevated arterial renin activity in spontaneously hypertensive (SH-) rats; this is in agreement with the results of Barrett, Eggena and Sambhi (41), but not with those of other investigators (42, 43, 44). Rosenthal (42) obtained higher enzymatic values in the subcellular arterial wall fractions of SH-rats. For DOCA-salt hypertensive animals, Thurston et al. reported normal arterial renin activity. They concluded that the increased vascular renin of experimental renal hypertension was not due to elevation in blood pressure, and they doubted the importance of arterial renin in DOCA-salt or spontaneous hypertension.

A II antagonists and A II antiserum

Thurston and Swales (45) also investigated the effect of A II antiserum and A II antagonists on one-clip-two-kidney hypertensive rats, at 3 weeks and 4 months after the operation. They observed that the application of an antagonist abolished the blood pressure elevation in rats with short-term hypertension. In the chronic state, however, blood pressure values dropped following the injection of antagonists or removal of the ischaemic kidney, although it did not return to normal. Thus, the authors concluded that the vascular RAS was involved in the maintenance of the hypertensive state, and that the ischaemic kidney sustained hypertension by means of the RAS.

The effect of the ACE inhibitor SQ 20881 (teprotide) and the A II antagonist P 113 (saralasin) on blood pressure and plasma renin activity was studied in rats with one-clip-two-kidney hypertension and subsequent bilateral nephrectomy (36, 46, 47). The researchers measured only a small decrease in blood pressure even though plasma renin disappeared with a half-life of 10 minutes. Following administration of the ACE inhibitor, a pronounced fall in blood pressure was observed, which diminished gradually. No additional effect was achieved when saralasin was applied prior to the inhibitor. The authors suggested that the vascular RAS maintained blood pressure even when plasma renin activity had decreased to undetectable levels.

They concluded that the vascular enzyme had a longer half-life than circulating renin and participated in control of blood pressure.

Plasma and aortic wall renin

In subsequent studies, the authors investigated the effect of varying salt intake on renin activity in both plasma and aortic walls of normotensive rats, and also in one-clip-two-kidney hypertensive animals (36, 48, 49, 50). In addition, some of the clipped animals were bilaterally nephrectomized. Aortic renin activity was measured following incubation at pH 5.3 and 6.5. Aortic and plasma renin activity measured at pH 6.5 increased in sodium-deprived, and decreased in sodium-loaded rats. The initially high renin levels of the hypertensive animals had decreased in the plasma to undetectable values one hour following bilateral nephrectomy, and in the vascular wall after 24 h, when incubated at pH 6.5. Based on these results, Swales assumed that under steady state conditions, plasma renin activity was a measure of aortic renin content (49). Vascular renin determined at pH 5.3 remained easily measurable even 24 h after bilateral nephrectomy. The authors postulated that the enzyme measured at pH 5.3 originated from vascular tissue, whereas that with pH optimum at 6.5 was derived from plasma. They assumed that the vascular RAS participated in the mechanisms responsible for the maintenance of blood pressure following bilateral nephrectomy.

Removal of the clip in Goldblatt hypertension resulted in a fall of blood pressure to normal levels within three hours, whereas aortic renin returned to normal after 24 h (51). Therefore, the investigators assumed that renal pressor systems other than the RAS were involved in the decrease of blood pressure after removal of the stenosis.

In conscious bilaterally nephrectomized rats, the effects of purified rat renin and saralasin on vascular and plasma renin activities were studied at 1, 3, 6 and 9 h after injection (52).

Blood pressure remained elevated up to 6 h and had returned to normal by 9 h. Saralasin abolished the blood pressure effect of renin when infused for 30 minutes, 2.5 h and 5.5 h after the injection. Aortic renin content followed the blood pressure behaviour, whereas plasma renin concentration returned to subnormal values within 3 h. The authors assumed that circulating the renin of renal origin was taken up by aortic tissue. The pressure response to exogenous renin in bilaterally nephrectomized rats was not found to be related to plasma renin activity; however, its duration was similar to aortic renin activity.

Subcellular fractions and renin

Rosenthal (42) compared renin activity from aortic homogenate, aortic subcellular fractions and plasma, and plasma renin substrate concentration in SH-rats (Wistar Kyoto strain) with their normotensive controls. The ratio of renin activity (supernatant to microsomal fraction) of the aorta was three- to fourfold higher for the hypertensive than for the normotensive animals. No significant difference was obtained for renin activity in total aortic homogenate and for plasma renin substrate concentrations. Plasma renin activity was slightly higher in the hypertensive animals. This is in agreement with the earlier studies of Dahlheim (53) and the more recent investigations of Murakami and coworkers (54).

In a further publication, Rosenthal (55) reported on the behaviour of aortic (homogenate and subcellular fractions) and plasma renin activity in normal and unilaterally nephrectomized rats. The surgically treated animals were separated into three sub-groups: one group was kept on a normal diet, the second was treated with D-aldosterone for 8 weeks, and the last group with spironolactone for 8 weeks; the two latter groups received sodium chloride solution (10 g./l) as fluid intake. Rosenthal observed no significant difference in renin activity for the spironolactone-treated animals when compared with both the normal and the nephrectomized controls. The aldosterone-treated rats developed hypertension within 3-6 weeks. This parallelled a decrease of plasma and renal renin activity, whereas total aortic renin content increased up to six-fold. The ratio of supernatant to microsomal fraction renin activity in the aorta increased significantly.

Previously, Hayduk et al. (25) had reported that acute aldosterone administration raised arterial renin significantly, whereas 8 days of treatment lowered the enzymatic activity. As mentioned elsewhere, Swales did not find any changes in arterial renin after treatment with DOCA-salt (40). A 4-week application of progesterone induced a significant decrease in arterial wall renin (25).

Intravenous infusions of renin

Garst and colleagues (43) also studied aortic renin activity and blood pressure in normal rats following intravenous infusion of purified rat renin. They observed that the increase in blood pressure caused by the application of renin corresponded to a significant elevation of arterial renin content. Furthermore, the authors investigated renin activity in the arterial wall and in plasma from the renal vein and femoral artery of SH-rats (Wistar Kyoto strain). No significant difference was found in 6 month-old hypertensive animals, whereas renin activity of the arterial walls was significantly increased and venous plasma renin significantly decreased, in 12 month-old hypertensive animals. A small reduction of plasma renin activity was found in the femoral artery.

Garst et al. performed similar experiments in one-clip-two-kidney hypertensive rats, in the acute as well as in the chronic phases. In both cases, arterial wall renin increased significantly. In the earlier hypertensive stage, plasma renin activity of the renal vein and the femoral artery were elevated, whereas later on, both values returned to normal or subnormal. These workers concluded that "arterial wall renin may play a role in maintenance of acute and chronic hypertension, and also perhaps of spontaneous hypertension of long duration in older animals".

Barrett, Eggena and Sambhi (56) investigated the biochemical characteristics of arterial wall renin in SH-rats, and studied its behaviour under different conditions, e.g. bilateral nephrectomy, varying salt intake, administration of several drugs (metolazone, hydralazine and propranolol). In addition, they determined the effect of ageing and the distribution of renin in segments of the arterial vasculature.

Arterial renin could not be differentiated from renal renin by Km values. The authors demonstrated that vascular renin is not identical with "pseudorenin" described by Skeggs and coworkers (57) or cathepsin D; this was done by determining aortic renin activity using several solvents, different substrates, and various pH values. The aortic enzyme was found to be freely dissociable (saline homogenisation) and to have an affinity for the renin inhibitor pepstatin. The highest specific activity of arterial wall renin was found in the renal artery, followed by the iliac artery, carotid artery, and the aorta.

Barrett et al. observed that the activity of arterial wall renin decreased with the duration of hypertension in SH-rats. In those animals which failed to develop hypertension, the vascular renin levels remained constant. In normotensive controls of the same strain, vascular renin activity did not alter with age, whereas plasma renin activity declined slightly. No significant change of arterial renin could be observed in SH-rats 24 h following bilateral nephrectomy; plasma renin, however, was reduced to undetectable values.

Sodium deprivation and renin

Sodium deprivation for 25 days stimulated arterial wall renin and plasma renin activity in SH-rats. The same enzymatic behaviour was observed in SH-rats as well as in normotensives treated with metolazone for 23 days; however, this diuretic lowered aortic and plasma renin activities when administered for one week only. Treatment with hydralazine for 23 days reduced aortic renin significantly, whereas plasma renin activity remained constant. The authors reported that in SH-rats, an induced fall of blood pressure was parallelled by a decline of vascular renin.

In a further study, Barrett et al. (41) tried to evaluate whether these two parameters were statistically correlated in hypertensive (SH) and normotensive rats between 7.5 and 8.8 months of age. A positive correlation was obtained for normotensive, and a negative one for hypertensive rats.

Aortic renin and age

The authors did not recognize any correlation between aortic renin content and age, either in hypertensive (SH) or in normotensive rats. A negative correlation was found in the case of SH-rats between total (active and inactive) plasma renin activity and age, whereas there was no linear correlation between arterial blood pressure and total, active or inactive renin.

Biochemical studies on aortic renin

Barrett and colleagues (58) biochemically studied aortic renin and compared its characteristics with A I forming enzymes from the plasma and renal cortex, by determination of pH optima, molecular weights (MW) and isoelectric points (pI) of the preparations. For aortic renin, a pH optimum between 7.0 and 7.5 was measured. The same optimum was obtained for plasma and renal cortical enzymes. An additional pH optimum was found below 5.0, which could be detected in plasma as well, but which had disappeared from plasma 30 h after bilateral nephrectomy. A pH optimum in the range between 4.0 and 5.0 had also been demonstrated by other investigators (57, 59, 60, 61, 62, 63).

The authors determined the MW of aortic renin to be 44,000 and found the same value for plasma and kidney cortex slices. In plasma, a further enzyme with MW of 150,000, and in the kidney, an additional one with MW of 38,000 were identified. Two isoelectric points were determined for aortic renin (pI 5.0 and 5.3); one of these (pI 5.0) could also be detected in plasma and kidney. The A I forming enzyme with pI 5.3 and MW of 44,000 was assumed to originate from aortic tissue.

ACE blocker studies

Asaad and Antonaccio (44) studied the effect of 8 days of treatment with the ACE blocker captopril, on blood pressure and renin activity in both aortic and venous tissues, and in the plasma of SH-rats and normotensive controls (Wistar Kyoto strain). They performed similar experiments in bilaterally nephrectomized SH-rats. The authors measured a significantly higher renin activity in the arterial wall of SH-rats as compared with the normotensive controls. This is in agreement with the results of Rosenthal (42), but not with those of Thurston et al. (40) and Barrett et al. (41). Asaad and Antonaccio found no difference between venous activities of hypertensive (SH) and normotensive rats. Following captopril treatment for 8 days, the blood pressure fell, although renin increased in plasma and in aortic and venous tissues in both animal groups. The rise in vascular renin was more pronounced in the normotensive rats. Positive correlations were calculated between aortic and plasma renin activities or blood pressure in SH-rats treated with captopril or left untreated. Plasma renin activity of SH-rats was barely detectable 24 h following bilateral nephrectomy, whereas aortic renin remained constant up to 4 h after extirpation of the kidneys; 65% of the enzymatic activity was still present 24 h later. Blood pressure rose after nephrectomy, but decreased when captopril was injected into the anephric animals. The authors suggested that the elevated aortic renin activity in SH-rats may play a role in the development or maintenance of hypertension; the blood pressure lowering effect of captopril on both nephrectomized and intact SH-rats might be explained by its ability to inhibit vascular A II formation. Vascular renin was not assumed to be of renal origin.

The Vascular RAS as a Whole

In order to study the vascular RAS as a whole, Rosenthal and colleagues tried to identify and characterise those components possibly involved in local A II formation (63, 64, 65). They investigated the isoelectric behaviour and measured the pH optima, and in some cases the molecular weights, of the enzymatic components of aortic tissue of normal rats. In addition, they studied venous tissue of aortic smooth muscle cells cultivated in vitro. Some experiments were also done on SH-rats.

pH optima and isoelectric points

Using aortic homogenate extracts and partially purified rat renin substrate, pH optima were determined at 7.5, 4.8, and a smaller one at pH 6.5. Following separation by the isoelectric focusing technique, two pH optima - one at about 7.5 and one below 4.7 were detected, which corresponded with the isoelectric points 5.6 and <2.0. The pH optimum at 7.5 was also found by Barrett and coworkers (58), who measured one between 7.0 and 7.5. However, the latter investigators observed the same pH optimum in plasma, renal aortic tissues. Thurston et al. (36) found two distinct optima at pH 4.5 and 6.5. Both are supported by the results of Rosenthal et al. Unfortunately, Thurston et al. measured neither the effect of pH on plasma renin below pH 5.0, nor on aortic tissue renin above pH 7.0. They suggested that the renin measurable at pH 6.5 was derived from plasma (48), and that the A I forming enzyme measured at a low incubation pH was not important for blood pressure maintenance (36). Dahlheim, Granger and Thurau determined a pH optimum of 6.5 for a renal renin preparation of the rat, purified according to Haas (66), and incubated with a homologous renin substrate preparation (67).

The pH value at about 4.7 was also found by Barrett et al. (58). These authors determined this pH optimum in both aortic tissue and plasma of non-nephrectomized rats. Recently, Haas and coworkers reported on an A I forming enzyme in plasma with a pH optimum at 4.7 (59, 60, 61, 62), which they first detected following immunization with renin (59). It remains to be seen in future studies whether this enzyme is identical with that of aortic tissue.

For arterial renin, Barrett et al. (58) determined two pI values (5.0 and 5.3), and assumed the enzyme with pI 5.3 to be of local origin. Rosenthal et al. measured an isoelectric point in the range between 5.45 and 5.75. The slightly different values of both groups possibly apply to the same enzyme.

The A I forming enzyme with pI below 2.0 was considered to be a compound partially denaturated by the isoelectric focusing procedure (64). However, the same pH optimum was found in aortic homogenate which was not submitted to isoelectric focusing. Therefore, another A I forming enzyme was assumed to be present in aortic tissue. The MW of this enzyme was estimated to be in the range of 17,000 to 20,000, so that it may be considered as a fragment of the original renin molecule. Galen and colleagues (68) reported on a comparable fractionation resulting in a form of renin with similar MW. The pI of aortic renin of SH-rats (Wistar Kyoto strain) was found to be identical with that of their normotensive controls. The aortic renin activity of SH-rats, determined following isoelectric focusing separation, was found to be much higher than that of their normotensive controls. Therefore, the authors assumed that a naturally occurring renin inhibitor was separated by the isoelectric focusing procedure.

Renin activity in venous tissue

Rosenthal and coworkers also characterized biochemically renin activity in venous tissue, and found different isoelectric behaviour (pI 4.35). Another pI with lower enzymatic activity was determined at 5.25, which corresponds to the value measured by Barrett et al. (58) for aortic renin. The different pI value found suggested that renin from venous tissue was not identical with that of the arteries. Further studies are needed in order to clarify whether the venous RAS must be considered an intrinsic one. Asaad and Antonaccio (44) demonstrated that venous renin was not elevated in SH-rats when contrasted with that of arteries. The authors consider this to be an indication that the influence of the RAS on the low and high pressure systems is not alike; moreover, they commented that interference with these systems, for example by therapeutic application of ACE inhibitors, does not affect pre- and afterload to the same extent.

Renin and angiotensin administration

Bock and Gross (69) administered renin or angiotensin to anaesthetized dogs, and produced a considerable, dose-dependent rise in central venous pressure. However, the authors assumed that a direct effect on smooth musculature of the veins could only partly account for this elevation.

For plasma and kidney cortex extracts, Rosenthal et al. found a pI value at 4.8

In aortic smooth muscle cells, pI values for A I forming enzyme were determined at 6.5 and also, although less pronounced, at 5.0 and 2.0. Also, two pH optima were measured for aortic smooth muscle cells: one at pH 5.0, and a smaller one between 6.5 and 7.0. Both values were in agreement with those found in total aortic homogenate. In smooth muscle cells, the enzymatic activity was highest at pH 5.0, whereas it was nearly equal at both pH optima in aortic homogenate.

Characteristics of ACE

Furthermore, Rosenthal and colleagues compared the biochemical characteristics of vascular ACE with those of different origin. The presence of ACE in vascular tissues had already been postulated (70, 71, 72, 73, 74, 75) and measured (76, 77, 78) by other authors. The pH optimum ranged between 8.0 and 8.5 for plasma and tissue homogenates from aorta, vena cava, aortic smooth muscle cells, renal cortex, lung, and testicular structures. In kidney cortex, an iso-ACE with a pH optimum between 6.0 and 6.5 was detected (79). For aortic, pulmonary and testicular tissue, aortic smooth muscle cells and plasma, the pI values were also in the same range (pI 4.5-5.5), whereas those found for renal cortex differed significantly. In vitro experiments with the specific ACE inhibitor MK 421 appear to indicate that vascular ACE is different from the plasma enzyme. However, this might be due to a different degree of activation of the blocker. The MW of aortic ACE was estimated between 650,000 and 710,000 (80), whereas that of plasma has been measured between 128,000 and 330,000 by various authors (81, 82, 83).

Aortic ACE activity of SH-rats was significantly higher than that of their normotensive controls. This is in agreement with the findings of Mizuno, Hata and Fukuchi (84). These authors studied the effect of sodium intake on the distribution of ACE in subcellular fractions of aortic tissue from hypertensive (SH) and normotensive rats. They also confirmed ACE levels to be elevated in SH-rats. Comparing the subcellular fractions, they found the highest enzymatic activity in the supernatant of both groups of animals; there was a marked reduction in each fraction following sodium loading. The authors suggested that vascular ACE participates in local control of vascular tone. Mizuno, Gotoh and Fukuchi (85) also studied the behaviour of vascular ACE in different models of experimental renovascular hypertension. Only in one-clip-two-kidney hypertensive rats, was ACE found to be elevated, in both total aortic homogenate as well as in the subcellular fractions.

Miyauchi and coworkers (86) compared specific ACE activities in several vascular tissues of the rabbit. They found the highest levels in the pulmonary artery, followed by the renal artery and vena cava; the lowest was in the aorta. Schweisfurth (87) measured specific ACE activities in different segments of arterial pulmonary vessels and observed enzyme levels to rise with decrease in diameter.

Rosenthal and coworkers (63, 64) identified and characterised ACE in aortic smooth muscle cells of the rat cultivated in vitro. The enzyme could be differentiated from that predominantly present in aortic tissue by its isoelectric behaviour. Johnson and Erdös (88) did not detect any ACE activity in smooth muscle cells from human umbilical veins. This may be due either to the difference of species or location, or to the sensitivity of the method employed. These authors consider ACE to be a marker for endothelial cells, located on the cell surface. This is in agreement with the findings of other authors (89, 90, 91). ACE was also identified by Rightsel and colleagues (92) in juxtaglomerular cells grown as monolayer cell culture.

A I degradation

According to Rosenthal and coworkers (65, 93), A I could also be degraded in vascular walls by an enzyme different from ACE. The pI value of this enzyme ranged between 3.6 and 3.9, and differed significantly from that of aortic ACE (pI 4.6-5.0). The pH optimum of this A I degrading enzyme was determined at about 7.75, and the molecular weight was estimated between 440,000 and 457,000, in comparison to 650,000-710,000 for aortic ACE (80). The enzyme could be blocked neither by the ACE inhibitor MK 421, nor by trasylol, and only up to 50% by EDTA. No activation occurred in vitro by sodium chloride. The specific activity of A I degrading enzyme was in the same range or even higher than that of ACE. Therefore, the A I present in vascular tissue can be degraded by at least two enzymes: ACE, and an A I degrading enzyme. Preliminary studies show that the Km value for the A I degrading enzyme is smaller than that of ACE (80).

A I degrading enzyme also differed from A II degrading enzyme(s) present in aortic tissue. The latter had one isoelectric point between 4.5 and 5.0, and another between 8.0 and 8.25. The pH optimum was found at 8.1.

A II degradation

Johnson and Erdös (88) reported on an A II degrading enzyme present in human endothelial cells cultivated in vitro. Up to now, the results do not allow any conclusions regarding the identity of these enzymes.

Based on their systematically performed studies, and on the Paton hypothesis (95), Kairallah and coworkers (94) assumed angiotensinases to be present at the site of the vascular angiotensin receptors. The assumption that angiotensin tachyphylaxis depends on vascular angiotensinase activity was questioned by Hollenberg, Barbero and Hinrichs (96).

A II degrading enzyme activity was well measurable in aortic smooth muscle cells cultivated in vitro. The main isoelectric point was found between 4.0 and 4.25, and the pH optimum at about 8.0. Compared with the other enzymes of the RAS measured, A II degrading enzyme activity was relatively high. It appears that this cellular enzyme is identical with the main A II degrading enzyme in aortic homogenate.

Further Scope for Research

The main biologically active component of the renin angiotensin system is the octapeptide A II. This substance is the most potent vasopressor known. It has been accepted for a long time that the RAS is affected by the autonomic nervous system. The assumption that an intrinsic vascular RAS mediates and possibly modulates nervous influences on the vascular receptors is obvious. This is supported by the fact that, in the meantime, more evidence has accumulated for the existence of an intrinsic vascular RAS. However, more experimental details are needed in order to definitely clarify its physiological or pathophysiological role.

Recently, the existence of intracellular angiotensin II formation has been suggested (64, 92). The question arises as to whether such a system might be involved in protein synthesis and/or mitochondrial oxidation; both can be of critical relevance and may open up new avenues of research.

Clinically, involvement of the intrinsic vascular RAS in essential hypertension would be of primary importance.

ACE and sarcoidosis

Excessive release of vascular ACE into plasma is known to occur in the acute state of sarcoidosis (97, 98). Since this enzyme is likely to originate from the endothelial cells of pulmonary and possibly also from other vasculature (99), it has to be clarified whether this enzyme belongs to the intrinsic vascular RAS, the subject of this survey. The disease can be treated successfully with corticosteroids (99). Little is known about the pathophysiology of sarcoidosis, and better knowledge of the physiological function of the vascular RAS would also be helpful to obtain further insight into this disease.

The future

Some important questions remain for future work. It has not been elucidated whether the compounds of the RAS demonstrated in the vascular walls are synthesized there, and to what extent the plasma components can penetrate into the vascular walls and are accumulated there. It is particularly important to know this in relation to renin substrate, since its presence within vascular tissue is an essential prerequisite for the efficiency of the intrinsic vascular RAS. In addition, it should be investigated which components are rate-limiting for local A II formation, and which other factors (electrolytes, enzymatic effectors, etc.) are likely to interfere. Do further enzymes exist, for example intracellularly? The demonstration of a potent A I degrading enzyme requires further investigations in relation to its physiological and pathophysiological significance. Thus, different iso-enzymes and other peptidases may possibly compete for the same substrates (angiotensinogen, angiotensin I, angiotensin II); moreover, other peptides (e.g. bradykinin) may be involved. The kallikrein-kinin system, which is connected to the RAS through ACE (kininase II), should not be ignored in this context.

Very little is known about the availability of naturally occurring inhibitors or activators. There is some evidence of the existence of such components; this has been assumed for a long time.

The existence of other extrarenal intrinsic renin angiotensin systems is likely - e.g. in the brain (100, 101). The most important intrinsic RAS appears to be that of the kidney. It can be assumed that these local systems are connected and/or may depend on each other, either through single components transported in the plasma, through other humoral systems, or perhaps through the autonomic nervous system.

The experiments performed up to the present, and which have been mainly on larger vessels, should be reproduced on smaller ones, possibly on arterioles which are the main influence on vascular resistance. It is known that the specific enzymatic activity of vascular renin and ACE increases with decreasing vascular diameter.

Conclusions

Assumptions related to the physiological role of the vascular RAS, and its possible participation in the pathogenesis of essential hypertension, arteriosclerosis, or other vascular diseases, have existed ever since the presence of renin was suspected in the extrarenal vascular wall (10). Today, after 40 years, our knowledge of the pathophysiological behaviour of the vascular RAS is more extensive, but the very first questions, whether the system participates in blood pressure regulation and in the pathogenesis of essential hypertension, still remain unsolved.

Acknowledgements

This work was supported by the Deutsche Forschungsgemeinschaft.

References

1. Tigerstedt, R., Bergman, P.G.: Niere und Kreislauf. Skand. Arch. Physiol. 8, 223-271 (1898).
2. Bingel, A., Strauss, E.: Über die blutdrucksteigernde Substanz der Niere. Deutsch Arch. klin. Med. 96, 476-492 (1909).
3. Hessel, G.: Über Renin. Klin. Wschr. 17(24), 843-849 (1938).
4. Schales, O.: Preparation and Properties of renin. J. Am. chem. Soc. 64, 561-564 (1942).
5. Braun-Menéndez, E., Fasciolo, J.C., Leloir, L.F., Munoz, J.M.: The substance causing renal hypertension. J. Physiol. 98, 283-298 (1940).
6. Page, I.H., Helmer, O.M.: A crystalline pressor substance (angiotonin) resulting from the reaction between renin and renin-activator. J. exp. Med. 71, 29-42 (1940).
7. Goldblatt, H.: The renal origin of hypertension. Charles C. Thomas Publisher, Springfield, Illinois (1948).
8. Jiménez-Dîaz, C., de la Barreda, P., de Molina, A.F.: La regulación quîmica de la presión arterial. Rev. Clin. Espan. 24, 417-419 (1947).
9. de la Barreda, P., de Molina, A.F., Jiménez-Dîaz, C.: Neurochemical regulation of the blood pressure. Bull. Inst. Med. Res. Madrid, 1, 53-63 (1948).
10. Jiménez-Dîaz, C.: Le rôle de la paroi artérielle dans la régulation neurochimique de la pression artérielle. Schweiz. med. Wschr. 38, 920-923 (1948).
11. de la Barreda, P.: Enzymic activities of the arterial wall and their modification by adrenalin, noradrenalin and vagal excitation. Bull. Inst. Med. Res. Madrid, 7, 17-32 (1954).
12. Dengler, H.: Über einen reninartigen Wirkstoff in Arterienextrakten. Arch. exp. Path. Pharmak.227, 481-487 (1956).
13. Skeggs, L.T., Marsh, W.H., Kahn, J.R., Shumway, N.P.: The existence of two forms of hypertensin. J. exp. Med. 99, 275-282 (1954).
14. Kahn, J.R., Skeggs, L.T., Shumway, N.P., Wisenbaugh, P.E.: The assay of hypertensin from the arterial blood of normotensive and hypertensive human beings. J. exp. Med. 95, 523-529 (1952).
15. Skeggs, L.T.: Angiotensin and allied substances. Proc. 21st Int. Congr. Physiol. Sci., Buenos Aires, 54-61 (1959).
16. Gould, A.B., Skeggs, L.T., Kahn, J.R.: The presence of renin activity in blood vessel walls. J. exp. Med. 119, 389-399 (1964).
17. Basso, N., Taquini, A.C.: Effect of bilateral nephrectomy on renin activity of blood vessel walls. Acta physiol. lat.-amer.21, 8-14 (1971).

18. Rosenthal, J., Boucher, R., Rojo-Ortega, J.M., Genest, J.: Renin activity in aortic tissue of rats. Can. J. Physiol. Pharmacol. 47, 53-56 (1969).

19. Genest, J., Simard, S., Rosenthal, J., Boucher, R.: Norepinephrine and renin content in arterial tissue from different vascular beds. Can. J. Physiol. Pharmacol. 47, 87-91 (1969).

20. Daum, A., Uehleke, H., Klaus, D.: Unterschiedliche Beeinflussung der Blutdruckwirkung von Renin und Angiotensin durch Aminopeptidase. Naunyn-Schmiedebergs Arch. exp. Path. Pharmak. 254, 327-333 (1966).

21. Schaechtelin, G., Regoli, D., Gross, F.: Quantitative assay and disappearance rate of circulating renin. Amer. J. Physiol. 206, 1361-1364 (1964).

22. Hayduk, K., Boucher, R., Genest, J.: Renin activity content in various tissues of dogs under different physiopathological states. Proc. Soc. exp. Biol Med. 134, 252-255 (1970).

23. Hayduk, K., Brecht, H.M., Vladutiu, A., Simard, S., Rojo-Ortega, J.M., Belleau, L., Boucher, R., Genest, J.: Renin activity and norepinephrine, cation, and water contents of cardiovascular tissue of dogs with congestive heart failure and ascites. Can. J. Physiol. Pharmacol. 48, 463-468 (1970).

24. Ganten, D., Hayduk, K., Brecht, H.M., Boucher, R., Genest, J.: Evidence of renin release or production in splanchnic territory. Nature 226, 551-552 (1970).

25. Hayduk, K., Ganten, D., Boucher, R., Genest, J.: Arterial and urinary renin activity. In: "Hypertension" 1972, Eds. Genest, J., Koiw, E., Springer Verlag, Berlin-New York, pp. 435-443.

26. Ganten, D., Ganten, U., Granger, P., Boucher, R., Genest, J.: Renin in heart muscle and arterial tissue. Verhandlungsberichte der deutschen Gesellschaft für Kreislaufforschung vol. 38, Herzhypertrophie, Steinkopf Verlag, Darmstadt, pp. 268-272 (1972).

27. Hayduk, K., Brecht, H.M., Vladutiu, A., Rojo-Ortega, J.M., Boucher, R., Genest, J.: Effects of sodium restriction on renin, norepinephrine, and cation content of cardiovascular tissues of dogs. Proc. Soc. exp. Biol Med. 135, 271-274 (1970).

28. Strewler, G.J., Hinrichs, K.J., Guiod, L.R., Hollenberg, N.K.: Sodium intake and vascular smooth muscle responsiveness to norepinephrine and angiotensin in the rabbit. Circulat. Res. 31, 758-766 (1972).

29. Brunner, H.R., Kirshman, J.D., Sealey, J.E., Laragh, J.H.: Hypertension of renal origin: evidence for two different mechanisms. Science 174, 1344-1346 (1971).

30. Brunner, H.R., Chang, P., Wallach, R., Sealey, J.E., Laragh, J.H.: Angiotensin II vascular receptors: their avidity in relationship to sodium balance, the autonomic nervous system, and hypertension. J. clin. Invest. 51, 58-67 (1972).

31. Swales, J.D., Thurston, H.: Generation of angiotensin II at peripheral vascular level: studies using angiotensin II antisera. Clin. Sci. Mol. Med. 45, 691-700 (1973).

32. Swales, J.D., Tange, J.D., Thurston, H.: Vascular angiotensin II receptors and sodium balance in rats; role of kidneys and vascular renin activity. Circulat. Res. 37, 96-100 (1975).

33. Weiser, R.A., Johnson, A.G., Hoobler, S.W.: The effect of antirenin on the blood pressure of the rat with experimental renal hypertension. Lab. Invest. 20(4), 326-331 (1969).

34. Bing, J., Poulsen, K.: Effect of anti-angiotensin II on blood pressure and sensitivity to angiotensin and renin. Acta path. microbiol. scand. Section A, 78, 6-18 (1970).

35. Bumpus, F.M., Sen, S., Smeby, R.R., Sweet, C., Ferrario, C.M., Khosla, M.C.: Use of angiotensin II antagonists in experimental hypertension. Circulat. Res. 32, Suppl. 1, 150-158 (1973).

36. Thurston, H., Swales, J.D., Bing, R.F., Hurst, B.C., Marks, E.S.: Vascular renin-like activity and blood pressure maintenance in the rat; studies of the effect of changes in sodium balance, hypertension and nephrectomy. Hypertension 1, 643-649 (1979).

37. Thurston, H., Swales, J.D.: Action of angiotensin antagonists and antiserum upon the pressor response to renin: further evidence for the local generation of angiotensin II. Clin. Sci. Mol. Med. 46, 273-276 (1974).

38. Swales, J.D.: Antagonists, inhibitors and antisera in the evaluation of vascular renin activity; the role of local generation of angiotensin II. In: "Drugs Affecting the Renin-Angiotensin-Aldosterone System", Eds. Stokes, G.S., Edwards, R., Prog. Biochem. Pharmacol. vol. 12, Karger, Basel, pp. 98-113 (1976).

39. Thurston, H.: Vascular angiotensin receptors and their role in blood pressure control. Am. J. Med. 61, 768-778 (1976).

40. Thurston, H., Hurst, B.C., Bing, R.F., Swales, J.D.: Vascular renin. In: "Frontiers in Hypertension Research", Eds. Laragh, J.H., Buhler, F.R., Seldin, D.W., Springer Verlag, New York, pp. 274-276 (1981).

41. Barrett, J.D., Eggena, P., Sambhi, M.P.: Aortic and plasma renin in the SHR and its relationship to spontaneous progression of hypertension. Jap. Heart J. 20, Suppl. 1, 313-315 (1979).

42. Rosenthal, J.: Arterial renin in spontaneously hypertensive rats. (SHR). Clin. Exp. Pharmacol. Physiol. Suppl. 3, 153-155 (1976).

43. Garst, J.B., Koletsky, S., Wisenbaugh, P.E., Hadady, M., Matthews, D.: Arterial wall renin and renal venous renin in the hypertensive rat. Clin. Sci. 56, 41-46 (1979).

44. Asaad, M.M., Antonaccio, M.J.: Vascular wall renin in spontaneously hypertensive rats: potential relevance to hypertension maintenance and antihypertensive effect of captopril. Hypertension 4, 487-493 (1982).

45. Thurston, H., Swales, J.D.: Comparison of angiotensin II antagonist and antiserum infusion with nephrectomy in the rat with two-kidney Goldblatt hypertension. Circulat. Res. 35, 325-329 (1974).

46. Thurston, H., Laragh, J.H.: Prior receptor occupancy as a determinant of the pressor activity of infused angiotensin II in the rat. Circulat. Res. 36, 113-117 (1975).

47. Thurston, H., Swales, J.D.: Blood pressure response of nephrectomized hypertensive rats to converting enzyme inhibition: evidence for persistent vascular renin activity. Clin. Sci. Mol. Med. 52, 299-304 (1977).

48. Thurston, H., Hurst, B.C., Bing, R.F., Swales, J.D.: Role of persistent vascular renin after bilateral nephrectomy in Goldblatt-two kidney hypertension. Clin. Sci. Mol. Med. 55, Suppl. 4, 23s-26s (1978).

49. Swales, J.D.: Vascular renin in hypertension. Hormone Res. 12, 65-78 (1980).

50. Swales, J.D.: Arterial wall or plasma renin in hypertension? Clin. Sci. 56, 293-298 (1979).

51. Brice, J.M., Russell, G.I., Bing, R.F., Swales, J.D., Thurston, H.: Surgical reversal of renovascular hypertension: changes in blood pressure, plasma and aortic renin. Clin. Sci. 62, 17p-18p (1982).

52. Loudon, M., Bing, R.F., Swales, J.D., Thurston, H.: Changes in blood pressure in relation to vascular and plasma renin injection in rats. Clin. Sci. 63, 001s-004s (1982).

53. Dahlheim, H.: Die Wirkung eines Angiotensin II-Antagonisten (Saralasin-Azetat) auf verschiedene Komponenten des Renin-Angiotensinsystems in mikrodissezierten Nieren-Glomeruli und im Plasma der Ratte. Therapiewoche 26, 7591 (1976).

54. Murakami, K., Suzuki, F., Morita, N., Ito, H., Okamoto, K., Hirose, S., Inagami, T.: High molecular weight renin in stroke-prone spontaneously hypertensive rats. Biochim. biophys. Acta 622, 115-122 (1980).

55. Rosenthal, J.: Effects of aldosterone and spironolactone on arterial renin in rats. Clin. Sci. Mol. Med. 51, 121s-123s (1976).

56. Barrett, J.D., Eggena, P., Sambhi, M.P.: Partial characterization of aortic renin in the spontaneously hypertensive rat and its interrelationship with plasma renin, blood pressure and sodium balance. Clin. Sci. Mol. Med. 55, 261-270 (1978).

57. Skeggs, L.T., Lentz, K.E., Kahn, J.R., Dorer, F.E., Levine, M.: Pseudorenin: a new angiotensin-forming enzyme. Circulat. Res. 25, 451-462 (1969).

58. Barrett, J.D., Eggena, P., Krall, J.F., Sambhi, M.P.: A comparison of physical characteristics of active renin isolated from aorty, plasma and kidney of the rat. Clin. Sci. 61, 671-678 (1981).

59. Haas, E., Lewis, LaV., Scipione, P., Koshy, T.J.: Angiotensin-producing enzyme I: formation by immunization with renin. ICRS Med. Sci. 8, 101 (1980).

60. Haas, E., Scipione, P., Lewis, LaV., Koshy, T.J.: Angiotensin-producing enzyme II: formation by activation of a proenzyme and separation of an inhibitor. ICRS Med. Sci. 8, 102 (1980).

61. Haas, E., Scipione, P., Lewis, LaV., Koshy, T.J., Kandaswamy, K.: Angiotensin-producing enzyme II: formation by activation of a proenzyme with plasmin. ICRS Med. Sci. 10, 733-734 (1980).

62. Haas, E., Lewis, LaV., Scipione, P., Renerts, L., Koshy, T.J.: Angiotensin-producing enzyme II of serum: five methods for the activation of proenzyme II to enzyme II. ICRS Med. Sci. 10, 44-45 (1982).

63. Rosenthal, J., Michailov, M.L., Pschorr, J., Pfeifle, B., Dahlheim, H.: Identification and characterization of components of the renin angiotensin system (RAS) in rat vascular tissues. 36th Annual Fall Conference of the Council for High Blood Pressure Research, 1982 (Abstract).

64. Rosenthal, J., Pfeifle, B., Michailov, M.L., Pschorr, J., Jacob, I.C.M., Dahlheim, H.: Identification of components of the renin angiotensin system in rat vascular tissue. Hypertension (in press).

65. Rosenthal, J., Pschorr, J., Jacob, I.C.M., Michailov, M.L., Pfeifle, B., Dahlheim, H.: Evidence for a potent angiotensin I degrading enzyme in vascular walls. Fifth Scientific Meeting of the Inter-American Society of Hypertension, Sao Paulo, 1983 (Abstract).

66. Haas, E., Goldblatt, H., Gipson, E.C., Lewis, LaV.: Extraction, purification and assay of human renin free of angiotensinase. Circulat. Res. 19, 739 (1966).

67. Dahlheim, H., Granger, P., Thurau, K.: A sensitive method for determination of renin activity in the single juxtaglomerular apparatus of the rat kidney. Pflügers Arch. ges. Physiol. 321, 303-315 (1970).

68. Galen, F.-X., Devaux, C., Guyenne, T., Menard, J., Corvol, P.: Multiple forms of human renin, purification and characterisation. J. biol. Chem. 254(11): 4848-4855 (1979).

69. Bock, K.D., Gross, F.: Venendruckänderungen nach Gabe von Renin, Angiotensin und Noradrenalin. Naunyn-Schmiedebergs Arch. exp. Path. Pharmak. 242, 188-200 (1961).

70. Hodge, R.L., Ng, K.K.F., Vane, J.R.: Disappearance of angiotensin from the circulation of the dog. Nature 215, 138-141 (1967).

71. Aiken, J.W., Vane, J.R.: The renin-angiotensin system: inhibition of converting enzyme in isolated tissues. Nature 228, 30-36 (1970).

72. Kreye, V.A.W., Gross, F.: Conversion of angiotensin I to angiotensin II in peripheral vascular beds of the rat. Am. J. Physiol. 220(5), 1294-1296 (1971).

73. DiSalvo, J., Montefusco, C.B.: Conversion of angiotensin I to angiotensin II in the canine mesenteric circulation. Am. J. Physiol. 221(6), 1576-1579 (1971).

74. Fei, D.T.W., Coghlan, J.P., Fernley, R.T., Scoggins, B.A., Tregear, G.W.: Peripheral production of angiotensin II and III in sheep. Circulat. Res. 46(6), Suppl. I, I135-I137 (1980).

75. Collier, J.G., Robinson, B.F.: Comparison of effects of locally infused angiotensin I and II on hand veins and forearm arteries in man: evidence for converting enzyme activity in limb vessels. Clin. Sci. Mol. Med. 47, 189-192 (1974).

76. Cushman, D.W., Cheung, H.S.: Concentrations of angiotensin-converting enzyme in tissues of the rat. Biochim. biophys. Acta 250, 261-265 (1971).

77. Brecher, P., Tercyak, A., Chobanian, A.V.: Properties of angiotensin-converting enzyme in intact cerebral microvessels. Hypertension 3, 198-204 (1981).

78. Mendelsohn, F.A.O., Lloyd, C.J., Kachel, C., Funder, J.W.: Induction by glucocorticoids of angiotensin converting enzyme production from bovine endothelial cells in culture and rat lung in vivo. J. clin. Invest. 70, 684-692 (1982).

79. Dahlheim, H., Schweisfurth, H.: Does the kidney contain its own angiotensin I converting enzyme? Pflügers Arch. ges. Physiol. 359 (Suppl.), 125 (1975).

80. Dahlheim, H.: Personal communication.

81. Das, M., Soffer, R.L.: Pulmonary angiotensin-converting enzyme antienzyme antibody. Biochemistry 15 (23), 5088-5094 (1976).

82. Soffer, R.L.: Angiotensin-converting enzyme and the regulation of vasoactive peptides. Ann. Rev. Biochem. 45, 73-94 (1976).

83. Stevens, R.L., Micalizzi, E.R., Fessler, D.C., Pals, D.T.: Angiotensin I converting enzyme of calf lung. Method of assay and partial purification. Biochemistry 11 (16), 2999-3007 (1972).

84. Mizuno, K., Hata, S., Fukuchi, S.: Effect of sodium intake on angiotensin-converting enzyme activity of aorta in rats. Clin. Sci. 61, 249-251 (1981).

85. Mizuno, K., Gotoh, M., Fukuchi, S.: Increased angiotensin-converting enzyme activity of aorta in two-kidney, one-clip Goldblatt hypertension in rats. Clin. Sci. 63, 331-332(1982).

86. Miyauchi, Y., Nishimura, K., Ueda, E., Kokubu, T.: Angiotensin-converting enzyme activity in the vascular tissue from rabbits. Biomed. Res. 2(4), 364-366 (1981).

87. Schweisfurth, H.: Lokalisation, Charakterisierung und physiologisches Verhalten des Angiotensin I-converting enzyme. MD Thesis, Medical Faculty of the University of Munich, 1975.

88. Johnson, A.R., Erdös, E.G.: Metabolism of vasoactive peptides by human endothelial cells in culture: angiotensin I converting enzyme (kininase II) and angiotensinase. J. clin. Invest. 59, 684-695 (1977).

89. Ryan, J.W., Ryan, U.S., Schultz, D.R., Whitaker, C., Chung,A.: Subcellular localization of pulmonary angiotensin-converting enzyme (kininase II). Biochem. J. 146, 497-499 (1975).

90. Caldwell, P.R.B-. Seegal, B.C., Hsu, K.C., Das, M., Soffer, R.L.: Angiotensin-converting enzyme: vascular endothelial localization. Science 91, 1050-1051 (1976).

91. Ody, C., Junod, A.F.: Converting enzyme activity in endothelial cells isolated from pig pulmonary artery and aorta. Am. J. Physiol. 232 (3), C95-C98 (1977).

92. Rightsel, W.A., Okamura, T., Inagami, T., Pitcock, J.A., Takii, Y., Brooks, B., Brown, P., Muirhead, E.E.: Juxtaglomerular cells grown as monolayer cell culture contain renin, angiotensin I-converting enzyme, and angiotensins I and II/III. Circulat. Res. 50, 822-829 (1982).

93. Rosenthal, J., Pschorr, J., Jacob, I.C.M., Michailov, M.L., Pfeifle, B., Dahlheim. H.: Further evidence for the existence of an intrinsic renin angiotensin system in extrarenal vascular tissue. Deutsch. Ges. f. Endocrinol. 27, Symposium (1983).

94. Khairallah, P.A., Page, I.H., Bumpus, F.M., Türker, R.K.: Angiotensin tachyphylaxis and its reversal. Circulat. Res. 19, 247-254 (1966).

95. Paton, W.D.M.: A theory of drug action based on the rate of drug receptor combination. Proc. roy. Soc. B 154, 21-69 (1961).

96. Hollenberg, N.K., Barbero, L.R., Hinrichs, K.P.J.: Angiotensin tachyphylaxis and vascular angiotensinase activity. Experientia 27, 1032-1034 (1971).

97. Lieberman, J.: Elevation of serum angiotensin converting enzyme (ACE) level in sarcoidosis. Am. J. Med. 59, 365-372 (1975).

98. Baur, X., Fruhmann, G., Dahlheim, H.: Follow-up of angiotensin-converting enzyme in serum of patients with sarcoidosis. Respiration 41, 133-138 (1981).

99. Baur, X., Fruhmann, G., König, G., Rienmüller, R., Knonsalla, M., Dahlheim, H.: Die Bedeutung des Angiotensin I-Converting-Enzyms für die Diagnose einer Sarkoidose. Klin. Wschr. 58, 199-206 (1980).

100. Ganong, W.F.: The brain and the renin-angiotensin system. In: "Central Nervous System Mechanisms in Hypertension", Eds. Buckley, J.P., Ferrario, C.M., Raven Press, New York pp. 283-291 (1981).

101. Weindl, A., Schweisfurth, H., Sofroniew, M.V., Dahlheim, H.: Distribution of converting enzyme in the rat brain: high activities in subfornical organ, area postrema, and choroid plexus. Acta Endocrinol. 85, Suppl.212, 158 (1977).

Subject Index

CUMULATIVE INDEX OF AUTHORS AND TITLES FROM VOLUMES 1, 2 AND 3

Bei Fragen zur Produktsicherheit wenden Sie sich bitte an:
If you have any questions regarding product safety,
please contact:

Walter de Gruyter GmbH
Genthiner Straße 13
10785 Berlin
productsafety@degruyterbrill.com